D0113230

The Conquest
of Epidemic Disease

*A Chapter
in the History of Ideas*

Charles-Edward Amory Winslow

The University of Wisconsin Press

To A. R. W.

"AND THE WHOLE IS WELL WORTH THINKING O'ER

WHEN THE AUTUMN COMES"

Published by
The University of Wisconsin Press
114 North Murray Street
Madison, Wisconsin 53715

The University of Wisconsin Press, Ltd.
1 Gower Street
London WC1E 6HA, England

First Wisconsin printing, 1980

Printed in the United States of America
ISBN 0-299-08240-7 cloth, 0-299-08244-X paper
LC 79-48055

This printing is by arrangement with Princeton University Press.

CONTENTS

PREFACE

THERE are many approaches to the study of medical history, each with its own individual appeal. It is interesting to know the personalities who made that history, the story of their careers, their habits of daily life, their relation to associates. There is charm in the study of the great books in which that history is recorded, the tale of printers and typography, of editions and colophons. To me, however, the most fascinating objective has been the history of ideas, the slow and gradual evolution of human thought. How did the leaders of science really visualize a given problem in a given century, what was their solution and what were the reasons which dictated that solution?

As a teacher of public health, the problem of the causation of epidemic disease has specially piqued my curiosity. Demons, miasms and germs are obviously the three concepts which have here dominated human thought; but there are many subsidiary questions which intrigue the imagination.

Analysis of the beliefs and practices of primitive peoples, for example, arouses distinct respect for the logic of the procedures designed to ward off or propitiate the demons—once the basic premise of personal malign forces has been granted. The Old Testament theory of pestilence as a punishment for sin emerges as a concept on a far higher spiritual and intellectual plane than that of demonic possession which dominates the New Testament. A middle ground between demonology and objective science, which I have called metaphysical medicine, postulates no anthropomorphic forces but moves in a field of abstract intellectual conceptions rather than in a world of physical fact. The qualities which are common to magic and science and those which distinguish these two points of view have direct bearing on our understanding of superstition in the world of today.

The fifth century B.C. in medicine, as in every other field of human thought, for the first time revealed the inspiring vision of a world no longer the playground of chaotic personalized forces but an orderly universe of law. That the actual chain of causation postulated by Hippocrates was incomplete or erroneous is of little moment. It was a chain which lay in the field of objective and observable fact, each link of which could be checked, each theory corrected, by submission to the test of controlled experience. Nor were the actual results of the new approach to be considered negligible. Greek hygiene and Roman sanitation were marked by significant contributions to the cause of public health.

With the fall of the classic civilization, there came a tragic recession under the terrible shadows of the Dark Ages—when, from A.D. 400 to 1000 no one in this field in Western Europe, outside the Arabic influence, contributed a single new thought to the stream of human knowledge—and the pendulum swung back toward primitive demonology. With the spread of leprosy in the sixth century, the practice of isolation was once more emphasized. The pandemic of bubonic plague which began in 1348 led to a widespread acceptance of the doctrine of contagion embodied in hundreds of Plague Tractates which represent the first great effort at popular health instruction. The epidemic of syphilis about 1500 accentuated this lesson and in the sixteenth century Fracastorius—the second great figure in the field after Hippocrates—elaborated a clear and convincing doctrine of contagion, even though he conceived of the contagious element as a gaseous emanation rather than a living organism.

In the seventeenth century Anastasius Kircher presented the first clear scientific statement of the concept of a "contagium animatum"; Redi gave the first valid experiments to disprove the theory of spontaneous generation; and Leeuwenhoek actually described the bacteria and protozoa. By 1700, the stage was set for a germ theory of disease.

At this time, however, there was no genius in medicine to synthesize these pregnant conceptions. On the contrary, Thomas Sydenham—well deserving of his title of the English Hippocrates for his notable application of scientific principles in clinical medicine—was by no means as good an epidemiologist as a clinician. He tended to ignore not merely the germ but the whole fact of contagion and led medicine back to an emphasis on mystical conceptions of unknown and unknowable atmospheric influences which was far more extreme than that of Hippocrates himself. The Greeks used the concept of an "epidemic constitution" of the atmosphere to explain individual phenomena which could not be understood on known objective grounds; Sydenham made it the whole basis of his epidemiological thinking.

It is fascinating to note how, for two millennia, laymen were generally contagionists and physicians were miasmatists. Nor was this due to traditionalism or prejudice on the part of the medical profession. The layman observed certain obvious phenomena and jumped at the conclusion of contagion. The physician, knowing more, was quite correct in denying that any *then-available* theory of contagion could explain the facts. Richard Mead, fine flower of urbane eighteenth-century medicine, harmonized the contagionistic and miasmatic views with a skill which, to my mind, makes him the third great epidemiologist in the lineage from Hippocrates.

The history of epidemiology is an excellent example of the relativity of scientific theory. Even physics today claims no absolute and uncondi-tioned laws but only deductions as to the validity of certain relations when other factors are constant. All that we can demand from a scien-tific "law" is that it shall "work" under specified conditions. The "great sanitary awakening" of the middle nineteenth century was based on the assumption that disease was generated by decomposing filth. Crude as this conception was, it had in it enough truth to work; for dirt, if not the mother, is the nurse of disease. When Chadwick and his followers cleaned up the masses of decomposing matter in which our forefathers lived (and died), the prevalence of typhus and typhoid and cholera was strikingly reduced.

From 1850 to 1890, the empirically-justified filth theory of disease was gradually transformed into a more complete formula. Snow and Budd, in England, proved the importance of water supply and direct contact by some of the most competent investigations in the history of epidemi-ology. At last came the unrivalled brilliance of Pasteur and the firm establishment of the germ theory of disease.

The structure of modern epidemiology was, however, not yet com-plete. Throughout the latter half of the nineteenth century, Pettenkofer at Munich carried on a gallant last-ditch battle for the local miasmatic factors in the production of pestilence. The germ theory, as developed by Pasteur, still left unsolved two major enigmas, the occurrence of cases among persons who had no contact with the sick and the failure of many persons in intimate contact with the sick to develop dis-ease. The first of these enigmas was solved by the demonstration of the importance of the well carrier and the insect host; the second by an understanding of the low viability of the disease germ and analysis of the modes of infection. With these buttresses, the germ theory of disease at last stood four-square—one of the outstanding achievements of the mind of man.

In the present volume, the story of this progressive stream of human thought has been told as far as possible in the actual words of the various participants and after a thorough analysis of all their surviving works. I am indebted, of course, to university and public libraries in the United States and Europe for source material and, particularly, to my colleagues, Harvey Cushing and John F. Fulton of Yale, and to my friend, Arnold C. Klebs of Nyon, Switzerland, for access to rare editions and unpublished manuscripts; also, to my colleague, G. Lincoln Hendrickson, for assistance in regard to complex problems of ancient and medieval Latinity; and to my Secretary, Miss W. A. Thompson, for invaluable aid in checking references and in proof-reading.

The work has turned out to be more lengthy than I had hoped, both for my own sake and for that of possible prospective readers. It may be of interest, however, as the consecutive story of an intellectual progress which has made possible one of the greatest practical triumphs in the history of the human race, the conquest of epidemic disease. Furthermore, the general advances (and the occasional retreats) in this field are, perhaps, of even greater significance in the light they throw on the human understanding. The paths which have led the intellect forward and those which have lured it into unprofitable bypaths have many analogous characteristics in diverse areas of thought. It is possible that the story of epidemiological thinking may throw light on the pitfalls of scientific analysis in other fields.

C.-E. A. WINSLOW

Yale School of Medicine
New Haven, Connecticut

THE CONQUEST OF EPIDEMIC DISEASE

CHAPTER I

THE WORLD OF DEMONS

"God by god flits past in thunder till his glories turn to shades,
God by god bears wondering witness how his Gospel flames and fades;
More was each of these, while yet they were, than man their servant seemed;
Dead are all of these and man survives who made them while he dreamed."

—SWINBURNE

As Osler reminds us, "Civilization is but a filmy fringe on the history of man"; and even through this fringe there penetrate the warp and woof of the ancient fabric.

If we could visualize the thinking of the entire human race since its beginnings, it is clear that the overwhelming majority of that race have held the belief that disease is caused by the malign influence of individual supernatural powers. These powers may be exercised by living persons (witches), by the spirits of the disembodied dead or by superhuman entities; but the principle remains the same. For brevity and convenience, we may group all three of these forms of personal malignity under the general heading of the Demonic Theory of Disease.

As thus defined, the demonic theory of disease is obviously an offshoot of the broader philosophy of animism which is so general a characteristic of primitive society. To quote Jastrow, "In its belief habits the human mind has emerged from jungle magic. Primitive explanations proceed upon the basis of a hidden virtue or *mana*, which assumes an over-world from which it derives. Sorceries, incantations, mystic ceremonies, magic prescriptions, totems, and taboos express the primitive supernatural; and it is all *psychic* in its pattern of operation. This is what is meant by animism—that the primitive world is a soul-world."

Or, in the words of Garrison, "The common point of convergence of all medical folk-lore is animism, i.e., the notion that the world swarms with invisible spirits which are the efficient causes of disease and death."

"In his attempts to interpret the ways of nature," Garrison tells us, "savage man, untutored because inexperienced, first of all confused life with motion. Like Mime in Wagner's 'Siegfried,' he was puzzled if not awed by the rustling of leaves in the forest, the crash and flash of thunder and lightning, the flicker and play of sunlight and firelight, and he could see no causal relation between a natural object and its moving shadow, a sound and its echo, flowing water and the reflections on its surface. Winds, clouds, storms, earthquakes or unusual sights and sounds in nature were to him the outward and visible signs of malevolent gods, demons, spirits, or other supernatural agencies."

The world, thus peopled with menacing spirits, was a place of terror. As an Eskimo Shaman told Rasmussen, "We do not believe, we fear." And, as always, fear found its natural reaction in barbarous cruelty. In ancient Scotland, Germany, Denmark, Italy and the Balkans—as well as in Africa, Polynesia, Borneo, India and Japan—legend tells us of the rite of human sacrifice to propitiate the spirits of the place when a new building was erected. Tylor in *Primitive Culture* relates the Thuringian tale that to make the castle of Liebenstein fast and impregnable, a child was bought for hard money of its mother and walled in. It was eating a cake while the masons were at work, and it cried out, "Mother, I see thee still"; then later, "Mother, I see thee a little still"; and, as they put in the last stone, "Mother, now I see thee no more."

In such a world, each type of disease was often interpreted as the handiwork of a particular evil spirit. In the folklore of Persia, there were 99,999 specific disease demons. The demon of scarlet fever was named Al and an ancient verse describes her:

> "Would you know Al? She seems a blushing maid,
> With locks of flame and cheeks all rosy red."

Tylor tells us that "when the great plague raged in Justinian's time, men saw on the sea brazen barks whose crews were black and headless men, and where they landed, the pestilence broke out."

The same author quotes from Hanusch the following dramatic description: "There sat a Russian under a larch-tree, and the sunshine glared like fire. He saw something coming from afar; he looked again— it was the Pest-maiden, huge of stature, all shrouded in linen, striding towards him. He would have fled in terror, but the form grasped him with her long outstretched hand. 'Knowest thou the Pest?' she said. 'I am she. Take me on thy shoulders and carry me through all Russia; miss no village, no town, for I must visit all. But fear not for thyself, thou shalt be safe amid the dying.' Clinging with her long hands, she clambered on the peasant's back; he stepped onward, saw the form above him as he went, but felt no burden. First he bore her to the towns; they found there joyous dance and song; but the form waved her linen shroud, and joy and mirth were gone. As the wretched man looked round, he saw mourning, he heard the tolling of the bells, there came funeral processions, the graves could not hold the dead. He passed on, and coming near each village heard the shriek of the dying, saw all faces white in the desolate houses. But high on the hill stands his own hamlet: his wife, his little children are there, and the aged parents, and his heart bleeds as he draws near. With strong gripe he holds the maiden fast, and plunges with her beneath the waves. He sank: she rose again, but she quailed before a heart so fearless, and fled far away to the forest and the mountain."

Hovorka and Kronfeld cite a poem by Taliesin which they consider a description of the plague demon.[1]

> Guess who this powerful creature is
> Who lived before the flood,
> Without flesh and blood
> Without bones and veins,
> Without head and foot.
> It becomes neither older nor younger
> Than it was in the beginning.
>
> .   .   .   .
>
> Almighty God, how white the sea grows
> When it comes near,
> Accompanied by great storms
> It comes from the sea.
> Great are the waves
> When it strikes the shore.
>
> It is in the field,
> It is in the wood,
> Without hand and foot,
> Without sign of age,
> And yet as old as five generations or periods,
> Yet older numberless years.
>
> It is as extensive
> As the surface of the earth
> Yet never was it born
> And no one has seen it.

[1] This traditional view of German scholarship is almost certainly erroneous. J. G. Evans, the greatest authority on medieval Welsh, considered this poem a Song of the Wind.

It wanders about
And comes not at a wish,
On the land, on the sea.
It is inevitable,
There is no other like it.
It has four sides.
It is incomparable.
It comes from four directions
And cannot be foreseen.
Its course begins across the sea of Marmora.

The Old English speech had a good word for epidemic disease, "on-flyge"—the on-flying.

Among all primitive tribes known to the ethnologist, the demonic theory of disease is the prevailing one. The following passage from Corlett on the American Indian will serve for races on a similar cultural level in every quarter of the globe. "With other primitive races he regards disease as a visitation of some ill-defined spirit or more material object that gained access to the body, and naturally the process of getting rid of, or eliminating, this malevolent influence or substance constitutes the art of medicine. . . . These spirits according to the Indian belief even of today hold in their hand the destiny of men; who afflict some and restore others to health, and who upon occasion let loose epidemics which, like thistle down, are borne on the wind and men fall like trees in the path of the hurricane. These spirits of the air and below must be placated by song and dance, by rattle and beat of drum as well as by sweet incense, the smoke of tobacco which bears their supplications aloft and are pleasing to the good spirits."

The demonic theory of disease though dominant was not necessarily all-inclusive. Speckmann says that, among the Zulus, "the cause of illness may be threefold. Either the medicine-man declares it to be caused by the *amadhlozi* (ghosts), in which case a sacrifice must be offered to them . . . or it is the work of a sorcerer. . . . The third possibility is that the witch-doctor should declare it to be an *ordinary* illness." Yet the area of "ordinary" illness was a narrow one. Our modern conception of chance is rarely present among primitive peoples. Every accident has to them a meaning and ordinarily an animistic one. In the words of Lévy-Bruhl, "the laws of nature are not conceived of by the Eskimo, even though he does actually take them into account in the various crafts and implements he has produced for his use. The natural order is masked by the incalculable action of a multitude of invisible powers and capricious influences."

In every part of the world the story is the same. Wong and Wu tell us that primitive man, in China, "attributed to all inanimate objects his own sentiments and passions, fancying them influenced by the same things in the same way. . . . Consequently health and disease were thought to be controlled by them and diseases, in particular, were regarded as the work of devils or were devils in temporary possession of the human body, which would only be cured of its infirmity when the intruders were evicted by the application of appropriate incantations, charms, and other superstitious practices.

"Indeed the number of these devils, as they increased down the ages, multiplied to such an extent that current Chinese traditions have almost one particular devil to each disease. For example, nightmares are supposed to be caused by the fox ghost, pains in the abdomen by the house god. The devil of neuralgia uses an iron band which he forces on one's head producing that terrible pain. The god of thunder employs a hammer and chisel to strike one down. There are water spirits to entice a person to the waters; the wicked devils to snatch away the souls of children; and the demons of malaria, three in number, one with a bucket of cold water to give the chills, another with a stave to set up the fever, and a third with a hammer with which to knock the head producing headaches." Even today, the Chinese peasant believes that devils lurk on every hand; and each act of life—marrying and burying, buying and selling, eating and sleeping, going in and out of a door—must be safeguarded by the use of proper charms and incantations. The motorist in China is frequently enraged by the coolie who dashes across the road just in front of the car and grins happily because he believes that he has succeeded in having the familiar demon who has been dogging his footsteps run over and destroyed.

Passing west to India, we find in primitive periods the same philosophy of disease. According to Garrison, "in the earliest Sanskrit documents, the Rig Veda (1500 B.C.) and the Atharva-Veda, medicine is wholly theurgic, and treatment consists of the usual versified spells and incantations against the demons of disease or their human agents, the witches and wizards." J. E. Harrison says that in the Vedic texts the word "bráhman" in the neuter means a "charm, rite, formulary, prayer" and "that the caste of the Brahmans is nothing but the men who have brahman or magic power."

In ancient Egypt, along with the development of a medical art based on empirical observation, we find the same magical theories and practices. Maspero says, in discussing the malign influence to which the Egyptians attributed disease, "Often though, it belongs to the invisible world, and only reveals itself by the malignity of its attacks; it is a god, a spirit, the soul of a dead man, that has cunningly entered a living person, or that throws itself upon him with irresistible violence. Once in possession of the body, the evil influence breaks the bones, sucks out the marrow, drinks the blood, gnaws the intestines and the heart and devours the flesh. The invalid perishes according to the progress of this destructive work; and death speedily ensues unless the evil genius can be driven out of it before it has committed irreparable damage. Whoever treats a sick person has therefore two equally important duties to perform. He must first discover the nature of the spirit in possession, and if necessary, its name, and then attack it, drive it out, or even destroy it. He can only succeed by powerful magic, so he must be an expert in reciting incantations and skillful in making amulets. He must then use medicine (drugs and diet) to contend with the disorder which the presence of the strange being has produced in the body."

A similar mixture of magic and empirical science appears in the great civilizations which grew up in the valleys of the Euphrates and the Tigris. "For the most part," says Garrison, "the Babylonian physicians regarded disease as the work of demons, which swarmed in the earth, air and water, and against which long litanies or incantations were recited." Persian practice, while involving many different ideological elements which will be discussed more fully in later chapters, included, also, a generous share of incantations against evil demons.

The Old Testament, on the other hand, is extraordinarily free from demonology. The phenomena of demonic possession and of witchcraft are recognized but they are peripheral rather than central in the general scheme of things and the practice of magic arts is always condemned. Saul who consulted a woman with a familiar spirit, the "Witch of Endor" (I Samuel 28 and I Chronicles 10), and Manasseh who "observed times, and used enchantments, and dealt with familiar spirits and wizards" (II Kings 21 and II Chronicles 33) were exceptional cases of reprehensible practice. We are told that "Thou shalt not suffer a witch to live" (Exodus 22:18) and in Deuteronomy 18 is a vigorous condemnation of anyone who "useth divination, or an observer of times, or an enchanter or a witch, or a charmer, or a consulter with familiar spirits, or a wizard or a necromancer."

Even among the Jewish people, however, the control of demonological practices was not easy. The 91st Psalm was used in Jerusalem as an incantation against evil spirits. According to Rappoport, "In later times, as a result of Babylonian and Persian influence, the demons gradually penetrated into the Folklore of the Talmud and the Apocryphal literature. . . . All kinds of diseases were attributed to the demons and almost everyone of these spirits had his particular function."

The Persian beliefs relating to the malign influences which might be exerted through the use of hair and fingernails are emphasized in Talmudic literature. "Men who throw away the parings of their fingernails are responsible for the destruction and death of their fellow men, for out of the second window of heaven emerge one hundred thousand evil spirits which rule over the fingernails of men, and when the parings are openly thrown away they are 'picked up by sorcerers who use them for all kinds of sorcery.' " In the Talmud, too, is a curious passage which one might almost twist into a foreshadowing of microbiology: "The evil spirits crowd the academies and are to be found by the side of the bride. They hide in the crumbs that we throw on the floor and in the water we drink; they are to be found in the diseases we contract, in the oil, in the vessels and in the air. No mortal could survive if he saw their number, for they are like the earth that is thrown up around a bed that is sown."

The dibbuk played a considerable part in later Jewish folklore and, in spite of protests of Maimonides and a vast majority of Hebrew leaders, some famous rabbis made a practice of the exorcism of demons.

Primitive medicine among the Greek people first developed along similar lines. Hippocrates, in discussing popular explanations of the behavior of epileptics, says, "if they imitate a goat, or grind their teeth, or if their right side be convulsed, they say that the mother of the gods is the cause. But if they speak in a sharper and more intense tone, they resemble this state to a horse and say that Poseidon [Neptune] is the cause. . . . But if foam be emitted by the mouth and the patient kick with his feet, Ares [Mars] gets the blame. But terrors which happen during the night, and fevers, and delirium, and jumpings out of bed, and frightful apparitions, and fleeing away—all these they hold to be the plots of Hecate, and the invasions of the Heroes, and use purifications and incantations, and, as it appears to me, make the divinity to be most wicked and impious." (Adams' translation)

The transforming power of clear and objective thinking banished demonology completely from the intellectual world in which the leaders of Greek thought lived and moved and had their being. That such an attitude permeated the entire people can, however, scarcely be assumed; and the votive tablets hung in the Greek temples can hardly have been purely symbolical. The story that Epimenides controlled the plague by taking white and black sheep to the Areopagus, letting them wander where they would, to be sacrificed by those who followed them to the local gods of the place where they ultimately stopped, is an interesting example of transference. Plutarch believed in demons as mediators between gods and men; and the employment of the wryneck or "iunx" in Greek magic is the origin of the "jinx," so dear to the sports writer of today.

On the other side of the Adriatic, we find that "Fever had three temples in Rome, and was supplicated as the goddess *Febris* and flatteringly addressed as *Febris diva, Febris sancta, Febris magna*. Foul odours were invoked in the name of *Mephitis*, to whom a temple was erected at a place where asphyxiating fumes emerged from the earth." Osler quotes a touching tablet erected by a mourning mother, inscribed:

Febri divae, Febri
Sanctae, Febri magnae,
Camillo amato pro
Filio meli effecto. Posuit.

"Le corna," the sign still made with the fingers in Italy to ward off the influence of "the Evil Eye," was a mystic gesture used by the Romans at the festival of the Lemuralia. Pliny refers to many practices of primarily magical type. For the cure of a fever, toe and fingernail parings of the sufferer are to be mixed with wax and attached before sunrise to another person's door. Vervain, for effective medicinal use "should be plucked about the rising of the dog-star when there is neither sun nor moon. Honey and honeycomb should be offered to appease the earth; then the plant should be dug around with iron with the left hand and raised aloft."

In the New Testament, we find an emphasis on demonology which is far stronger than that of the more ancient Hebrew prophets. It is true that idolatry and witchcraft are denounced as among the works of the flesh (Galatians 5:20); but the theory that disease is caused by evil spirits and must be controlled by exorcism is overwhelmingly dominant.

It has been noted that Rappoport attributes a similar progressive trend toward demonology among the Jews to foreign influence; but there seem to be much more fundamental forces at work. It appears that in India, in Egypt, as well as among the Jews and the Christians, an early phase of emphasis on broad moral principles and universal law degenerated into a later phase of animism. The peak of Egyptian scientific medicine was reached in 2000 B.C., with a later reaction toward magic under the Hyksos kings. Wong and Wu tell the same story for China; magic supplanted a more rational philosophy under Taoism, superstition reaching its highest point during the Han and T'ang dynasties. The passage from the classical to the medieval world in Europe was marked by a similar transition. It seems that in each of these great civilizations the early vision of a universe of moral and natural law was too severe a challenge to the halting human spirit.

Be this as it may, the universal theory of disease in the New Testament is that of demonic possession. From the fourth chapter of St. Matthew on, we find numerous references to the healing of the sick and the casting out of devils; "and they brought unto him all sick people that were taken with divers diseases and torments, and those which were possessed with devils, and those which were lunatick, and those that had the palsy; and he healed them." There are sixteen other references to such healings in Matthew, nineteen in Mark and twenty in Luke. The most interesting case is, of course, that of the devils expelled from their two human victims into the herd of Gadarene swine when "behold, the whole herd of swine ran violently down a steep place into the sea" (Matthew 8; Mark 5; Luke 8). This is an interesting reminder of the concept of transference.

Nor was the power of casting out devils solely a divine prerogative, for it was specifically conferred upon the disciples. "And when he had called unto him his twelve disciples, he gave them power against unclean spirits, to cast them out, and to heal all manner of sickness and all manner of disease" (Matthew 10:1). "Heal the sick, cleanse the lepers, raise the dead, cast out devils" (Matthew 10:8). Healing by the apostles is described in Acts 3, 5, 14, and 27. It was so successful that "they brought forth the sick into the streets, and laid them on beds and couches, that at the least the shadow of Peter passing by might overshadow some of them" (Acts 5:15).

Nor was the power of exorcism even confined to the elect. "And John answered and said, Master, we saw one casting out devils in thy name;

and we forbade him, because he followeth not with us. And Jesus said unto him, Forbid him not; for he that is not against us is for us" (Luke 9:49-50).

With this background of New Testament demonology, the tendency of religion and science to revert to animism developed unchecked with the decay of the Greco-Roman civilization in Europe. The elements of superstition which had persisted through classical times were carried into the Christian civilization, reenforced and extended. The Temple of Romulus, a place of healing for young children was replaced by the Church of St. Theodorus, still used for the same purpose in the nineteenth century.

Magic comes regally into her own again with Apuleius of Madaura in the second century. He tells us that

"By magic's mutterings swift streams are reversed, the sea is calmed, the sun stopped, foam drawn from the moon, the stars torn from the sky, and day turned into night." The violent, secret, and occult power of witches was widely accepted and omens, incantations and the use of magical materials became more prominent. The "magi" or magicians and their methods were discussed in detail and justified by religious analogies. Apuleius says, "If, as I have read in many authors, *magus* in the Persian language corresponds to the word *sacerdos* in ours, what crime, pray, is it to be a priest and duly know and understand and cherish the rules of ceremonial, the sacred customs, the laws of religion?"

In the third century, Celsus denounced Christ, his Christian followers and the Jewish people, from whom their religion sprang, as magicians; but Origen, in answering him, urged that Christian and heathen miracles could be distinguished by their motives and results. There grew up an extensive literature on the difference between sacred and profane practices. The Neo-Platonists drew a sharp contrast between divine theurgy and human magic, the first being considered as a divine mystery or revelation, the other as a mere human art or contrivance. So St. Augustine says that the miracles of Christians "were wrought by simple confidence and devout faith, not by incantations and spells compounded by an art of depraved curiosity." One is obviously tempted to paraphrase the famous epigram, "Orthodoxy is my doxy, heterodoxy the other fellow's doxy" by saying, "Theurgy is my magic, magic is the other fellow's theurgy."

The conversion of Cyprian, an ardent student and practitioner of magic who repented and became bishop of Antioch, illustrates from this standpoint merely substitution of one form of magic for another. Calling upon God and making the sign of the Cross replaced other incantations. Yet such an analysis would not be altogether fair. Not only was the motivation different (the object of theurgy always being beneficent, that of magic generally malefic), but there was a distinct difference in intellectual atmosphere. When Iamblichus drew a distinction between divine revelation and human contrivance, he had a dim conception of the difference between a universe of spiritual law and one of willful machination. It is of extraordinary interest to note that underlying the general acceptance of the power of magic, there was a vague recognition that its phenomena were in some sense transient, evanescent, unreal. Yet it is true that the demonic theory of disease was at this period the dominant one. Augustine tells us categorically that "all diseases are to be ascribed to demons"; and the therapeutic methods appropriate to such a diagnosis were widely prevalent. Marcellus the Empiric in the fifth century, recommends the following treatment of stomach and intestinal troubles. "Press abdomen with left thumb and say, 'Adam, bedam, alam, betur, alem botum.' Repeat 9 times, touch the earth with same thumb and spit, say charm 9 times more, again for a third series of 9, touching the ground and spitting 9 times also."

Alexander of Tralles in the sixth century quotes Galen (whether correctly or not) as saying: "Many consider incantations merely as old wives' tales, a belief which I, myself, long shared. Gradually, however, I have come to the conclusion from evidence of their operation that they do have power. I have learned their value in the treatment of scorpion stings and also in the case of bones which had become stuck in the throat and which have been coughed up at once as a result of incantations. The magic formulae accomplished their object."

We all recall how Gregory the Great received assurance of the cessation of the plague in Rome by the vision of the Angel sheathing his sword, commemorated on the spot by the Castle of St. Angelo. The same Gregory gives us a delightfully intimate picture of demonology in the following tale:

A female servant in a monastery ate a lettuce in the garden without making the sign of the Cross, and became possessed of a demon. When the abbot was summoned the demon excused himself by saying "What have I done? I was just sitting on a lettuce when she came along and ate me." The abbot however indignantly drove him out, with no consideration of the extenuating circumstances.

In the same text, Pope Gregory relates the story of Basilius, who by magic arts suspended a whole monastery in mid-air; but was never able to injure anyone in it—an excellent example of the conception that demonic power was a curiously unreal and limited one. Nevertheless Basilius was duly burned to death in Rome by the zeal of the good Christian people.

According to Singer, the nadir of the human intellect in Europe was reached in the tenth century. In the next three hundred years there was a mighty flowering of intellectual and artistic energy, yet the replacement of supernaturalism by rationality was a slow and tedious process. The mighty Abelard, in the twelfth century, believed in demons and occult forces.

Hildegard of Bingen in the twelfth century fully recognizes magic but makes the True Worship of God reply to the claims of magic, "You, moreover, O Magic Art, have the circle without the center, and while you investigate many problems in the circle of creation . . . you have robbed God of His very name." She herself describes elaborate procedures of counter-magic, involving herbs plucked and dried at certain hours and under certain aspects of the sun, and a wheaten loaf with a cross cut in the crust and over which specific religious incantations have been said.

In the thirteenth century, we find so keen and rational a mind as Arnold of Villanova accepting the existence of demons, though he does not believe they can be controlled by magicians. Yet he recounts supernatural cures effected by priests, including his own relief of 100 warts in 10 days.

The Malleus Maleficarum, or Hammer for Witches was prepared with the approval of the Pope in 1489 as a compendium of anti-demonological procedure.

The sixteenth century, with the advent of Vesalius and Copernicus, is generally considered as marking the beginning of the modern scientific age. Yet it was in this century that Martin Luther said, "I would have no pity on these witches; I would burn them all."

In the seventeenth century, indeed, there was a world-wide stimulation of the practice of witch-hunting. Tylor says that this general period "can show the good Sir Matthew Hale hanging witches in Suffolk, on the authority of Scripture and the consenting wisdom of all nations; and King James presiding at the torture of Dr. Fian for bringing a storm against the King's ship on its course from Denmark, by the aid of a fleet of witches in sieves, who carried out a christened cat to sea."

Matthew Hopkins, the "Witch Finder General," travelled from shire to shire of England in 1644, receiving a fee for each conviction secured. Two unfortunates who were believed to have caused the death of the Earl and Countess of Rutland and their children by means of the evil eye were put to death at this period. Sir Thomas Browne, in a trial before Sir Matthew Hale in 1664, testified to his belief in witchcraft, although he thought the phenomena in the particular case in question explicable by natural causes.

On our own side of the water, the Salem witchcraft mania and Increase Mather's tract on "Providences" belong to the same wave of superstitious terror.

The ceremony of the "Royal Touch" for "King's Evil" was one of the last official survivals of magic procedure. It was combined with prayers and the gift of a gold coin (incantation and talisman, as well as the mystic power of personality); and Charles II is said, between May 1662 and April 1682, to have administered this treatment to 92,107 persons. Browne, Boyle and Newton believed in the practice which was continued into the reign of Queen Anne, and Samuel Johnson was "touched" by her in his boyhood.

Occasional psychic epidemics of demonology have of course occurred in even more recent times. Tylor relates the case of "George Lukins of Yatton, whom seven devils threw into fits, and talked and sang and barked out of, and who was delivered by a solemn exorcism by seven clergymen at the Temple Church at Bristol in the year 1788." In the village of Morzine, near the Lake of Geneva, there was an epidemic of demoniac possession in 1861 which affected 110 persons.

Beliefs so widespread in space and time, so profoundly influential on the behavior of mankind are not unworthy of study. We are dealing, here, not with casual childish superstitions but with a phase of human thought which in certain civilizations has been crystallized into a well-knit philosophy and a complex system of "applied science." Let us accept, for the moment, the assumptions underlying this system and consider its logical development upon those premises.

The cardinal assumption involved is that disease is caused by the malign influence of individual supernatural powers, excluding by such definition the related theory that disease is a punishment for sin and, also, all forms of magic which do not explicitly involve a personalized demonic influence. These two alternative philosophies will be discussed in later chapters.

The active malefic powers may, as we have seen, be of various kinds. First of all, they may be exerted by living human beings, as in the case of witchcraft or the "malicious animal magnetism" of Mary Baker Eddy. Lévy-Bruhl points out that the primitive believes "firstly, that serious illness and death *are*, most frequently, the result of bewitchments; and secondly, that malevolent dispositions of their own accord, and without the subject in whom they are present being conscious of it, may exert a malign, and even fatal influence."

This latter concept, that of evil effects of subconscious ill-wishing, has often tragic effects. Among many savage peoples, all the members of a family in which a death has occurred fall automatically under suspicion.

Secondly, the bewitchment may be the work of the souls of the departed, as in the belief of the natives of Annam that the souls of those who have died of smallpox and plague are likely to pass into the bodies of their friends.

Thirdly, the active forces may be non-human spirits often associated with animals or plants. Among the Creek and Choctaw Indians, "the animals, birds, fish, reptiles, and insects cause disease to afflict mankind because man killed and trampled on them. Each of these abused creatures obtained revenge by creating a certain disease to plague men" (Corlett). In the sacred writings of the Persians the demons of disease were associated with the fly, in Teuton folklore with the wriggling worm. Certain tribes of the Malay Peninsula believe in "hantu kayu," "tree-demons" which frequent every species of tree, and afflict men with diseases; some trees are noted for the malignity of their demons (Tylor).

So much for the fundamental etiological causes of disease; we come next to their *modus operandi*. This, in its simplest form, consisted in the entrance of the spirit into the body of the victim. We still use phraseology reminiscent of this concept in connection with mental disease. We say a person acts "like one possessed." Sometimes a contrary idea of soul-kidnaping or soul-theft comes into the picture as when we say someone is "out of his head." Here, it is clearly the function of the medicine-man to recapture and restore the lost vital principle. It was an obvious logical view that disease must be due to addition or subtraction, to the presence of a foreign agent or the absence of something necessary to health (somewhat like our own recognition of infections and deficiency diseases). The idea of possession was, however, much more conspicuous than that of soul-kidnaping.

Frequently, the cause of a malady was not primarily "possession" by the demon but the introduction by the demon into the body of some harmful element. Corlett says: "The idea concerning the cause of disease and of death which was most widespread in the New World was that which supported the belief that some unfriendly individual had caused a small material object to enter another person's body. The extraction of this object was the main job of the medicine man. This removal was most frequently accomplished by sucking on the irritated or aching spot directly with the mouth, or by means of a tubular stone or pottery pipe. . . . The disease or pain-causing object might be a small stick, a piece of bone, an insect, a pebble, a splinter, an arrow, a maggot or a bit of hair. After sucking out the object which caused the pain and illness, the medicine-man usually showed it to the patient, relatives or friends, after which it was destroyed or retained by the shaman for personal use."

Carelessness on the part of the victim was recognized as a predisposing cause in demonological theory. Particularly, inattention to the disposal of partly consumed food or of the hair cuttings and nail-parings played directly into the hands of malign spirits. The natives of Queensland burned all food left over from meals to prevent sorcerers from using it to work injury upon them. Among certain American Indians, the parings of finger and toenails of a child or of a dead person were similarly burned to avoid control over the soul of the individual concerned.

Sticker gives an extraordinarily interesting account of the theories of the ancient Persians and correlates these theories with their pastoral habits. Commenting particularly on the Vendidad he says that no people who had lived in well ordered cities would see the menace and contamination proceeding from a dead body—the specter of decay—in the image of an insolent and importunate fly; would ever and always dread this fly-symbol as the agent in the spread of disease from man to man and from man to dogs, and would make the fly alone of the multiform vermin which beset dogs and men and the earth, the symbol of decay. "They would not keep in the house the bodies of dogs and men which had died during the winter until the spring permitted their delivery to carrion-eating dogs and birds, thirty steps from the fireside, thirty steps from water, thirty steps from planted land. It would not have occurred to them to punish the burying of dogs and men in the all-absorbing soil or the burning of bodies in the heaven-born fire which destroys evil spirits, vermin and impurity as the greatest of crimes; to see in burial mounds places for the nightly gathering of demons from which emanate sicknesses and skin diseases and fevers and other six or seven-fold evils. They would not consider a burial which commits to the vultures and jackals the destruction of the corpse and of the menace which it harbors as the only burial which is permissible and pleasing to God. They would not keep the woman at the time of her monthly bleeding, the wife in child-bed, the mother in child-bed fever like a corpse thirty steps from fire, thirty steps from water, thirty steps from cultivated land and three paces from a righteous man; nor would they call the womb itself after a still birth a burial ground."

It is obvious that in such a philosophy there was a basis of primitive demonology, colored by metaphysical analogies and perhaps modified and overlaid with empirical experience of the danger of infection from flies, from sick people, from dead bodies. Ultimately, the whole was crystallized into a rigid religious system.

As Sticker says: "Law and belief stiffened into a dead formula. The Magus reverences fire to such an extent that he protects it against the whole world about, even by covering the mouth and nose against his own impure breath; he denies to the faithful the use of the holy destroyer for expiation and purification. He cares more for the purity of water than for the cleanliness of man; the hierarchy dethrones King Balasch or Kawat because he has built himself a bath-house; it forbids to the Jews in their median exile the use of the required acts of purification. The Magus protects the purity of the earth from dead bodies; but he also requires that clippings of hair and parings of nails should be buried, two hand-breadths deep in hard soil, one span deep in soft soil— ten steps from the true believer, twenty steps from fire and water and the altar—so that the hands of evil spirits might not make of them spears, arrows or sling-stones and so that these impurities might not generate vermin, lice, meal moths and clothes moths. The Magus uses the sacred word 'ahuna vairya' as the best protection, the most powerful invocation for curse and ban. The Magus claimed for himself alone the right of purification; only when poured by his hands, only when used according to his ritual, only when accompanied by his formulas, did the urine of cattle or water become purifying agents; but in his hands a drop only was sufficient."

Assuming the demonic cause of disease, the principles of therapeutics were reasonably obvious. You could buy off the evil spirit; you could frighten it away; or you could escape it by trickery.

Tylor says, "Disease being accounted for by attack of spirits, it naturally follows that to get rid of these spirits is the proper means of cure. Thus the practices of the exorcist appear side by side with the doctrine of possession, from its first appearance in savagery to its survival in modern civilization; and nothing could display more vividly the conception of a disease or a mental affection as caused by a personal spiritual being than the proceedings of the exorcist who talks to it, coaxes or threatens it, makes offerings to it, entices or drives it out of the patient's body, and induces it to take up its abode in some other."

The first of the three types of treatment mentioned above is propitiation of the demon. It is well illustrated by the following practices, cited by Hovorka and Kronfeld. In times of epidemic, certain tribes in Bengal erected a wooden scaffold and hung on it a vessel filled with blood as a sacrifice to the *genius epidemicus*. The Tunguses and Buriats when smallpox was prevalent set before their huts milk, tea and meat and begged the disease for this service to spare their homes. The Winnebago Indians hung dogs on trees or poles outside their dwellings for the same purpose. In the Indian Archipelago, according to Tylor, "the personal semi-human nature of the disease-spirits is clearly acknowledged by appeasing them with feasts and dances and offerings of food set out for them away in the woods, to induce them to quit their victims, or by sending tiny proas to sea with offerings, that spirits which have taken up their abode in sick men's bowels may embark and not come back."

From this type of dealing with demons there derives the whole magical and theurgic ideology of sacrifice. The horrible cult of foundation sacrifices cited in an earlier paragraph survives in modern Greece in the practice of killing a lamb or a black cock on the initiation of a new building. The Asiatic habit of introducing a subtle imperfection into every artistic design is the symbol of a similar propitiation. So is the propitiatory sacrifice of the first fruits of the harvest. So perhaps is the trick of "touching wood" after a dangerously hopeful prediction.

The second type of therapeutic or prophylactic treatment is *exorcism* or the repelling of the evil spirit by *force majeure*. The natives of the Andaman Islands set up poles smeared with black beeswax, the odor of which was supposed to be distasteful to the demon, illustrating the concept of repelling the demon instead of propitiating him. The natives of

Togoland fixed before their houses poles decorated with leaves to drive away the smallpox. Garrison says, "Whether North American Indian or Asiatic Samoyed, he does his best to frighten away the demons of disease by assuming a terrifying aspect, covering himself with the skins of animals, so as to resemble an enormous beast walking on its hind legs, resorting to such demonstrations as shouting, raving, slapping his hands, or shaking a rattle, and pretending (or endeavoring) to extract the active principle of the disease by sucking it through a hollow tube. To prevent future attacks, in other words, to keep the demon away for the future, he provides his patient with a special fetish or amulet to be worn or carried about his person."

Sometimes the principle of exorcism is applied not directly but indirectly by invoking the power of a friendly spirit to overcome a hostile one. The fairy tales of all nations are full of illustrations of this technique, as are the legends of the healing power of the saints throughout the ages. Kerler has compiled a bulky volume on the patron saints related to medicine. St. Roch was invoked in the case of plague; St. Guy, St. Vitus and St. With in chorea; St. Avertin, St. John and St. Valentine in epilepsy; St. Hubert in rabies; St. Anthony, St. Benedict, St. Martial, and Ste. Genevieve in ergotism. In reviewing cures supposed to be effected by the saints at the present time, Tylor says, "it is plain that in our time the dead still receive worship from far the larger half of mankind."

The third type of procedure was *evasion*, the tricking of the demon in some way. Rappoport cites the medieval Jewish practices of writing on the door of a house, "The epidemic has already passed here" and of locking the door and throwing away the key. Equally naive is the following charm used in Holstein:

> "Fieber bleib aus
> R R ist nicht zu Haus"

The Jews in medieval times changed a sick person's name in order to bring about a speedy recovery; and the Chinese, in a time of epidemic, change the calendar and celebrate the feast of another season of the year with great pomp in order to deceive the *genius epidemicus* and convince him that the period of his power is over.

A particularly unfortunate method of deceiving (or bluffing) the demon is the belief of the Assiniboine Indians, described by Lowie that "smallpox has eyes and sees who is afraid of it. Hence it is best to stay near those smitten with smallpox, to use the same pipe, eat from the same dish, wrap onesself in the same blanket, and to show in other ways that one is not afraid of the disease."

The procedures so far described have been aimed directly at the personalized spiritual cause of the disease. There is another group of therapeutic procedures directed against the disease itself, corresponding to what we should today call "symptomatic treatment." This, as pointed out in an earlier paragraph, is perhaps the dominant conception among the North American Indians, but is common throughout the world. As pointed out by Tylor, "In Australia, the native doctor fastens one end of a string to the ailing part of the patient's body and by sucking at the other end pretends to draw out blood for his relief." Again, "Among those strong believers in disease-spirits, the Dayaks of Borneo, the priest, waving and jingling charms over the affected part of the patient, pretends to extract stones, splinters, and bits of rag, which he declares are spirits; of such evil spirits he will occasionally bring half a dozen out of a man's stomach, and as he is paid a fee of six gallons of rice for each, he is probably disposed (like a chiropodist under similar circumstances) to extract a good many."

One therapeutic practice which is extraordinarily widespread is that of *transference*. Among the Babylonians, images were constructed and buried, after the disease had been transferred to them. The miracle of the Gadarene swine involves the same idea, as does the concept of the "scape-goat," and the use of a quickly-running stream for the washing away of disease, as described in the Talmud and by Pliny. Pliny also relates that intestinal disease may be transferred to puppies which have not yet opened their eyes by pressing them to the body and giving them milk from the patients mouth; also that a cough may be disposed of by spitting in a frog's mouth.

The following procedure outlined by Gilbert of England in the thirteenth century involves many magical conceptions but is chiefly transference. In a case of epilepsy, when the patient falls to the ground, all his clothes except his shirt should be removed and placed at his feet. The nails of all his fingers and toes should next be clipped and wrapped in a cloth. A long white thorn is then to be split and the patient dragged feet first through the cleft as far as his middle. The thorn should then be cut into small bits and placed with the nail parings. Next the patient's hair should be cut in three places. These clippings of hair and the knife used in the operation are then to be added to the other paraphernalia wrapped in the cloth, and the whole is to be buried underground, and the following words uttered: in the patient's right ear, "Christ conquers"; in his left ear, "Christ reigns"; and to his face, "Christ commands."

The mystically-minded Sir Kenelm Digby described the following remedy for fever and ague: "Pare the patient's nails; put the parings in a little bag, and hang the bag around the neck of a live eel, and place him in a tub of water. The eel will die, the patient will recover."

In Sodersleben in 1788, "the head of the village would take a child suffering from smallpox into the woods after sunset and drive a nail from a black stallion into a tree after rubbing it with blood or pus from a wound or a sore of the patient." The same practice is perhaps illustrated by an exhibit in the museum of the Smithsonian Institution. It is a section of a tree grown on government grounds near the Naval Hospital at Norfolk, Va. The tree had been tapped, human (Negro) hair inserted, the hole plugged and sealed with clay. Rings showed that fifty years had passed since this was done. Whitebread suggests that this represents an attempt either to cure headache by transference or to cause pain in some enemy.

Another very common transference procedure is described by the same author as used for the cure of warts: Rub the warts with a cinder; the cinder is then to be tied up in a paper and dropped where four roads meet; the warts will be transferred to whomever opens the parcel.

The Bosnian prophylactic against the fever, cited by Hovorka and Kronfeld involves chiefly propitiation but also transference. An old shoe is filled with salt, bread and garlic. Early in the morning, before sunrise, even before the birds begin their song, one seeks the banks of a river and cries out, "O Schulze aus dem Dorfe, O Pfarrer aus dem Pfarre, O Wolf aus dem Walde! Wenn ihr selbdritt zusammenkomt und dieses Frühstück einnehmet, dann soll euch das Fieber packen." The shoe with its contents is then thrown into the water; and the operator returns home without looking behind him.

Hovorka and Kronfeld, with German thoroughness, list thirty-one different types of sympathetic magic, including the following procedures for disposing of disease by transference—washing off, spitting out, feeding to animals, burial, casting into water, burning, or baking, tying or untying and driving nails into trees.

Finally, after this analysis of the basic principles of demonological therapeusis, we may review some of the more important elements in the demonologist's *materia medica*. We shall find, of course, that polypharmacy is the rule rather than the exception; yet, however they may be commingled, at least five different types of medicinal agents may be recognized.

The first of these agents are *human beings* possessed of certain inherent powers over the forces of evil. This is exemplified by the expulsion of demons in the New Testament where, as Osler says, "the cure is simple—usually a fiat of the Lord, rarely with a prayer, or with the use of means such as spittle. They are all miraculous, and the same power was granted to the apostles—'power against unclean spirits, to cast them out, to heal all manner of sickness and all manner of disease.'" Through the ages, and down into our own times, saints and holy men of the church have exercised the gift of healing.

Among the American Indians, the medicine-man was possessed of direct personal power over disease demons. He was specially "called" to his profession by some unusual experience, such as a dream, or he obtained his power by inheritance or purchase or initiation. In the folklore of many peoples we find the idea that the fasting, the virgin, the chaste and the unclothed possess a peculiar virtue. In a famous medieval treatise "The Herbarion" is the following procedure for obtaining medicinal plants: "The person plucking the herb and uttering the incantation must be barefoot, ungirded, chaste, and wear no ring. The plant is adjured not only 'by the living God' and 'the holy name of God, Sabaoth' but also by Seia, the Roman goddess of sowing."

In later times, we find that the blood of certain families in the west of Ireland (the Cahills, Keoghs and Walshes) was held to be an infallible remedy for erysipelas or toothache. Finally, the Royal Touch for scrofula, depending on a power peculiar to the King or Queen, persisted, as we have seen, into the eighteenth century.

A second sort of procedures may be grouped under the head of *ceremonies*, special acts by which ordinary human beings may attain power which they do not inherently possess (as in making the sign of the Cross). Such procedure usually involves other types of medication (the use of sacred objects and incantations) which will be discussed in succeeding paragraphs; but the observance of a complex prescribed ritual may be considered as constituting a distinct element. The medicine dances of the American Indians, with their use of horrifying masks and dress and with the accompaniment of noises of drums and rattles to affright the demon are examples of this methodology. Similar practices are found, of course, among many primitive peoples and are conspicuous in Chinese folklore.

In classical and medieval times the use of ritual ceremony was common in connection with the gathering of medicinal herbs, as in the passage from Pliny cited above.

Many sacrificial and propitiatory religious rites come under this same heading of ceremonial medical procedures. A somewhat bizarre case is cited by McKenzie as a common treatment of whooping cough in Britain. "The child is drawn, naked, nine times over the back and under the belly of an ass, three years old, on three mornings running. Three hairs are cut from the belly and back of the animal respectively, and put into three spoonfuls of milk drawn from the teats. This must stand for three hours, and then the child has to drink it in three draughts. The ceremony would, of course, be incomplete without the incantation, and this is to the effect that as Christ placed the Cross on the ass's back when He rode into Jerusalem, so rendering the animal holy, if the child touches the place whereon He sat, it will cough no more."

We must go back to the Persians, however, for the most extravagant development of ritual medicine. Sticker summarizes from the Vendidad the following procedure for removing spiritual-corporeal contamination.

Zarathustra says: "O creator of the earthly things, thou Holy One, can a man be purified if he has touched the carcass of a dead dog or the corpse of a dead man?—Ahura Mazdah answers: Certainly, O holy Zarathustra.—How?—In case the corpse has already been eaten upon by carrion-devouring dogs or carrion-devouring birds, then he will be purified by washing with the urine of the cow and with water. But in case the corpse has not been eaten upon, then the polluted ones should go to an orthodox man who knows how to say the proper words, who searches the holy word in orthodox fashion and who is entrusted with the laws of purification of Mazdah. He will measure off a space of nine fathoms in all four directions, there where there is the least amount of water and plants, thirty paces from the fire, thirty paces from water, and thirty paces from the holy bundles of sacrificial branches, three paces from orthodox men; there he will dig three holes, two fingers deep after the beginning of summer, four fingers deep after the beginning of the icy winter, each one one pace or three feet away from the other. Then the purifier should wash his own body with cow's urine, not with water; he should bring the dogs of Ahura Mazdah dragging them by the forelegs. Then he should dig three more holes, wash his own body with cow's urine, not with water, and wait until the points of hair on the crown of his head become dry. For a third time he should dig three holes in the earth, three paces or nine feet from the first ones, then cleanse his own body with water, not with urine; first the hands; because if the hands remain unwashed, then he will pollute the whole body. Thereupon he who is to be cleansed should approach the holes and the priest should pronounce the words of purification, whereupon the polluted person always answers with the same words. The priest should first wash his hands for him with cow's urine, then bathe his forehead from an iron or lead vessel which is fastened to a cane, saying: 'O creator, when the good waters flow on the forehead, upon which part shall the specter of decay, the Nasow, this Drug, come a-flying?' Ahura Mazdah answers: 'Upon the saddle between the eyebrows shall this she-devil and phantom come a-flying.' And when the good waters flow upon the saddle between the eye-brows, where then does the specter of decay come a-flying?—On the back of the head . . . on the face . . . on the right ear . . . on the left ear . . . on the right shoulder . . . on the left shoulder . . . on the right armpit . . . on the neck . . . on the back . . . on the right breast . . . on the left breast . . . on the right side of the ribs . . . on the left side of the ribs . . . on the right buttock . . . on the left buttock . . . on the inside surface of the upper thigh the specter of decay will then come a-flying. If it is a man then you shall wash him at first in back and then in front. If it is a woman then you shall wash her first in front and then in back . . . on the right thigh . . . on the left thigh . . . on the right knee . . . on the left knee . . . on the right calf . . . on the left calf . . . on the right anklebone . . . on the left anklebone . . . on the right instep . . . on the left instep. . . . And when the good waters flow on the left instep, upon which part then does this she-devil, this phantom come a-flying? Under the soles she will be tossed down, like the wings of a fly. Then you shall wash with propped up toes and lifted heels, the right sole . . . wash the left sole. Then she will be tossed down under the toes; you see her like the wings of a fly. With propped up heels and raised toes you shall wash the right toes . . . the left toes. . . . Then the specter of decay will be tossed in the northern direction in the form of an abominable fly, the knees stretched forward, rump erected, covered over and over with spots like the loathsome vermin. . . ."

A third type of magico-medical procedure, therapeutic or prophylactic, involves the use of *material objects* possessed of peculiar virtue. These may be tied to the body as ligatures, worn as suspensions (amulets), carried as talismans (the horse-chestnut and the rabbit's foot) or set up in the home (the fetish or ikon) or village (the totem pole).

As to the type of materials utilized, Garrison says, "Amulets include a motley array of strange and incongruous objects, such as the bits of crania excised in prehistoric trephining, objects of nephrite, Egyptian scarabs, the grigris of African savages, the voodoo fetishes of Haiti and Louisiana, teeth from the mouths of corpses, bones and other parts of the lower animals, the

> Finger of birth-strangled babe,
> Ditch-delivered by a drab

of the Weird Sisters in Macbeth, rings made of coffin-nails, widows' wedding rings, rings made from pennies collected by beggars at a church porch and changed for a silver coin from the offertory, 'sacrament shillings' collected on Easter Sunday, and the ikons and scapularies blessed by the dignitaries of the church."

Sometimes, it is obvious that the amulet or charm possesses an essentially sacred character, as in the ikon or the reliquary of a saint, or a minute copy of the Koran worn by Mohammedans. The medicine bundles of the Plains Indians and the medicine bags of the Pawnees have a similar significance.

In many instances, the virtue of the curative and protective materials lies in their rarity as in the case of the horn of the unicorn which played a considerable role in medieval pharmacy. Rings made of coffin-nails and other objects associated with the dead may sometimes fall under this heading. The various semi-precious stones undoubtedly owe their power to their rarity. The bezoar stone (assumed to be a calculus) was obviously possessed of virtue because stones could get into a body only by magic. The use of a silver bullet to kill a witch is another illustration of the power of the rare and the unusual.

Certain elements in the primitive pharmacopeia clearly owe their selection to the idea of repelling the evil spirit—excrement, parts of snakes and other noxious animals and the like. The practice of fumigation involves this psychological element, along with others. Possibly the carrying in the pocket of an onion for protection against cholera (practiced in Munich in 1854) and the wearing of a bag of camphor to ward off influenza (prevalent in Connecticut in 1918) have a similar origin.

Very frequently it is obvious that the healing virtue of objects is associated with analogies in form, or color, similarity of names or association of ideas, which suggests curative power. Here, demonological concepts merge with those of metaphysical science, which will be considered in a later chapter; at present, we shall consider only those practices which more or less clearly suggest a demonic etiology, although the line of demarcation is never a sharp one.

The therapeutic use of water to wash away disease or its prophylactic value in blocking the way of demons is a case in point. Under certain circumstances, the concept of purification has merely a symbolic spiritual significance. In other cases it is associated with the removal of physical contamination and may be considered a rational practice. In others, as in the healing of Naaman the Syrian and in the general recognition of the Jordan, the Nile, the Ganges and the Tiber as seats of the Gods, it is apparent that an animistic procedure is involved.

The therapeutic value of blood, flesh and saliva is probably associated with the concept of human power, that of iron with its material strength. Tylor suggests that the latter concept may date back to the end of the Stone Age. Among the Jews, a knife or other pointed instrument was placed under the pillow of the pregnant woman to protect her against demons. Copper and mercury were worn as amulets against cholera as late as the nineteenth century; and the nailing up of a horseshoe for "luck" is an innocuous present-day survival.

Whitebread lists, among many others, the following amulets and charms in the Smithsonian Collection, most of which involve an obvious association of ideas.

> Peony root (epilepsy)
> Horse-chestnut (rheumatism)
> Scarlet silk thread (nose-bleed)
> Rabbit's foot (rheumatism)
> Mistletoe (epilepsy)
> Part of harness of a horse (sprains)
> Spider in a nutshell (ague)
> Madstone (rabies)
> Carnelian and other red stones (hemorrhage)

Color furnishes the association of ideas in two of these instances. Similarly, in the England of Edward II and also in Japan, smallpox was treated by red hangings and curtains about the bed (an interesting but probably accidental anticipation of Finsen); while red-cloth suspensions for scarlet fever are recent in England.

The horse-chestnut perhaps suggests the nodules of rheumatism and the motion of the spider in a nutshell the shivering of ague.

Anything worn by a horse should naturally restore locomotion. The Winnebago Indians made their medicine pouches of otter skin because the otter is so wise. And Sir Thomas Browne in his analysis of "Vulgar Errors" cites the use of the right foot of a frog wrapped in a deer-skin for the gout. Surely the *right* foot of a jumper in the skin of a runner should provide the necessary stimulus.

The widespread use of the mandrake for magical purposes is probably primarily related to the resemblance of this root to the human body.

A fourth important element in such *materia medica* was the use of *words* in the form of ejaculation or more elaborate incantation. As Jastrow says "Folk-mind and doctrinal mind are impressed with the power of words." The employment of holy names is one of the simplest of such procedures and the greeting of a sneeze with "God bless you" or "Gesundheit" is a vestigial practice of the same kind.

Much more elaborate verbal charms may be recited to ward off or cure disease, or to ensure the efficacy of medicinal remedies. Pliny describes how the Magi plucked their healing herbs with a statement of what they were to be used for. In primitive Chinese medicine, written charms played a major role. They might be hung on the wall or used as suspensions or burned and the ashes administered to the patient.

Sometimes the charms were purely occult as in the sacred formula cited by Hovorka and Kronfeld as in use in 1785.

> S A T A N
> A D A M A
> T A B A T
> A M A D A
> N A T A S

Quintus Serenus Sammonicus, a noted physician of Rome in the second and third centuries, gives the following recipe usual for fevers: "Write several times on a piece of paper the word, 'Abracadabra' and repeat the words in the lines below, but take away letters from the complete word and let the letters fall away one at a time in each succeeding line. Take these away, but keep the rest until the writing is reduced to a narrow cone. Remember to tie these papers with flax and bind them round the neck." After wearing the charm for nine days, it had to be thrown over the shoulder into a stream running eastward.

Often, magical folklore and religious invocation were inextricably mingled. Hovorka and Kronfeld cite two excellent examples, as follows:

Among the Ruthenians it was a custom to place on the table a vessel of glowing coals, a broom, an oven rake and a little grain, and to chant the following incantation:

> In the name of God the Father, Son, and Holy Ghost, Amen.
>> Plague, mighty Plague,
>> Demon, mighty Demon,
>> Out of the fire,
>> From the water
>> From the wind
>> Go from God's servant—away,
>> Christened, consecrated and baptized,
>> From his red blood,
>> From his yellow bones,
>> From his white body,
>> Go away over the rapid-flowing Dniester,
>> Beyond the blue lake,
>> Out to the open river.

A Bohemian mode of preventing malaria was as follows: One goes at sunrise into the fields without having washed or combed the hair. On the way one must not turn around and must not speak to anyone who may be met. Then one kneels down in the field, spreads the arms out, invokes the Holy Cross without making the sign, says three Paternosters and three Aves without Amen, and then repeats the following invocation

>> Lord Jesus Christ, why do you tremble so?
>> Have you perhaps a fever?
>> I have none and will have none,
>> And whosoever thinks of my sufferings
>> He also will have no fever.

A purely religious medical incantation is the *Lorica* (coat-of-mail) of Gildas the Briton which Singer dates at about the year 600. It begins with the statement that "Gildas made this lorica to drive out those demons who pestered him." It invokes divine aid as follows:

> "Help, O oneness of Trinity,
> have pity O threeness of unity,
> I beseech thee to help me who am placed
> in peril as of a mighty sea,
> So that neither the pestilence of this year
> nor the vanity of the world may suck me under"

After enumerating the various hierarchies of angelic beings it continues: "O God, with thy inscrutable saving power defend all my parts, deliver the whole trunk of my body with thine own protecting shield that foul demons may not hurl, as is their wont, their darts at my flanks." For more than twenty lines, the specific parts of the body to be protected are then enumerated, closing with the final covering clause "and other members the names of which I have perchance omitted."

There is perhaps a fifth principle which may be distinguished, that of *sacred numbers, times, seasons* and *directions*. Many instances have been already cited of the virtue associated with such numbers as 3, 7, and 9. The concept of favorable days exercised a far-reaching influence on medieval medicine. The significance of right and left, the facing of Christian churches to the east, omens from the flight of birds all illustrate the significance of orientation. "The German cottager declares that if a dog howls looking downward, it portends a death; but if upward, then a recovery from sickness. . . . So to the negro of Old Calabar, the cry of the great kingfisher bodes good or evil, according as it is heard on the right or left" (Tylor).

Many of these practices belong to metaphysical rather than demonological medicine; but in others we may clearly trace the thread of supernaturalism.

It is as difficult to separate prophylaxis from therapeutics in primitive as in modern medicine; but we may consider very briefly certain communal procedures adopted in the presence of epidemics, which clearly belong in the field of public health practice.

Hovorka and Kronfeld mention three types of such procedures. The first of these is the flight of the population. The natives of Coram leave their villages and subsist for months in the impenetrable forest in order to escape contact with the spirit of smallpox. A second procedure is to remove the sick from the neighborhood of the well. On the island of

Rias smallpox cases are permitted to remain in their homes so long as cases are few; but when an epidemic breaks out they are sent out from the village and a special shelter provided for them. A third practical measure is external quarantine. This was probably first designed to exclude the *genius epidemicus* but later was extended to exclusion of human beings.

Into such practices, it is easy to read a perception of the principle of contagion. It is very probable that they were indeed fortified by empirical experience through a process of what has been called "super-natural selection." Yet, in view of their general setting, it is probable that they were primarily demonological in origin, as Hovorka and Kronfeld suggest.

It is interesting, as a foreshadowing of the concept of contagion, to note how general was the belief that the demons of epidemic disease came from some other country—just as syphilis in 1500 was known as "the French disease" and influenza in 1918 as the "Spanish" influenza. The plague-woman of Slavonia was always a stranger to the village. The plague, as described in the invocation quoted in an earlier paragraph "began across the sea of Marmora."

Methods of quarantine differed widely in detail. The Dayaks of Borneo hung a red string across the stream below their dwellings and fastened thereon red and white flags. This was a sign that no one could pass. Sometimes the quarantine warning was not symbolic as in the above case, but contained a written warning to outsiders to keep out, as was the practice in Sumatra. Tylor cites a Malay tribe as "placing thorns and brush in the paths leading to a part where smallpox had broken out, to keep the demons off; just as the Khonds of Orissa try with thorns, and ditches, and stinking oil poured on the ground, to barricade the paths to their hamlets against the goddess of smallpox, Jugah Pennu." A delightfully simple quarantine procedure employed in China is to surround the dwelling by small staggered brick walls, since evil spirits move only along straight lines.

A somewhat different principle of demonological quarantine (suggesting propitiation rather than exorcism) is attributed by McKenzie to native public health authorities in the South Sea Islands who put a stop to epidemics by providing a boat with rudder, sails, anchor, provisions, and a flag to take the demon away from the island.

Corlett, in discussing the Pueblo Indians describes an annual "spring clean-up," when respiratory diseases are prevalent, in which the whole village participates. "Disease and witches are whipped away with eagle plumes. Even the animals are included in this general curing ceremony. Just before dawn and the departure of the people, everyone is given a swallow of a powerful medicine. The head doctor thanks everyone and hopes that all sickness has been dispelled and all witches dispersed."

Goldenweiser says of the Iroquois, "In addition to their activities as visiting physicians, some of the societies practice ceremonial rites or exercise elaborate medicinal functions of a more generalized kind. . . . The False-faces (a medicine society) twice a year . . . drive away the disease spirits and act as do our health officers for the public good."

Similar special ceremonies against pestilence were held in China in spring and fall under the Chan dynasty; and Osler says, "In times of epidemic the specialists of Wu-ism, who act as seers, soothsayers and exorcists, engage in processions, stripped to the waist, dancing in a frantic, delirious state, covering themselves with blood by means of prick-balls, or with needles thrust through their tongues, or sitting or stretching themselves on nail-points or rows of sword edges."

Child hygiene is one of the most important aspects of public health. Therefore, for the protection of the infant, whose resistance against malign influences is so small, the inhabitants of the Central Celebes have the following procedure, described by A. C. Kruyt: "In Onda, when a child is taken out of the house for the first time, the mother puts some ashes and some ylong-ylong grass on every step of the stairs. The ashes neutralize any uncleanness that the steps may have suffered from the many people passing up and down them, and the grass checks the evil by smothering it. By these two methods, the magic power which may be lurking there is prevented from injuring the baby."

All in all, it seems clear that what Reinach calls "the strategy of animism" was a reasonably compact and purposeful set of procedures, following quite logically from the basic etiological assumptions involved.

These assumptions, and the practices derived from them, are by no means limited to past ages or to remote regions of the earth. The *New York Times* of January 24, 1926, described the following episode in France. "Today began at Melun, near Paris, the trial of the twelve religious devotees, ten of them women, who nearly killed the Curé of Bombon several weeks ago when, with sticks and stones, they tried to drive the devil out of the body of the poor man.

"Their accusation against him was that when migrating birds flew southward over Bombon the priest filled them with disease, so that when they passed over Bordeaux, 500 miles away, they caused to grow poisoned mushrooms of lascivious shapes and noxious odor, which gave the residents on the banks of the Gironde shameful diseases in various forms."

The same paper for January 6, 1929, contained an account of the trial at York, Pennsylvania, of John Blymyer, "powwow doctor," John Curry and Wilbur Hess accused of murdering Nelson Rehmeyer when he resisted efforts to obtain a lock of his hair to use as a charm. The statements of the accused centered largely about a charm book published in 1856 which had the following precious attributes: "Whoever carries this book with him, is safe from all his enemies, visible or invisible; and whoever has this book with him, cannot die without the Holy Corpse of Jesus Christ, nor drown in any water, nor burn up in any fire, nor can any unjust sentence be passed upon him." In this latter case the local coroner told a reporter, "At least half of the 60,000 residents of the city of York believe in witchcraft and as for the county's rural population of 90,000, they not only believe in witchcraft, but guide the minutest details of their lives by it."

Reed reminds us that every year nearly a million people go on pilgrimage to Lourdes; and quotes the story of the shrine at Malden, Mass., where 847,000 people came in a period of three weeks in 1929 to be healed at the grave of a miracle-working priest, until the church authorities put a stop to the episode.

Finally, the Lynds in *Middletown* give us the following picture of a completely typical community of the Middle West:

"A number of citizens have gone in recent years to 'the old nigger out in ————,' an outlying village, who is alleged to drive disease down through a patient's feet into the ground by waving his hands before him. Some people still treasure incantations for curing erysipelas and other ills, carefully passed down from generation to generation, always to one of the opposite sex. A downtown barber regularly takes patients into a back room for magical treatment for everything from headache to cancer. Some people still believe that an old leather hatband wrapped about each breast of the mother at child-birth will prevent all forms of breast trouble. An old leather shoe-string wrapped about a child's neck will prevent croup; 'Our little boy had croup' said a working class woman, 'and I'd forgotten about this cure, but I got a leather shoe-string, and the boy got well.' Assafoetida worn about the neck prevents the catching of contagious diseases; 'Our little girl wore one bag and played day after day with children who had whooping-cough and never caught it' said another worker's wife. If one rubs a wart with a bean picked at random from a sack of beans and then drops the bean back into the sack the wart will disappear. Some people believe in curing a stye by rubbing a wedding ring on the eye, in carrying a copper wire about the wrist or a buckeye in the pocket to prevent rheumatism—copper rheumatism rings may still be purchased—or in the magical potency of flannel."

In view of its continuing impact upon present-day society, as well as for its theoretical interest as a chapter in the history of human thought, our long analysis of demonological medicine may perhaps be considered justified.

CHAPTER II

THE WRATH OF GOD

"For now I will stretch out mine hand, that I may smite thee and thy people with pestilence."—EXODUS 9:14

"If thou wilt diligently hearken to the voice of the Lord thy God, and wilt do that which is right in his sight, and wilt give ear to his commandments, and keep all his statutes, I will put none of these diseases upon thee, which I have brought upon the Egyptians; for I am the Lord that healeth thee."—EXODUS 15:26

THE ideology we have so far been considering is based on the conception that disease is due to diverse individual supernatural powers operating in a spirit of wilful malignity. There is a second conception of disease which resembles the first in that it visualizes a world governed by supernatural rather than natural forces but differs sharply from it in other respects. This is the ideology which interprets disease as an expression of the wrath of an essentially righteous god animated by an innate necessity for the punishment of sin. The way to deal with malign spirits is by exorcism, evasion or sacrificial propitiation. Neither exorcism nor evasion can operate against a supreme being; and propitiation is not efficient in itself but only as a token of repentance and a pledge of amendment. The sacrifice of Isaac has a quality quite different from the black cock killed to appease an evil spirit. Both intellectually and morally, the theory of divine wrath is immeasurably superior to the nightmares of animism; for it involves the concept of a universe of law, although the law is spiritual rather than material.

Even among very primitive peoples, this higher conception of suffering as due to one's own sin rather than to demonic malignity is to be found mixed with a baser animism. J. Singer says "The crudest notion of taboo is the naive belief that contact with objects both sacred and unclean leads to physical consequences both evil (disease) and fatal (death). On a higher level of culture the crude belief has been modified by the conception of wrath or anger of the deity who may or may not punish the sinner. The risk of physical punishment is incurred by violating a taboo. On a more rational level the avoidances are religious or ritualistic conventions interpreted as part of a religious discipline or as symbolic of moral and spiritual values." Lévy-Bruhl cites numerous instances in which confession of sin is a fundamental element in primitive rites of purification. Similarly Corlett points out that among the American Indians, violation of taboo often involved the interpretation of sickness as a punishment sent by just and not malign gods. He describes this principle as of special prominence in the medico-religious ideology of the Aztecs and Peruvians.

We may read the same interpretation into the fact that in the Egyptian Pantheon, Sekhmet was the sender of plagues and pestilences and at the same time the patron-goddess of medicine. So, in Greece, Apollo caused disease by his arrows but also presided over its cure. When the same god chastises and restores, we have passed out of the world of naive demonology.

Among the Semitic peoples, the concept of disease as punishment for sin reached its apogee. Even in Babylonian medicine, which was primarily built on demonology, the thought of disease as associated with bodily impurity or sin enters into the picture. In Persian dualism, with disease and demonic possession due to Ahriman and medicine and surgery deriving from Ahura Mazdah, we pass a little further along the road. There is a foretaste of the Hebrew scriptures in the following passage from the Persian writings quoted by Sticker: "Who is it that robs me of my prosperity and my increase, that brings sickness to me and ruin? Surely it is the teacher of false doctrines, who without authority usurps the place of the purifier; away goes good fortune and abundance, health and well-being, prosperity and growth and increase, the sprouting of herb and of grass; none of these blessings will return until the false teacher is overthrown and until obedience to orthodox authority is again duly honored in the land for three days and three nights long by gleaming fire, by strewn sacrificial branches, by the established carousals."

It is in the Old Testament, however, that this concept comes to full flower. The existence of magic and divination, as pointed out in Chapter I, is clearly recognized as in the following passages:

"Thou art wearied in the multitude of thy counsels. Let now the astrologers, the star-gazers, the monthly prognosticators, stand up, and save thee from these things that shall come upon thee" (Isaiah 47:13).

"My people ask counsel at their stocks, and their staff declareth unto them" (Hosea 4:12).

Yet even such mildly magical practices are always condemned.

"And they shall no more offer their sacrifices unto devils, after whom they have gone a whoring" (Leviticus 17:7).

"Neither shall ye use enchantment, nor observe times" (Leviticus 19:26).

"A man also or woman that hath a familiar spirit, or that is a wizard, shall surely be put to death" (Leviticus 20:27).

"Forasmuch as thou hast sent messengers to enquire of Baal-zebub the god of Ekron, is it not because there is no God in Israel to enquire of his word? therefore thou shalt not come down off that bed on which thou art gone up, but shalt surely die" (II Kings 1:16).

Even as an object of condemnation, however, the role of magic in the Old Testament is a minor one. In sharpest contrast with the prevailing demonology of the New Testament, as well as with Babylonian and Persian ideology, the overwhelming mass of references to disease in the Old Testament, from beginning to end, involve the higher concept of punishment for sin and the nobler gospel of righteousness as its only remedy.

This distinction seems so important that a citation of some of the chief texts may be justified. Their cumulative effect is overwhelming.

"And the Lord plagued Pharaoh and his house with great plagues because of Sarai Abram's wife" (Genesis 12:17).

"I will even appoint over you terror, consumption, and the burning ague" (Leviticus 26:6).

"If ye walk contrary unto me, and will not hearken unto me; I will bring seven times more plagues upon you according to your sins" (Leviticus 26:21).

"When ye are gathered together in your cities, I will send the pestilence among you" (Leviticus 26:25).

"So the plague was stayed from the children of Israel" (Numbers 25:8).

See also Numbers 31:16 and I Samuel 4:8, also 5:6 and 5:9.

"And the Lord will take away from thee all sickness, and will put none of the evil diseases of Egypt, which thou knowest, upon thee; but will lay them upon all them that hate thee" (Deuteronomy 7:15).

"That there be no plague among the children of Israel" (Numbers 8:19).

"The Lord smote the people with a very great plague" (Numbers 11:33).

"Even those men that did bring up the evil report upon the land, died by the plague before the Lord" (Numbers 15:37).

"The Lord shall smite thee with a consumption, and with a fever, and with an inflammation, and with an extreme burning" (Deuteronomy 28:22).

"But the Spirit of the Lord departed from Saul, and an evil spirit from the Lord troubled him" (I Samuel 16:14). "And it came to pass, when the evil spirit from God was upon Saul, that David took an harp and played with his hand; so Saul was refreshed and was well, and the evil spirit departed from him" (I Samuel 16:23). Note that, as in the later case of Job, the demonic possession was ordained by God and was cured by refreshing Saul's spirit, not by direct exorcism.

"So the Lord sent a pestilence upon Israel from the morning even to the time appointed; and there died of the people from Dan even to Beer-sheba seventy thousand men." After David had made appropriate burnt offerings and peace offerings, "the Lord was intreated for the land, and the plague was stayed from Israel" (II Samuel 25).

"And the Lord smote the king, so that he was a leper unto the day of his death" (II Kings 15:5).

Asa "was diseased in his feet, until his disease was exceeding great; yet in his disease he sought not to the Lord, but to the physicians. And Asa slept with his fathers" (II Chronicles 16:12-13).

So Uzziah was stricken with leprosy in punishment for his sin (II Chronicles 26).

One exception is of special interest. Satan smote Job with boils, but *only by the permission of the Lord* (Job 2).

The protecting power of God is beautifully expressed in the 91st Psalm.

"Thus they provoked him to anger with their inventions; and the plague brake in upon them. Then stood up Phinehas and executed judgment; and so the plague was stayed" (Psalms 106:29-30).

"And I will smite the inhabitants of this city, both man and beast; they shall die of a great pestilence" (Jeremiah 21:6).

"Behold I will send upon them the sword, the famine and the pestilence" (Jeremiah 19:17-18; also 33:36, 38:2, 42:17 and 22, 44:13. See also Ezekiel 6:11-12, 7:15).

According to Rappoport, the same point of view is characteristic of the later history of the Jewish race. He says: "The folklore of the Jews is distinguished from that of other nations, primitive and even civilized, by its *monotheistic* and *ethical* background. There is hardly a belief, a custom or a superstition, a legend, a folktale or a folksong, even if imported from abroad, that does not reflect the Jewish conviction of the existence of one God or does not teach a moral lesson."

In the New Testament, on the other hand, this majestic conception of disease as a penalty for sin is almost wholly absent until we come to Revelation where St. John the Divine repeats the message of the ancient Hebrew prophets in the text:

"Therefore shall her plagues come in one day, death and mourning and famine; and she shall be utterly burned with fire; for strong is the Lord God who judgeth her" (Revelation 8:8).

Martin Luther, in the sixteenth century, said that, "pestilence fever, and other severe diseases are naught else than the devil's work." Cotton Mather, in the seventeenth century, defined disease as "the scourge of God for the sins of the world." Here are two concepts which indicate a fundamental difference of outlook. Throughout the ages these two distinct supernatural explanations of disease have survived, battling with each other and with conceptions of a different type. Hovorka and Kronfeld tell us that at the time of the plague epidemic in Bombay (1896-1897) both Mohammedans and Hindus agreed that evil spirits were at work. These revealed themselves to one Mohammedan woman in the shape of four gigantic female figures with bloody teeth and fleshless bones and wrapped in white garments. To ward off their influence, the Mohammedans hung paper talismans inscribed with sacred formulae in the streets. The Hindus, on the other hand, considered the visitation as a punishment inflicted by the god, Siva, for the sins of his people.

There is a world of difference between the conceptions discussed in the present chapter and the preceding one. In dealing with social and international problems, our attitude is still essentially that of demonology. Some day, perhaps, we shall—in these fields, too—attain the moral elevation of the Hebrew prophets if not the intellectual clarity of the Greek philosophers.

CHAPTER III

METAPHYSICAL MEDICINE

"Chacune de nos conceptions principales, chaque branche de nos connaissances, passe successivement par trois états théoriques différents; l'état theologique, ou fictif; l'état metaphysique, ou abstrait; l'état scientifique ou positif."
—COMTE

THE term "magic," as we have seen in earlier chapters, is used in various senses. In the medieval church, it was distinguished from the supernatural powers exercised by the saints by its malign motivation and by a certain illusory and limited quality in its results. Among scientific thinkers, it has been characterized by its inherent fallacy. It is "the other fellow's religion" and "the other fellow's science."

If, however, we consider the problem from the standpoint of "the other fellow" and attempt to understand his attitude—which is a main purpose in the present study—the distinction is less obvious. Whitebread cites a definition of "magic" as the "pretended art of producing supernatural effects by bringing into play the action of supernatural or spiritual beings, of departed spirits, or of the occult powers of nature." For the believer in magic, we must drop out the word "pretended"; for, to him, the phenomena are real. And the word "supernatural" does not, to him, connote something dubious, as it does to us. And "occult" means merely "hidden" or "secret." Most of modern science is highly occult to the average man or woman.

Magic, like science, is a practical means of controlling the course of life by a supposed knowledge of its laws. In each instance, the believer conceives himself to be attaining his ends by rational means; and in each case, he can adduce what seems to him valid experimental evidence in favor of his procedures. Pareto points out that the person who tells you that when a cock crows at midnight there will be a death in the household considers that he is using the same kind of reasoning as when he tells you that when a cock is placed with the hens egg-laying will follow. If you cite instances where a midnight cock-crow was not followed by fatal results, he points out that hens are sometimes infertile.

Thorndike, in discussing the thinking of the Middle Ages, is undoubtedly right in his contention that "Magic and experimental science have been connected in their development, that magicians were the first to experiment; and that the history of both magic and experimental science can be better understood by studying them together."

For an understanding of the psychology of magic we must, I think, dismiss the concepts of malignity and illusoriness as criteria. Magical procedures may be used for good purposes, as in the text cited from the Gospel according to St. Luke in Chapter I; and the test of illusoriness is, after all, only one of volume of experience.

It may perhaps be profitable to forget the emotional overtones of such words as "magic" and "science" and analyze the actual practices of mankind—with regard to the control of communicable disease—from the standpoint of their underlying ideologies. The same action may be performed with quite different attitudes of mind. The savage might use the blood of a recovered patient to cure diphtheria because such blood was an acceptable sacrifice to the demon of the disease. The believer in the occult might do the same thing because of an assumed relation of sympathy—mysterious, but nōt supernatural. The scientist might employ exactly the same practice to neutralize diphtheria toxin.

The ideology involved is, indeed, more important than the practical results attained in a particular instance. In a given case, blood supposed to possess sympathetic properties might succeed and blood supposed to contain antitoxin might fail. The scientist should, however, be a trail-maker rather than a treasure hunter. The right road will lead others to the promised land, even if the pathfinder does not proceed far himself; while a single concrete achievement, if obtained by accident, may be important in itself but open up no future possibilities. Jenner's happy discovery was of great immediate value, but Pasteur's methodology revealed a new world.

We have reviewed two basic ideologies, with regard to the causation of disease—that of the World of Demons, animistic and amoral, and that of the Wrath of God, monotheistic and involving a universe governed by moral law. Between these two philosophies and that of modern science lies another, which has been confused by most writers—even by Thorndike—with the demonological and religious theories, but which seems to deserve separate recognition.

This third ideology is distinguished from animistic and religious theory in that *it does not explicitly assume the influence of any supernatural being*, either demonic or divine. Belief in the power of the stars over human life, as we shall see, has generally carried no supernatural implication whatever. The ideology in question is distinguished, on the other hand, from physical science in that *it does assume the influence of occult forces* which lie beyond the framework of the known physical universe. This distinction is much more nebulous than the former. The framework of the known physical universe changes and expands. If Rhine's method of card-reading were proved—which, apparently is not the case—it would have to be transferred from the occult to the physical sphere. Whenever sufficient evidence accumulates, science, by its very nature, must expand to include the phenomenon concerned. The distinction we are here considering is therefore a shifting one; yet at any given moment in history we can recognize beliefs which, while not involving any supernatural connotation, lack valid objective experimental proof. As a rule, such beliefs are characterized by rationalization rather than observation. They involve primarily logical relations, associations of ideas, emotional motivations. Frequently, they depend on similarities of appearance or merely verbal analogies. They operate in a world of ideas rather than in that of observed facts. They merge with supernaturalism on the one hand and with physical science on the other; but they involve a central attitude which is distinctive and important in the history of human thought.

This type of ideology, I propose to call *Metaphysical Science*, even at the cost of arousing the wrath of the philosophers. It is inappropriate in the sense of the official definition of metaphysics as including the science of being and the theory of knowledge; but it is, I think, true to the common usage of the term as the science of the supersensible—the "transphysical science" of Albert the Great. It conforms to the classifications of Comte, cited as our chapter heading. In any case, it matters little what terms one uses, if they are defined; and by "Metaphysical Science," I mean, "a body of theory assumed to depict natural laws but involving principles foreign to the accepted body of experimental science," usually of a logical rather than an observational nature.

A borderline example of this type of metaphysical operation is divination. It is a practice clearly related to supernatural concepts and commonly accompanied by prayers and incantations. Divination by dreams is generally, but not always, associated with definitely spiritual forces; and the trivialities of the ouija board are in essence demonic. On the other hand, the search for omens derived from dissection of animal organs is distinctly colored by conceptions of cosmic law. The art of hepatoscopy, practiced as early as 3000 B.C. and developed to such a high degree in Babylonia, was conceived as a science rather than a magic art.

Seneca accepted all forms of natural divination, from flight of birds, organs of animals, astrology, thunder. "Only Seneca holds that every flight of a bird is not caused by a direct act of God, nor the vitals of the victim altered under the axe by divine interference, but that all has been prearranged in a fatal and causal series."

The use of the divining-rod for water-finding has very recently received serious attention from scientists of considerable standing. In all these fields, one can recognize primary associations of ideas, and obvious emotional symbolisms, crystallizing into a complex and artificial pseudo-science, as in card-reading, telling fortunes from tea leaves, palm-reading and phrenology.

Far more influential and more persistent in the higher fields of human thought—and, particularly, in relation to epidemiology—was the group of practices related to astrology. This art dates back at least to a Sumerian boundary stone of 1185 B.C. (bearing the signs of the Zodiac) and was a fundamental basis of Chaldean medicine. It was prominent among the Mohammedans and, in the New World, among the Aztecs. Two of Galen's treatises are devoted to astrology, and he informs us that "if Hippocrates said that physicians should know physiognomy, they ought much more to learn astrology, of which physiognomy is but a part." Astrology was always taught in medieval times as a part of astronomy, in the Quadrivium.

So, Roger Bacon, probably writing about the year, 1268, says: "Purgations, venesections and other evacuations and constrictions, and the whole of medical practice, are based on the study of atmospheric changes due to the influence of the spheres and stars. Wherefore a physician who knows not how to take into account the positions and aspects of the planets can effect nothing in the healing arts except by chance and good fortune. This is taught by medical authorities such as Hippocrates, Galen, Rhazes . . . and similarly experienced physicians, who know astronomy, clearly teach this by infallible proofs." Similarly James Yonge in 1422 writes, "As Galian the full wies leche Saith and Isoder the Gode clerk hit witnessith that a man may not perfitely can the sciens and craft of Medissen but yef he be an astronomoure."

Even into the seventeenth century horoscopes were cast to determine a favorable time for bleeding and purging.

Astrology probably began as a phase of animism. Garrison says "Another superstition derived from Chaldean astrology was the belief that the heavenly bodies influence disease. The sun, moon, stars, and planets were regarded as sentient, animated beings, exerting a profound influence upon human weal and woe."

According to Windelband, even for Aristotle the stars were "beings of superhuman intelligence, incorporate deities, . . . and from them a purposive rational influence upon the lower life of the earth seemed to proceed."

Yet, in parallel with this animistic concept there grew and increased quite a different conception—that of the stars, not as personal agents but as mirrors and indices of universal law. This attitude seems to me so far the prevailing one that I classify astrology on the whole as metaphysical science rather than demonology.

M. Jastrow is, I think, justified in concluding that "The basis on which the modified Greek system [of astrology] rests is likewise the same that we have observed in Babylonia—a correspondence between heaven and earth, but with this important difference, that instead of the caprices of the gods we have the unalterable fate controlling the entire universe— the movements of the heavens and the life of the individual alike."

Al-Kindî, in the ninth century, gives an elaborate explanation of the force of the stars (and also the power of the mind through words) as an influence exerted through the emission of rays. Such an influence was illustrated in medieval texts by comparison with the attraction of a magnet and the reflection of rays by a mirror—analogies of exertion of force at a distance which are clearly scientific in their underlying attitude.

The fundamentally fatalistic concept of astrology was repugnant to the more extreme advocates of free will and the difficulty was surmounted with amusing ingenuity by Hebrew authorities cited by Rappoport. Four famous Rabbis in the Talmud "declared that Israel formed an exception and was not subject to the influence and power of the planetary system." Another Rabbi of the Talmud reconciled the two tendencies, when he declared that "a man distinguished by his piety could render the stars and the planets subject to himself, though otherwise he would be subject to them."

One interesting corollary of astrology was the concept of the macrocosm and the microcosm. The idea that the human body and the physical universe exhibit a mystic parallelism was a characteristic conception of metaphysical science which exerted a powerful influence upon medieval medicine.

Another derivative of astrology was belief in the relation of unusual celestial phenomena (such as comets and eclipses) to human well-being. Among the Eskimos, eclipses were held to foretell the coming of an epidemic; and during its period the women would invert their cooking dishes to avoid dangerous emanations from the eclipsed moon (Corlett). This conception of a relation between cosmic marvels and disease outlasted all the rest of the pseudo-science of astrology; and was held (as we shall see in later chapters) by the leaders of the medical profession up to the end of the eighteenth century.

A third major influence in the area of metaphysical science was the vast group of practices associated with the idea of "sympathetic magic." Heraclitus was, perhaps, the first to give philosophic form to the concept of the inherent sympathies and antipathies of natural objects; and it was well stated by Giovanni Baptista Porta, as follows: "By reason of the hidden secret of things, there is in all kinds of creatures a certain compassion as I may call it, which the Greeks called sympathy and antipathy, but we term it more familiarly their consent and their disagreement."

Here, as in the case of divination and astrology, the roots of the practice lie in the soil of demonology and resemblances to the practices of "transference" are many and obvious. Yet it seems to the writer that, while transference is essentially animistic, the general color and texture of thought regarding sympathy warrant its classification as metaphysical science.

The beginnings of this mode of thinking may be noted among primitive peoples. Thus, the Cherokees place a flint arrowhead in a decoction to be used as a vermifuge to convey to the medicine the cutting quality of the stone. Among the Mayas, Corlett finds much evidence of the concept of sympathy; "A skin eruption resembling the stings of wasps was treated with a poultice made from the crushed nests of wasps and other stinging insects. Vines bearing a certain resemblance to snakes were employed to cure snake-bite; jaundice was cured by decoctions of yellow grubs, seeds or plants, while the vomiting of blood was treated with preparations based on plants or seeds of a red color."

The mystical virtues of blood—and of red ochre, which was its special symbol—are described in detail by Lévy-Bruhl.

The medical practice of Egypt included such procedures as the use of the hair of a black calf to prevent grayness and of the organs of generation to stimulate strength. (It may be noted that, however ineffective such practices may have been, they were quite as scientific in underlying attitude as our use of hormones; in 1941, preparations of male sex hormones were widely used in England for the treatment of shell shock.) Among the Persians, white pigeons were chased away because of a supposed relation to the white spots of "leprosy"; and these same spots were treated with colored plants using the following incantation: "Thou art born in the night, plant—dark, black and gloomy; O thou dyer, color that which is pale, the gray, that which is spotted wilt thou cause to disappear from this man; the original color restore to him; chase far away the white spots."

The streaked rods with which Jacob produced ringstraked cattle by maternal impressions is, of course, another example of the power of sympathy.

Pliny cites innumerable procedures of this kind, some with approval and some without. A few instances may be cited as follows:

To cure an epileptic, drive an iron nail into the spot where his head rested when he fell in a fit. (This is a borderline case, perhaps transference rather than sympathy.)

The use of organs of goats and gazelles to treat eye diseases, because these animals never have ophthalmia. (This is analogous, in psychological approach, to the use of hormones.)

Invincibility is promised the wearer of the head and tail of a dragon, hairs from a lion's forehead, a lion's marrow, the foam of a winning horse, a dog's claw bound in deerskin and the muscles, alternately, of a deer and a gazelle. (This is not endorsed but quoted as a practice of the Magi.)

Treatment of thighs chafed by horseback riding with the foam from a horse's mouth.

Cure of the bite of a mad dog by organs of the animal. (These last two are apparently approved by Pliny himself.)

As a protection against nocturnal fevers, two bed-bugs bound to the left arm in wool stolen from shepherds; for diurnal fevers the wrapping should be of russet cloth instead.

Even Galen is by no means free from this type of medicine. He recommends that for the extraction of a tooth from the upper jaw, it should be surrounded with the worms found in the tops of cabbages; for a lower tooth, the worms on the lower parts of the leaves should be used. It is clear, however, that he is thinking in terms of metaphysical science rather than demonology. In advocating the treatment of epilepsy by a suspension of peony root about the neck, he suggests that particles from the root may be drawn in by the patient's breathing or may alter the properties of the surrounding air.

St. Augustine, who did not believe in ligatures and suspensions, carries the analysis a little further. He says that it is one thing to say, "If you drink the juice of this herb, your stomach will not ache," and it is another thing to say, "If you suspend this herb from your neck, your stomach will not ache. For in one case a healing application is worthy of approval, in the other a superstitious significance is to be censured."

Clearly, both Galen and Augustine were thinking—within the limitations of their knowledge—in scientific and not magical terms.

The powers of the magnet had great vogue in medieval times, but were certainly conceived as physical effects. Paracelsus tells us that treatment with the magnet "can cure a flux from the eyes, the ears and the nose; a magnet can cure jaundice, fistula, ruptures of all kinds, and dispel both jaundice and dropsy." He carries us further toward the borderline of magic when he suggests that bits of magnetic substance be impregnated with mummy material and deposited with seeds in rich earth the seeds having "a congruity with the disease." As the plants grew, they would absorb the disease.

One of the most famous and influential applications of the principle we are considering was the "powder of sympathy" proposed in 1663 by Sir Kenelm Digby, one of the first members of the Royal Society and a man of the greatest eminence in his day. This powder was copperas; and it was used to cure a wound by applying it to the sword by which the wound was caused. In our own times the maxim *similia similibus curantur* of homeopathy is a survival of the same idea. The vogue of vomiting, purging and bleeding was distinctly colored with the metaphysical concept of eliminating an occult influence.

The *materia medica* of metaphysical science (according to our definition of that term) were simpler than those of demonology. Sacred persons and incantations find no place in it, although it must be remembered that we are making a distinction between two attitudes of mind which are often present in the same individual at the same time. When an herb is plucked with incantations, for instance, both science and animism may be involved.

From this arbitrary viewpoint the remedies of metaphysical science are chiefly material objects and, predominantly, perhaps, those objects supposed to possess the occult virtue of sympathy. One of the most striking examples of this mode of thinking is the Doctrine of Signatures, of Paracelsus, according to which divine providence had provided a cure for each disease and labelled it with a form or color or markings to indicate its use. This conception is, of course, centuries older than Paracelsus. Very primitive peoples use red flowers for anemia and yellow for jaundice. Jastrow lists the following examples; euphrasia for eye-diseases because of an eye-like spot on its corolla; saxifrage for the stone because it sends its roots over rocks and crumbles their surface; nettle tea for nettle rash; quaking grass for ague; toads for warts; snails (because of their coiled structure) for ear-ache. He adds "It is still the Chinese practice to prescribe the roots of plants for foot-trouble, the stems and middle parts for chest ailments, and the flowers and upper leaves for headaches."

In Pliny, we find innumerable examples of the same idea. Thus, ophites, a marble with serpentine streaks, was used for snake-bite; an herb on which grew small lumps, for stone in the bladder. Of this remedy he says, "In the case of no other herb is it so evident for what medicine it is intended; its species is such that it can be recognized at once by sight without book knowledge." In exactly similar fashion, Galen reports the cure of warts by myrmecia, a plant bearing wart-like lumps.

The elaboration of this conception is well illustrated by the Treatise of Signatures written by Crollius in 1669, which includes, for example, the following analysis: "Walnuts have an entire signature of the head; the exterior rinde or herby encompassment, of the pericranium: wherefore salt of the rindes, for wounds of the pericranium is a singular remedy. The interior hard rinde, or wooddy shell, of the cranium. The thin skin encompassing the kernel, of the skin and membranes of the brain. The kernel hath the figure of the brain itself: Therefore it is also helpful to the brain. For if the kernel beaten be moistened with the quintessence of wine, and applied to the crown of the head, it comforts the brain and head wonderfully."

A second important group of remedies (snake flesh, excrement, etc.) were related to the idea of *repellency*, which merges with the demonological practices of exorcism. The following methods mentioned by Pliny as said to be effective in treating malaria are certainly heavily tinged with animism: The dust in which a hawk has rolled is put in a bag and tied with a red thread and worn around the neck of the sick person. Or, the longest tooth of a black dog, or a certain kind of wasp which flies alone, and which one must catch with the left hand. It must be the first one seen in the year. Or the head cut from a living viper or the heart taken from it is wrapped in a linen cloth; or the nose of a mouse and the points of its ears are placed in a red cloth—the mouse must be released again; or the right eye of a living lizard and its head, cut off afterward, wrapped in a goatskin. Another method is to bind on the body the heart torn from a living snake or four joints of a scorpion's tail together with the sting, in a black cloth; the sick person must not see the scorpion or the person who puts on the bandage for three days, and must hide the remedy after twelve days. Or to roll a caterpillar in a linen cloth, tie it three times with a thread provided with three knots, and the one who takes this remedy must say why he does it.

Yet it is also clear that primitive emotional animism is often overlaid and modified by rationalizations which make the user of such procedures believe that they are scientific. Galen's belief in the therapeutic value of viper's flesh is justified by the following anecdote: "When Galen was a youth in Asia, some reapers found a dead viper in their jug of wine and so were afraid to drink any of it. Instead they gave it to a man near by who suffered from the terrible skin disease elephantiasis and whom they thought it would be a mercy to put quietly out of his misery. He drank the wine but instead of dying recovered from his disease."

In Sir Kenelm Digby's day people carried about with them a living toad or a spider shut up in a box because those creatures soaked up the pestilential vapors "which otherwise would infect the party." Theriac, made from vipers' flesh, was eliminated from the British Pharmacopoeia in the middle of the eighteenth century by the College of Physicians by a majority of only one vote. As late as 1862, a Dr. John Hastings of London wrote a pamphlet upon the "Value of the Excreta of Reptiles in Phthisis and Some other Diseases" (McKenzie).

Sometimes the association of ideas involved in the selection of remedies was much more naive than in the use of signatured or repellent drugs. One of the wildest feats of the imagination was perhaps that of Quintus Serenus Sammonicus, a Latin physician of the third century, who advised as a remedy for quartan ague the placing of the fourth book of Homer's Iliad under the sufferer's head! Porta, in the sixteenth century, however, ran him a close second when he suggested that appropriate therapeutic effects might be produced by music played on instruments constructed of the wood of medicinal plants.

Such associations of ideas often bring in—as in demonology—the occult significance of times, seasons, numbers. The metaphysical thinker might pluck his herbs before sunrise or at a certain stage of the moon with no thought of propitiating spirits but in the belief that at such times the plant possessed a special natural virtue. Pliny's emphasis on such numbers as 3, 7 and 9 (thrice seven centipedes diluted with Attic honey for asthma) were certainly based in his mind on occult scientific principles rather than animism. The persistence of the conception of "critical days" for bleeding and purging, etc. (on which the great thinker, Roger Bacon wrote a special tract) was another metaphysical— but not in the least an animistic—concept.

The attempt has been made in these first three chapters to distinguish what seem to the writer to be three fundamentally different norms of human thought, whose recognition is vital to an evaluation of man's reasoning about disease. As a corrective for this logical classification, it is essential to keep always in mind the fact that in any given period of history these three attitudes (and, later, more rigidly scientific attitudes) are inextricably mingled. A particular set of procedures may be conceived clearly and simply as a means of repelling demons. Many of them persist as habitual occult practices, when the immanence of the demons has largely disappeared from consciousness. Some become justified in the minds of their practitioners by association of ideas which bring them clearly into the field of metaphysical science. A few (as in the case of the healing rays of the Sun-God) may actually be proved to have direct scientific efficacy. At different intellectual levels of the population, we find—even today—all these modes of thinking in operation; and, in all but the most rigidly scientific we may detect them in the same individual (as when an eminent physician interests himself in water-finding by the divining-rod).

Thorndike, who is perhaps our leading authority on this relation between magic and medicine in medieval times says, that "many secrets of nature still remained undiscovered in our period, and hence it is not surprising that the conception of occult virtue in nature, of occult influence exerted by animals, herbs, and gems, or by stars and spirits, still prevailed to such an extent among men of the highest scientific attainments then possible. How potent this connection was, has been shown by the continued use of amulets, of ligatures and suspensions, by the general belief in fascination, physiognomy, number mysticism, and divination from dreams. Some still countenanced the occult force of words, figures, characters, and images, or of this and that rite, ceremonial, and form. Especially surprising is the prevalence of lot-casting under the pseudo-scientific form of geomancy. But others had begun to doubt the efficacy of some or most of these things. Animism had pretty much had its day; necromancy and the notory art received relatively little attention, although the church appears to have rather encouraged them by insisting upon the existence and power of evil spirits. But even the fathers and theologians made the point that demons work their marvels largely through their superior knowledge of natural forces. Much more in science and medicine have we seen the notion of spiritual force displaced by that of occult natural virtue, and use made of natural substances rather than of incantations. Some of our authors would explain the results achieved by incantations entirely by the force of suggestion."

In our own days magic persists chiefly in relation to the mysterious and alluring field of electro-magnetic force. Mesmer, who had been granted his medical degree at Vienna in 1766 for a thesis on "The Influence of the Planets on the Human Body," substituted "animal" magnetism for the cruder concepts of Paracelsus and exerted a world-wide influence, reenforced and magnified by Mrs. Eddy and the Christian Scientists. Even in the twentieth century, things electrical still have a strong hold on the metaphysical imagination as evidenced by the cult of Abrams and the much more respectable (but equally unfounded) Dessauer treatment of disease with ionized air.

Such metaphysical science as we have considered in the present chapter is never considered to be "magic" by its practitioners; it is, as Tylor says, "a sincere but fallacious system of philosophy, evolved by the human intellect by processes still in great measure intelligible to our minds." It is a system of philosophy which is even today largely dominant in the field of the social sciences as recently demonstrated by Thurman Arnold and Stuart Chase. Above all, Pareto in his tremendously significant *Treatise on General Sociology*, has given us a most helpful analysis of the psychological factors underlying this type of thinking.

Magical practice can be differentiated from scientific practice only by the ultimate test of quality and quantity of objective evidence. There is, however, a distinct psychological difference between magical and scientific thinkers. In any generation there will be found some individuals (Pliny or Sir Kenelm Digby) who are inclined toward the occult, and others (Galen or Arnold of Villanova) who exhibit a minimum of this tendency. The difference is not one of intelligence or formal education· We all know people of limited intellectual opportunity who are hard-headed and skeptical, others of brilliance and culture who pursue with avidity every newest fad of pseudo-medicine. The distinction is, I believe, rather one of *balance* between the reason and the emotional desires.

The devotee of magic, in any generation, is the impatient person, who desires passionately an immediate escape from his dilemma; for magic offers a short-cut, a single panacea, a quick release by some all-powerful formula or physical device. The title of Jastrow's book, *Wish and Wisdom* admirably embodies the central antithesis involved. When "wish" outruns "wisdom" we have resort to magic. Or in Freud's terminology, thinking by the "pleasure principle" dominates thinking by the "reality principle." It was not by accident that William Jennings Bryan so frequently began his perorations with the phrase, "I like to believe."

The spirit of science on the other hand, involves two fundamental mental attitudes, and those two attitudes may be characterized by the terms humility and faith. By humility I mean realization of the fact that we live in a universe of laws and that progress—even survival—is attainable only by conformity to those laws. A truism, perhaps. When someone told Carlyle that Margaret Fuller was a great woman because "she accepts the universe," the old man growled, "Gad, she'd better." Yet the world is today full of people and of nations who refuse to accept the universe, who believe that that universe can be turned inside out and upside down by such figments of the imagination as "the Nordic inheritance" and "the German will."

The second fundamental attitude of the scientist is faith—faith that by learning how the laws of nature work, rather than by defying them, those laws can be molded to the uses and the purposes of man. "Ye shall know the truth, and the truth shall make you free." In the past century the whole physical background of human life has been transformed in the light of this doctrine. Comfort and ease and luxury have been brought within the potential reach of the peoples of the earth by applications of physics and chemistry and engineering, while hygiene and sanitation have lifted more than half of the burden of sickness and death from the shoulders of the human race.

CHAPTER IV

THE UNIVERSE OF NATURAL LAW

*"I too think that these diseases are divine, and so are all others, no one being
more divine or more human than any other; all are alike and all divine. Each
of them has a nature of its own, and none arises without its natural cause."*
—HIPPOCRATES

OSLER approaches the subject of Greek science with the following
glowing exhortation: "Let us come out of the murky night of
the East, heavy with phantoms, into the bright daylight of the
West, into the company of men whose thoughts made our thoughts, and
whose ways made our ways,—the men who first dared look on nature
with the clear eyes of the mind." The sharpness of the contrast is somewhat overdrawn, since in the valleys of the Nile and the Euphrates there
was much scientific medicine mingled with superstition. In the Old
Testament, as we shall see in a succeeding chapter, there was a keener
recognition of certain natural laws of sanitation than we can find among
the Attic philosophers. The assumption that superstition is necessarily
of the East and science of the West is certainly unfounded.

It is true, however, that even the earliest glimpses we can catch of the
Greek people exhibit a freedom from primitive demonology which is astounding. Sticker says that "for a long time superstitious ideas mix with
the growing natural ideas as shown among the Danaeans and Achaians as well as among the surrounding nations." We find a poetically
illumined remnant of the specter of disease in the life-like description of
the pest which Homer gives in a few verses in the beginning of the Iliad:
Called upon by the priest Chryseis concerning the outrage committed by
Agamemnon against Astynome, the daughter of Chryseis, Apollo, the
blazing god of light, strides angrily over the top of the Idaean mountain
range in the south of the Trojan country. "On his shoulder he carries the
silver bow, in the quiver the unfailing arrows, his countenance darkens
as the night; he descends far from the swift ships of the Achaeans and
shoots the first arrow amid the terrible sound of the silver bow. First the
mules and swift-footed hounds fall. But soon Apollo aims his sharp mis-
siles at the men. For nine days the people die, and unceasingly the funeral pyres burn. We will understand the Homeric picture if we know
that every year when the summer is far advanced, when the sun has at-

tained to the highest vault of heaven and then falls behind again, and when Sirius rises on the horizon early in the morning at milking time, in order to outshine all of the stars, that then strong fevers increase on the coastlands and on the islands of the eastern Mediterranean, intermittent fevers, brain-fever, relapsing fever, and continuous fever, and that then these fevers of the hot dog-days become deathly in many years to the miserable mortals" (G. Sticker). Centuries after Homer's time the dog-star was still fearfully worshipped on the island of Cos, the birthplace of Hippocrates; and Phoebus Apollo is the pest-bearer and god of death as well as the protector against plagues and god of healing in Roman times even as in the time of the Greeks.

Yet, after all, this is poetic imagery, not medical science. It is much more important to note, as Gomperz has pointed out, that "there is no mention in the Iliad of medical incantations. Weapons are drawn out of the bodies of wounded heroes, the flowing blood is staunched, and the wounds are smeared with ointments; exhausted warriors are restored with wine, pure or mixed, but there is not a single word about any kind of superstitious customs or spells."

Garrison is correct when he concludes that among the early Greeks, we find a genial polytheism, with many local tutelary medical gods, underlain by a much less conspicuous stratum of demonology concerned with the propitiation of the Chthonian deities of the earth and the underworld. These darker aspects of thought, however, tended to be sublimated into higher and nobler forms under the clarifying and constructive genius of the Greek mind. The Erinnyes became symbols of divine law, and propitiatory rites of purification merged into spiritual catharsis.

The more primitive instincts died hard. Hippocrates cites current Greek theories as to the supernatural causes of disease; and as late a classical writer as Pliny is full of magical prescriptions. On the whole, however, it is clear that among the earliest Greeks of whom we have record all authoritative thinking had passed beyond the world of demons into a more spacious and more orderly world where—if disease were of supernatural origin at all—it came as an evidence of the Wrath of God and not as the result of irresponsible spiritual malice.

The role of the gods in medicine clearly persisted—as will be noted in a later paragraph—among the people throughout the whole period of Attic civilization. By the fifth century B.C., however, it had been discarded by the intellectual leaders in favor of a philosophy which marked perhaps the most important turning-point in the whole history of human thought.

We have noted in earlier chapters that primitive races may recognize "ordinary" diseases as well as those caused by ghosts and sorcerers; and it is obvious that the veriest savage takes natural causation into account in many of the actions of his daily life. Yet the area of "ordinary" phenomena among such people is a limited one and the abstract conception of laws of nature rarely if ever enters his consciousness. The theoretical conception "that the universe is a rational system, working by discoverable laws, seems to have first appeared as a definite belief among the Ionian Greeks in the sixth century B.C." (C. Singer); and the fifth century was characterized by a supreme effort to cast off the incubus of supernatural influence in every field of thought.

The Hebrews gave us a universe of moral law; but the Greeks clearly visualized for the first time in human history a universe of natural law. In Osler's words, "Whether a plaything of the gods or a cog in the wheels of the universe—that was the problem which life offered to the thinking Greek; and in undertaking its solution he set in motion the forces that have made our modern civilization." As Marcellin Berthelot has justly said, "Ce furent les Grecs qui . . . fondèrent . . . la science naturelle, dépouillée de mystère et de magie, telle que nous la pratiquons maintenant." This achievement was incomparable and unique.

The immediate practical results of the application of this new conception were necessarily somewhat meager, for the trail of science is a long one. Much toilsome collection of facts was necessary before the true laws of the operation of the universe could be approximated. Many Greek thinkers, intoxicated with their dazzling vision, were too hasty in their generalizations. Philosophy tended to replace religion as an abstract determinant and the very brilliance of Greek generalizations acted for centuries as an obstacle to that study of the actual facts of nature which these generalizers preached. In the hands of lesser men who substituted ideas for observations, natural science degenerated into metaphysical science. The doctrine of sympathies and antipathies enunciated by Heraclitus formed a basis for a new sympathetic magic.

Yet it is vitally important to distinguish between the essence of the Greek method of thought and its abuse. As Gomperz says, "It is one thing to make an erroneous hypothesis, it is quite another thing to make an unscientific hypothesis which is entirely or partially incapable of verification." This is the real essence of the matter. If disease is postulated as caused by gods or demons, scientific progress is impossible. If it is attributed to hypothetical humors, the theory can be tested and improved; and, by the gradual processes of observation, the humors may be resolved into the hormones. The conception of natural causation was the essential first step. It marks incomparably the most epochal advance in the intellectual experience of the race.

In the development of Greek theories of the natural universe, medicine played a notable part. Gomperz traces the triumphs of the Greek intellect to three main sources, the metaphysical and dialectical discussions of the Eleatic philosophers, the semi-historical method of Hecataeus and Herodotus and the schools of the physicians, whose leaders "aimed at eliminating the arbitrary element from the view and knowledge of nature."

It is natural, therefore, that concepts of health and disease should correspond closely to theories of the physical universe as a whole; and these theories were based on the conception of "the four-fold root of all things" voiced by Empedocles but, according to Jones, first clearly stated by Polybus.

Four elementary properties, hot, cold, moist and dry, operated throughout this universe and mutually paired combinations of the properties constituted the four basic substances of which that universe was built. To each of these substances, there corresponded one of the four basic "humors" of the human body.

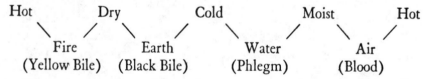

Hot	Dry	Cold	Moist	Hot
Fire	Earth	Water	Air	
(Yellow Bile)	(Black Bile)	(Phlegm)	(Blood)	

The life process was supposed to be animated by a vital atmospheric principle, the "pneuma," a theory expounded at a very early date by Anaximenes, the Ionian. "Our soul being air, holds us together."

Health consisted in a proper balance between the four humors, while disease was caused by an undue preponderance of one or more of them. Each of these humors is embedded as a sort of verbal fossil in our language; for a "sanguine" man is one who has too much blood in his composition, a "phlegmatic" man, one who has an excess of phlegm; a "bilious" man, one who has too much yellow bile; while "melancholy" is merely the Greek for a superabundance of black bile.

These conceptions seem to represent somewhat deep-seated trends of human thought, for we find in Asia almost exactly similar theories of disease. Wong and Wu tell us that while empirical medicine based on the use of drugs dates back in China to 3000 B.C., and while demonology persisted even among native physicians up to modern times, a philosophical concept of the universe, much like that later developed in Greece, was evolved in China in the eighth century B.C. The world as these early thinkers conceived it was governed by a dualistic principle, the Yang and the Yin, and was composed of five elements—water, fire, and earth (as with the Greeks)—and metal and wood—two distinct elements (instead of the air of the Greeks). Later Buddhism adopted the four Greek elements (fire, earth, water and wind) and considered disease as due to six main causes:

1. Disturbance of the four elements
2. Immoderation of food and drink
3. Wrong methods of meditation
4. Sinful desires
5. Evil influences
6. Devils and demons

Similarly, Hindu physiology was based on a theory of seven primal constituents of the body, health consisting in a normal quantitative relationship of these primary constituents, disease in a derangement of their proper proportions.

To return to the Greeks, the theory of the four humors offered a plausible explanation of diseased conditions arising within the body itself as a result of its inherent characteristics or as the influence of personal habits. In the field of epidemiology, with which we are primarily concerned, something more was necessary. When a plague suddenly broke out and spread through a whole population, some cause must be present, outside of the individual but operating on the community as a whole. Where could one look for such a locally universal factor save in the ambient air? Hence, it was inevitable that Greek thinkers should seek to account for such phenomena by changes in the atmosphere; and since the atmosphere obviously did exhibit varying properties of hotness, dryness, cold and moisture, the correspondence between these external properties and those within the body itself offered a reasonable explanation of epidemic disease. Hence the major emphasis on season and climate which characterizes the Hippocratic writings—an emphasis which is again paralleled in the early medical writings of China.

As Sticker says, "The acceptance of epidemics born in the air is impressed everywhere upon the observing person where the plague of intermittent fever increases its victims each year; then a reflective people tries to escape the bad air, malaria, by means of preventive precautions against certain winds which prove to be fever-bearing; living above the wind, arranging of doors on the side of the house away from the harmful wind, and especially at the setting-in of the west wind, avoidance of night air and coats with head coverings are some of the precautions. But in some places the recognition gains ground that the bad mist does not develop in the air itself, but arises out of stagnant waters and especially decaying swamps; one is protected against the malaria which is born in the water and other plagues which develop in the water by placing the home far from the water, upon elevated places and by the erection of sleeping towers. In Greek antiquity we find the conscious attention to the choice of the place of residence and arrangement of the home with reference to the danger of fever. In the Ionian philosophers there grows along with the beginnings of astronomy and general knowledge of the earth the necessity of understanding the plagues in natural terms. Thales of Miletus, who predicted the eclipse of May 28, 585 B.C., or else someone of his school, Democritus of Abdera, explains the origin of great pests by poisoning of the air by the dust of the comets of perished worlds. The scientific school of Pythagoras in south Italy searches for the cause of the pest again on the earth itself and thereby better corroborates the experiences concerning the behaviour of stationary as well as wandering plagues."

So Plutarch states that Empedocles delivered a certain region from the plague by closing the mountain gorges through which hurtful winds blew down into the plains.

As the physicians were influenced by the theories of the philosophers, so we find the philosophers (particularly the Pythagoreans) often treating of medical matters. Alcmaeon of Croton, who was closely connected with the Pythagorean school, described health as a balance between "opposites," and Philolaus in 440 B.C. discusses bile, blood and phlegm as causes of disease. The mutual interplay, of course, had its bad as well as its good side. From Pythagoras comes the emphasis so unfortunately laid by medicine on auspicious numbers and critical days for many centuries to come.

Against the abstract metaphysical theories of the philosophers, there came about 500 B.C. a reaction among medical thinkers which was of momentous significance. It revealed itself particularly in the medical school of Cos, and its earliest manifestation was in the tract "On Ancient Medicine" which is generally considered as pre-Hippocratic in origin. Here we find an inspiring attack on speculative nature-philosophy and an appeal for return to the safe road of observation and experimentation. Those blind leaders of the blind who had "misled the art of medicine from its ancient track and started it on the road of hypothesis" were challenged in vigorous terms, and the abstract conceptions of "hot" and "cold," "moist" and "dry" were denounced as meaningless and misleading. In their place the ancient author calls for a simple, rational attack on individual specific conditions of disease. Great emphasis is placed on diet, and the physician is conceived in essence as an expert dietitian for the sick.

In all this we have a forecast of the famous saying of John Hunter to Jenner, "Don't think. Try." This saying expresses only a half-truth. The scientist should *both* think and try; and medical research today often suffers from a lack of analytical thinking. In the fifth century B.C. and the eighteenth century A.D. the emphasis of the ancient Coan and the London surgeon was pertinent and timely. And this wholesome criticism of metaphysics at last reached its climax in Hippocrates. G. Sticker truly says, "The natural philosophy and interpretation of nature which was divorced from experience, such as the speculative philosophers of the Age of Pericles loved, seemed to the physician Hippocrates to be the greatest danger for true science and practical art. With all the sharpness possible he calls medical thinking back from meditation and speculation to observation and experience, from the imagined to the tangible and from heaven to earth."

This greatest personality in the history of medicine is but a shadowy figure from an historical standpoint. Baissette has given us a highly romantic biography; but one which is a work of imagination rather than scholarship. He tells us that Hippocrates was of the family of the Asclepiads, initiated into the full rights of the medical priesthood at the age of thirteen years. He describes his Wanderjähre in Egypt and other countries, his practice in Athens and conquest of the plague there by burning aromatic spices in the streets. He discusses the request of Artaxerxes for his services and the refusal of that request by the Athenian Senate and the patriotic physician himself. He describes in detail Hippocrates' departure from Athens and his later travels, his visit to Democritus and his death at the age of 109 years while sleeping under a pine tree.

All these details are apocryphal; but it does seem probable that there was a famous physician of the name. Aristotle speaks of "the great Hippocrates" and Plato refers to him in "Protagoras" and in "Phaedrus." In the latter, Phaedrus remarks, "Hippocrates the Asclepiad says that the nature, even of the body, can only be understood as a whole." Aristophanes not only mentions Hippocrates but implies a widespread familiarity with the Hippocratic Oath. Most authorities accept the fact that he was born on the island of Cos in 460 B.C., and the date of his death is generally given as between 375 and 377 B.C. Jones describes him as the son of Heraclides, trained by his father and by Herodicus. He accepts the story of his wide travel and the legend that his help was sought by Perdiccas of Macedonia and Artaxerxes of Persia.

Thus, Hippocrates lived at the very peak of the greatest period of Greek history. He was a contemporary, or a near-contemporary of Pericles, of Aeschylus, Sophocles, Euripides and Aristophanes, of Socrates and Plato, of Zenophon, Herodotus and Thucydides, of Pindar and of Phidias.

The standing of the physician in this brilliant society was a high one, and the centers of medical enlightenment appear to have been the two rival medical schools of Cos and of Cnidos, schools which have ever since stood for two sharply opposing viewpoints. Cnidian medicine laid great stress on disease, classifying particular maladies with enormous elaboration, emphasized diagnosis, used purges, milk and whey as practically its only remedies. Coan medicine was preoccupied with the patient rather than the disease, adapted its treatment to assisting the individual patient to overcome his individual difficulties by cooperation with the *vis medicatrix naturae*, and developed prognosis to a high degree. The brilliant triumphs of German nineteenth century medicine were in the spirit of Cnidos, while the preoccupation with the individual patient is a Coan tradition which has come down to us through Padua and Leyden and Edinburgh.

However legendary Hippocrates himself may be, the writings attributed to him constitute a definite historical fact, and they present us with a vivid picture of the teachings of the Coan school. It is generally accepted that the Hippocratic corpus represents what has survived of the library of the school at Cos. All commentators are agreed that the most characteristic of these treatises (such as "Airs, Waters and Places")

THE UNIVERSE OF NATURAL LAW — 61

date from the latter part of the fifth century B.C. and that many of them bear internal evidence of having been composed by the same hand. Gomperz thinks that they were all written before the year 400, while Jones and Garrison think some may date as late as 300 B.C.

In this series of treatises we find clearly outlined that courageous conception of a universe of causation which has been noted in an earlier paragraph as the characteristic and outstanding contribution of Greek genius to the stream of human thought. A quotation from "Airs, Waters and Places" has been used as a text for this chapter; and the same problem of natural as opposed to supernatural causation is discussed more fully in the essay on epilepsy, "The Sacred Disease." The following quotation is from Jones's translation,

"I. I am about to discuss the disease called 'sacred.' It is not, in my opinion, any more divine or more sacred than other diseases, but has a natural cause, and its supposed divine origin is due to men's inexperience, and to their wonder at its peculiar character. Now while men continue to believe in its divine origin because they are at a loss to understand it, they really disprove its divinity by the facile method of healing which they adopt, consisting as it does of purifications and incantations. But if it is to be considered divine just because it is wonderful, there will not be one sacred disease but many, for I will show that other diseases are no less wonderful and portentous, and yet nobody considers them sacred. For instance, quotidian fevers, tertians and quartans seem to me to be no less sacred and god-sent than this disease, but nobody wonders at them."

After discussing various suggestions for treatment, he continues;

"III. Accordingly I hold that those who attempt in this manner to cure these diseases cannot consider them either sacred or divine; for when they are removed by such purifications and by such treatment as this, there is nothing to prevent the production of attacks in men by devices that are similar. If so, something human is to blame, and not godhead. He who by purifications and magic can take away such an affection can also by similar means bring it on, so that by this argument the action of godhead is disproved. By these sayings and devices they claim superior knowledge, and deceive men by prescribing for them purifications and cleansings, most of their talk turning on the intervention of gods and spirits. Yet in my opinion their discussions show, not piety, as they think, but impiety rather, implying that the gods do not exist and what they call piety and the divine is, as I shall prove, impious and unholy.

"IV. For if they profess to know how to bring down the moon, to eclipse the sun, to make storm and sunshine, rain and drought, the sea impassable and the earth barren, and all such wonders, whether it be by rites or by some cunning or practice that they can, according to the adepts, be effected, in any case I am sure that they are impious, and cannot believe that the gods exist or have any strength, and that they would not refrain from the most extreme actions. Wherein surely they are terrible in the eyes of the gods. For if a man by magic and sacrifice will bring the moon down, eclipse the sun, and cause storm and sunshine, I shall not believe that any of these things is divine, but human, seeing that the power of godhead is overcome and enslaved by the cunning of man. But perhaps what they profess is not true, the fact being that men, in need of livelihood, contrive and devise many fictions of all sorts, about this disease among other things, putting the blame, for each form of the affection, upon a particular god. If the patient imitate a goat, if he roar, or suffer convulsions in the right side, they say that the Mother of the Gods is to blame. If he utter a piercing and loud cry, they liken him to a horse and blame Poseidon. Should he pass some excrement, as often happens under the stress of the disease, the surname Enodia is applied. If it be more frequent and thinner, like that of birds, it is Apollo Nomius. If he foam at the mouth and kick, Ares has the blame. When at night occur fears and terrors, delirium, jumpings from the bed and rushings out of doors, they say that Hecate is attacking or that heroes are assaulting. In making use, too, of purifications and incantations they do what I think is a very unholy and irreligious thing. For the sufferers from the disease they purify with blood and such like, as though they were polluted, blood-guilty, bewitched by men, or had committed some unholy act. All such they ought to have treated in the opposite way; they should have brought them to the sanctuaries, with sacrifices and prayers, in supplication to the gods. As it is, however, they do nothing of the kind, but merely purify them. Of the purifying objects some they hide in the earth, others they throw into the sea, others they carry away to the mountains, where nobody can touch them or tread on them. Yet, if a god is indeed the cause, they ought to have taken them to the sanctuaries and offered them to him. However, I hold that a man's body is not defiled by a god, the one being utterly corrupt, the other perfectly holy. Nay, even should it have been defiled or in any way injured through some different agency, a god is more likely to purify and sanctify it than he is to cause defilement."

And, finally, comes this magnificent passage;

"XXI. This disease styled sacred comes from the same causes as others, from the things that come to and go from the body, from cold, sun, and from the changing restlessness of winds. These things are divine. So that there is no need to put the disease in a special class and to consider it more divine than the others; they are all divine and all human. Each has a nature and power of its own; none is hopeless or incapable of treatment. Most are cured by the same things as caused them. One thing is food for one thing, and another for another, though occasionally it does it harm. So the physician must know how, by distinguishing the seasons for individual things, he may assign to one thing nutriment and growth, and to another diminution and harm. For in this disease as in all others it is necessary, not to increase the illness, but to wear it down by applying to each what is most hostile to it, not that to which it is accustomed. For what is customary gives vigour and increase; what is hostile causes weakness and decay. Whoever knows how to cause in men by regimen moist or dry, hot or cold, he can cure this disease also, if he distinguish the seasons for useful treatment, without having recourse to purifications and magic."

Hippocrates' general rational approach is once more admirably illustrated in three sentences from the "Precepts";

"I approve of theorizing also if it lays its foundation in incident, and deduces its conclusions in accordance with phenomena."

"For a theory is a composite memory of things apprehended with sense perception."

"But conclusions which are merely verbal cannot bear fruit."

Nowhere in the accepted corpus is there a trace of supernaturalism. There is only scorn for priestly physicians and their temple sleep; and the author tells us that the true art of divination "consists in divining things which are hidden by interpreting things which are known." In some treatises the fallacies of metaphysical abstraction do creep in (as in emphasis on the number seven in "On the Muscles"). In general, the discussion moves wholly on the plane of concrete, objective reality. Throughout every page runs the conception of disease as due to natural causes, those causes being disturbances of the composition of the material constituents of the body, related to atmospheric and climatic conditions. The function of the physician is to give nature a chance to repair the damage and restore a normal balance by advising an appropriate regimen.

Treatment, therefore, consisted in a regime of purging, bathing, diet and rest. In "Breaths," the author says, "Medicine in fact is subtraction and addition, subtraction of what is in excess, addition of what is wanting." Special emphasis is laid on diet in the four books on "Nutriment." Work, the author says, consumes what exists and food and drink replenish the void thus created. Food is an entity having power. It is dissolved in moisture and the "Power of nutriment reaches to bone and to all the parts of bone, to sinew, to vein, to artery, to muscle, to membrane, to flesh, fat, blood, phlegm, marrow, brain, spinal marrow, the intestines and all their parts; it reaches also to heart, breath, and moisture."

Passing to that phase of medicine with which we are here more directly concerned, we find that Hippocrates classifies disease as acute or chronic, the acute group being further subdivided into chest complaints and those of a typho-malarial nature. In the "Regimen" he says: "Now the acute diseases are those to which the ancients have given the names of pleurisy, pneumonia, phrenitis, and ardent fever, and such as are akin to these, the fever of which is on the whole continuous. For wherever there is no general type of pestilence prevalent, but diseases are sporadic, acute diseases cause many times more deaths than all others put together."

As to the causation of fevers, he says in "Breaths": "I will begin in the first place with the most common disease, fever, for this disease is associated with all other diseases. To proceed on these lines, there are two kinds of fevers; one is epidemic, called pestilence, the other is sporadic, attacking those who follow a bad regimen. Both of these fevers, however, are caused by air. Now epidemic fever has this characteristic because all men inhale the same wind; when a similar wind has mingled with all bodies in a similar way, the fevers too prove similar. But perhaps someone will say, 'Why then do such diseases attack, not all animals, but only one species of them?' I would reply that it is because one body differs from another, one air from another, one nature from another and one nutriment from another. For all species of animals do not find the same things either well or ill-adapted to themselves, but some things are beneficial to some things and other things to others, and the same is true of things harmful. So whenever the air has been infected with such pollutions as are hostile to the human race, then men fall sick, but when the air has become ill-adapted to some other species of animals, then these fall sick."

"Airs, Waters and Places," perhaps the greatest of the Hippocratic writings, is essentially a treatise on epidemiology and gives us a clear conception of the basic Greek theory of the controlling influence upon mass-diseases of wind, waters and seasons.

Hippocrates tells us (and in this treatise more than perhaps any other we hear his authentic voice) that "on arrival at a town with which he is unfamiliar, a physician should examine its position with respect to the winds and the risings of the sun." In another place, he says, "the contribution of astronomy to medicine is not a very small one but a very great one indeed. For with the seasons men's diseases, like their digestive organs, suffer change."

Hot winds cause poor appetite, derangement of the digestive organs, flabby physique; in women they lead to fluxes and barrenness; in children, to asthma, epilepsy and convulsions; in men, to dysentery, diarrhea and ague, with pleurisy and pneumonia rare. Cold winds make men sinewy, spare and costive; they conduce to pleurisies and acute diseases.

Passing to waters, we are told that cold and frosty waters cause colds and sore throats. Rain water is ideal and so is water from high places and earthy hills, while springs from rocks are dangerous and melted snow and ice very bad. Most fascinating is the notation that marshy stagnant water is associated with "large stiff spleens and hard, thin, hot stomachs, while their shoulders, collar-bone and faces are emaciated; the fact is that their flesh dissolves to feed the spleen." And, again, with marshy waters "in the summer there are epidemics of dysentery, diarrhœa, and long quartan fever."

As to season, we learn that a rainy spring will be followed by fever and dysenteries in summer, and that the solstices, the equinoxes, the time of rising of the Dog-Star and Arcturus and the time of the setting of the Pleiades are specifically dangerous periods.

The broad distinction between the intestinal and malarial fevers of summer and the respiratory diseases of winter; the recognition of danger from those waters which we now know are most likely to be polluted (springs in rocky soil and wash from melting snow at times of thaw); and the description of the symptoms of malaria as associated with marshy waters (even though the relation is not one of ingestion as Hippocrates thought): these are indeed masterpieces of epidemological observation.

In the first and third books of "Epidemics," which are generally accepted as of Hippocratic origin, is a valuable detailed notebook of clinical case histories with their preceding and accompanying atmospheric "constitutions." Malaria and continued fevers (typhoid and dysentery) predominate, with some reference to phthisis which appears to have been of the rapid and fatal type which we associate with a non-immune population. The other books of "Epidemics" which are generally regarded as apocryphal, contain many references to the influence of comets and earthquakes—a type of causative influence almost wholly lacking from the true Hippocratic writings.

If the cause of epidemics were due to corruption of the atmosphere, the obvious remedy was to correct the atmospheric disorders. There is no indication of such a public health procedure in those Hippocratic writings which have survived; but one of the most persistent of Hippocratic legends attributes to this physician (along with Acron and Empedocles) the practice of controlling epidemics by lighting great fires in the streets. Sticker says of Hippocrates, "In the great pest in the year 420 which came over Greece from the north out of Illyria and Paionia, he is supposed to have given the advice to the Thessalonian cities and also to Greece to light great wood fires in all of the infected and endangered areas and to feed the fires with fragrant wreaths and flowers and perfumed ointments. He himself went through Thessalonia, Phocis and Boeotia to Athens with his sons and pupils in order to direct the carrying out of his advice and to lend medical aid. He sent his oldest son to the Peloponnesus. His visit brought results. The Athenians decided in the year 419, in recognition of his services, to confer upon him the great ordination of Demeter and Persephone, as previously had been done to his ancestor on his mother's side, the Zeus-born Hercules. They sent him a golden crown and publicly announced the crowning at the next Panathenaean festival."

Throughout all the Hippocratic discussions, as Adams has said, "not the least reference to contagion, in any shape, is to be found." That such references may have existed in treatises which are now lost is, of course, possible; and it is of great interest to note that in the work known as "Pseudo-Aristotle" (Problems, vii, 8), while fevers were expressly stated to be non-infectious, phthisis and ophthalmia were, as definitely, listed as contagious.

It is highly significant in this connection to note that the diseases clearly described in the existing Hippocratic treatises are malaria, dys-

entery, diarrhea and other continued fevers—in other words, those diseases where the factor of contagion was masked by the influence of
insect carriers and water-borne infection—diseases which remained in
the class of miasmatic or pythogenic disorders until the end of the nineteenth century. There is no similarly obvious description of smallpox or
measles where the factor of contagion plays an easily recognizable role.
One is tempted to speculate on the possibility that other Coan manuscripts which were not preserved may have dealt with this side of the
picture. If so, such manuscripts must have been lost before the time of
Galen, who takes up the problem exactly where the existing Hippocratic
treatises laid it down.

Jones, in his penetrating analysis of the Coan writings, justly calls
attention to the necessary limitations of this great dawning of the scientific spirit in medicine. He says, "The Greek knew that there were certain collections of morbid phenomena which he called diseases; that
these diseases normally ran a certain course; that their origin was not
unconnected with geographical and atmospheric environment; that the
patient, in order to recover his health, must modify his ordinary mode of
living. Beyond this he knew, and could know nothing."

The achievements of Hippocrates, in spite of such obstacles, are well
summarized by Garrison who says: "All that a man of genius could do
for internal medicine, with no other instrument of precision than his
own open mind and keen senses, he accomplished, and, with these reser-
vations his best descriptions of disease are models of their kind today. To
him medicine owes the art of clinical inspection and observation, and he
is, above all, the exemplar of that flexible, critical, well-poised attitude of
mind, ever on the lookout for sources of error, which is the very essence
of the scientific spirit."

It would, of course, be a mistake to assume that the spirit of Hippocrates permeated the whole of the Greek people. In any civilization, as
Lewis Mumford points out, there is a dominant prevailing stage of
thought, below which are survivals of past attitudes, and above which
are mutations which anticipate the future. No doubt demonology was
present in the lower strata of Athenian society, while the philosophers
and the physicians enjoyed the vision of a new day. But the general tone
of thought with regard to health and disease may perhaps best be
gauged by the actual technique of the great institutions maintained for
the conduct of the healing art. It was characterized by a mixture of
scientific practice with the propitiation of divine (though not demonic)

supernatural powers. By the time of Alexander, there were 300 to 400 temples dedicated to the worship of Asklepios. These temples, of which one of the most magnificent was at Epidaurus, were semi-religious, semi-hygienic watering places. Included in their practice were pious meditation, physiotherapy, physical education, massage, diet and mental hygiene. They combined some of the characteristics of Cauterets and of Lourdes. The priests were usually asclepiads or gymnasts; but the rite of the "incubation sleep" in which the gods revealed to a patient the secret of his disease (described by Aristophanes in "Plutus" and by Pater in "Marius the Epicurean"), and the votive offerings left by convalescents, clearly point to a religious motive. As Osler says, "Access to the shrine was forbidden to the unclean and the impure, pregnant women and the mortally afflicted were kept away; no dead body could find a resting-place within the holy precincts, the shelter and the cure of the sick being undertaken by the keepers of inns and boarding-houses in the neighbour-hood. The suppliants for aid had to submit to careful purification, to bathe in the sea, river or spring, to fast for a prescribed time, to abjure wine and certain articles of diet, and they were only permitted to enter the temple when they were adequately prepared by cleansing, inunction and fumigation. This lengthy and exhausting preparation, partly die-tetic, partly suggestive, was accompanied by a solemn service of prayer and sacrifice."

Yet, above this theme of religio-scientific medicine, sounded the mag-nificent overtones of Coan rationalism; and it was these overtones which were to be amplified throughout the centuries to come in the symphony of modern science. We have heard their first prelude in Cos; we must listen to them once more as they were sounded six centuries later by Galen of Pergamos, the last, as Hippocrates was the first, of the great figures of classical medicine.

Here we are dealing with a definite historical figure and not with a symbolic legend. We know much about his life, much from his volumi-nous and highly subjective writings, about his temperament and habits. Galen was born at Pergamos in Asia Minor between A.D. 129 and 131, the son of Nikon, an architect and mathematician. Like all scholars of his time, he travelled widely, studying at Alexandria, Corinth and Smyrna and in 157 or 158 returned to practice in his native city where he received appointment as surgeon to the school of the gladiators. In 161 or 162 he migrated to Rome, whence he returned to Pergamos in 166. His depar-ture from the imperial city appears to have been influenced by professional jealousy and bitter quarrels with his medical colleagues, in which he seems to have borne his full share as evidenced by his remark that "the only difference between robbers and physicians is that the former practice on the mountains and the latter in Rome." (Malicious commentators hint that the desire to escape from an epidemic of plague was also a motive in his return to Pergamos.) He is believed to have attended Marcus Aurelius on one of his campaigns, and by 169 we find him once more established in Rome as medical attendant on the heir apparent, Commodus. He died, apparently still high in the imperial favor, between A.D. 198 and 201.

After Hippocrates, Galen was probably the greatest figure in the history of medicine. More than that, his voluminous writings formed the major channel through which the whole body of Greek medical thought found its way down to succeeding generations. He was, to medicine, what Aristotle was to natural science in general. As Daremberg says, "Galien a régné en maître à peu près absolu jusqu'au XVIII° siècle."

The volume of Galen's writings which has survived is enormous in spite of the fact that many of his books were lost in a fire which destroyed a bookshop on the Via Sacra in the year 192. His mind was encyclopedic, and Brock not unjustly compares the scope of his vision with that of Leonardo or Goethe. He wrote dogmatically and authoritatively; and for this reason his hand lay too heavily upon the minds of lesser men in succeeding generations. Yet, as Thorndike says, that it was his dogmatism rather than his empiricism which ruled and sterilized medical thought for a thousand years was the fault of medieval medicine and not of Galen. His tract, "On the Medical Sects," in which he analyzes the respective approaches of the Dogmatist, Empiricist and Methodist schools of the day, displays Galen, himself, as a follower of the sound middle road.

He was a thoroughgoing rationalist. As Thorndike says, "while Galen might look upon nature or certain things in nature as a divine work, he would not admit any supernatural force in science or medicine, or anything bordering upon special providence." Most important of all, he was an observer and an experimenter. Having learned all that the ancients have said, one "must judge the same and put it to the test for a long, long time and observe what agrees with visible phenomena and what disagrees, and so accept the one and reject the other." Finally, he avoided the Hunterian extreme as well as that of the nature-philosophers; for he says, "Reason alone discovers some things, experience alone discovers some, but to find others requires both experience and reason."

It is a fundamental error to consider Galen as merely a compiler. He was a keen and original thinker, an acute observer and the founder of experimental physiology. As Daremberg has said, "On a trop oublié Galien observateur, pour ne songer qu' à Galien systématique."

Galen was the greatest anatomist of antiquity and dissected animals, including apes. He was an experimental physiologist, demonstrating the effects of injury to the brain and of section at various levels of the spinal cord, and proving that the arteries contain blood and not air. Payne calls him "the founder of the physiology of the nervous system"; and Garrison says that "Galen's experiments on the physiology of the nervous, respiratory, and circulatory systems were the only real knowledge for seventeen centuries."

He made a substantial beginning at pathology (as in the treatise on "Affected Parts"); and was a keen and observant clinician. He laid much greater emphasis on the use of drugs than did Hippocrates, taking special journeys and spending considerable sums to obtain certain specifics and maintaining considerable pharmaceutical stores of his own. He claims however to restrict his account of medicinal simples to those which he had personally tested and his discussion of "critical days" is also supposed to be based on direct experience. He stresses care in dosage, careful control of the progress of the patient by observation of the pulse, and other clinical signs.

In personal hygiene, he was a notable pioneer, and his classification of the factors affecting health completely dominated thinking in this field for many centuries. His "Naturals" were the inherent properties of the body which made for health; his "Non-Naturals" were those conditions favorable to health which were not "natural" or inherent—essentially the conduct-factors of personal hygiene; and his "Contra-Naturals" were those conditions inimical to health. His subdivisions of the first and third of these general classes were metaphysical, and, to me, meaningless; but the classification of the chief Non-Naturals as Food, Fresh Air, Sleeping and Waking, Exercise and Rest, Repletion and Evacuation and the Passions and Affections of the Mind stands today as the best summary of the factors in personal hygiene which can be formulated.[1]

[1] This classification is briefly, and only incidentally, alluded to in *Ars Medica*, Kühn, Vol. I, p. 367. It is fully elaborated in a later treatise entitled "Galeni de Oculis a Demetria Translatus Nuper e Variis Mendis Expurgatus" which is to be found in "Galeni Librorum Septima Classis

Finally, Galen had an extraordinary grasp of the principles of mental hygiene. His treatise, "That the Qualities of Mind Depend on the Temperament of the Body" is a remarkable demonstration of the dependence of emotional factors on physical status; and "On the Knowledge and Cure of Mental Affections" is full of common sense, and lays a sound basis for psycho-therapeutics.

Passing to our own field of epidemiology, Galen's general view of the etiology of disease is, of course, based on the general Greek doctrine of unbalance between the four basic properties of hot, cold, moist and dry—in the human body and in the ambient atmosphere. His interest in such problems is, however, relatively slight. In the index of Kühn's edition, which occupies an entire volume of that monumental work, there is but one reference to the word "*epidemia*," two references to "*epidemici*," and one to "*contagiosi*." It is perhaps significant of the difference between the Greek and the Roman mind that Hippocrates is intrigued by problems of causation while Galen—Roman in environment if Greek by race—is almost exclusively preoccupied by the immediate practical problems of diagnosis and treatment. One is essentially a philosopher, the other an experimenter and clinician.

It is a strange anomaly that Galen, the second greatest figure in the history of medicine, should never have been completely translated into any modern language. The standard edition of Kühn in Greek and Latin occupies twenty volumes and the text is obscure and difficult and even such scholars as Payne and Thorndike confess the incompleteness of their knowledge of its contents. My colleague, Professor G. L. Hendrickson of the Latin Department of Yale, has been good enough to work with me in a search for references to the causation of epidemic diseases, with results which, though meager, are, we believe, reasonably representative. The most important of these references are as follows:

In "Medical Definitions" a pestilence is described as "a disease which attacks all, or the greater number, arising from corruption of the air with the result that great numbers perish" and again, "pestilence is a modification of the air such that the seasons of the year do not preserve their proper order" (XIX, 391).[2] In other words, a pestilence is an unusual mass-epidemic.

Curatium Methodum." Giunta Press, 1576, Vol. IV, p. 185. This is, according to Professor G. L. Hendrickson, a Renaissance production in which Galen himself, and Paul of Aegina (seventh century) are cited; but so far as we are aware it is the earliest full statement of the doctrine of the naturals, the non-naturals and the contra-naturals.

[2] References are to volumes and pages of Kühn.

The atmospheric cause of such epidemics is discussed in the "Letter on Theriac to Pison."

"For the plague, like the assault of some wild beast, attacks not only a few individuals but even destroys whole states. A disastrous change in the character of the air making it prone to corruption is brought about; and human beings, since they cannot from the necessity of breathing avoid the peril, draw in the air through the mouth like a poison. Therefore I praise Hippocrates, that man who deserves all praise, who cured that plague which attacked Greece from Ethiopia in no other way than by a change and alteration of the air in order to make it breathable. When therefore he had bidden fire to be kindled throughout the whole of Athens he caused not only the ordinary fuel to be placed upon it but also wreaths and flowers and sweet smelling unguents" (xiv, 280).

Here is the traditional miasmatic theory, which is stated again in the "Comments on Hippocrates." Putridity of humors is the cause of acute fevers, favored by filthy living conditions (xvi, 417). Epidemic diseases (as distinguished from those which are endemic) are due particularly to the influence of the ambient air. When many sicken and die at once we must look to a single common cause, the air we breathe (xvii a, 1). Putrid humors are caused by the constitution of the atmosphere (xvii a, 686). Throughout the "Comments" are also numerous references to the influence of season and weather (xvii a and xvii b).

In the "Dogmas of Hippocrates and Plato" the influence of season is again stressed and it is pointed out that the continued and ardent fevers, tertians and quartans, and diarrhea occur in summer; that the same diseases, and particularly quartan and splenic fevers, prevail in autumn; and that in winter we expect pleurisy, pneumonia and other respiratory diseases (v, 694).

The "Letter to Glaucon on the Therapeutic Method" again notes quartan fever as autumnal, quotidian as characteristic of damp climates and the winter season and contains reference to astronomical conditions in many of the case histories cited. It also emphasizes the influence upon the ephemeral fevers of contributory causes, such as fatigue, excessive drinking, anger, chagrin and other violent emotions, insomnia and extremes of cold or heat (xi, 6).

By far the most significant passages, however, are to be found in the First Book of "Characteristic Differences Between Fevers." Here, we read, "That a pestilential condition of the air produces fever is well known to any intelligent person; as it is known that it is dangerous to be associated with those who are suffering from the plague; or that there is obvious danger of contagion from cases of skin disease or ophthalmia. It is also dangerous to associate with those who are afflicted with consumption and in general with all those who are breathing forth putridity which causes the houses in which they lie sick to smell offensively" (xii, 279).

It is stated that "In a pestilential condition of the atmosphere, the air taken in in breathing is the principal cause [of fevers] (vii, 289). . . . The initial cause of putridity [of the air] is either a multitude of dead bodies which have not been burned, as happens commonly in war; or an exhalation from swamps or stagnant waters in the summer time; and sometimes excessive heat of the surrounding air is the starting point, as for example in the pestilence which invaded Athens (vii, 289-90). . . . But remember throughout that no external cause is efficient without a predisposition of the body itself. Otherwise external causes which affect one would affect all; all would fall ill at the rising of the dog-star and all would perish of the plague. But as has been said the largest share in the origin of diseases is the predisposition of the body of the one who shall fall a victim to it. Let us assume for example that the circumambient air carries certain seeds of plague; that, of the bodies that share (breathe) it, some are already filled with corruption and are ready of themselves to suffer putrefaction, others are free from such corruption and pure. Let us assume too that, in the former, there is present already general obstruction of the pores, so-called plethora, an inactive life given over to drinking, high living and sexual indulgence; that in the others which are pure and free from corruption there is wholesome transpiration through pores that are neither obstructed nor constricted, that they take moderate exercise and lead a temperate life; supposing all this, which of these two types will probably be affected by the breathing of air which is favorable to putrefaction?" (vii, 291-292).[3]

In these few scattered passages, we have a remarkably clear picture of the classical concept of the etiology of epidemic disease; and this concept involves three major factors.

First in importance—with Galen as with Hippocrates—is the factor of an epidemic constitution of the atmosphere. This corruption of the

---

[3] Professor Hendrickson finds the confusion of this passage as it stands in the Latin version to be due to misunderstanding of a corrupt word in the Greek text.

atmosphere is associated with climate and season; with miasms arising from putrefaction of dead bodies, filthy living conditions (*squalor*) and swamps; and in some degree with astronomical phenomena (such as the rising of the Dog-Star). That this pestilential state of the air produces fever "is well known to any intelligent person" since "when many sicken and die at once we must look to a single common cause, the air we breathe." Upon this factor was based the only practical method of controlling epidemic disease, the practice of correcting the epidemic constitution by fumigation, as Hippocrates is supposed to have done at Athens.

A second factor was individual predisposition, associated with inherent bodily properties as influenced by such unhygienic practices as fatigue, dietetic excesses, emotional strain, extreme cold or heat. Just as it was logically essential to assume the epidemic constitution of the atmosphere to explain mass epidemics, so it was necessary to invoke individual predisposition to account for the fact that even mass epidemics are not universal in their incidence—"otherwise external causes which affect one would affect all."

Finally, certain diseases—of which ophthalmia, skin diseases, phthisis and plague are specified—are recognized as contagious so that "it is dangerous to associate with those who are afflicted." It is of the greatest interest to note that two of these four diseases are the ones mentioned in the "Pseudo-Aristotle." Galen had added only skin diseases and plague.

Here, in the second century A.D., were the three factors of atmospheric influence, individual predisposition, and contagion which were to dominate scientific thinking up to the time of Pasteur. For more than sixteen hundred years the history of epidemiology is a story of a shifting emphasis on these three basic conceptions.

CHAPTER V

PRIMITIVE CONCEPTS OF CONTAGION

"Appalling too was the rapidity with which men caught the infection; dying like sheep if they attended on one another; and this was the principal cause of mortality."—THUCYDIDES

Among primitive peoples, we find many practices which suggest the idea of contagion; and this is very natural, since the conception of disease as caused by a specific demon has analogy with—and may merge into—the conception of a physical transmissible cause. In Chapter I, we have noted the flight from a village where an epidemic is in progress (Coram); the exclusion of the sick from the community (island of Rias); and the establishment of a quarantine against both spirits and men (Borneo). The following passages from Lévy-Bruhl bring this phenomenon out more clearly.

He tells us that, according to Mrs. L. Parker, "If blacks go visiting, when they leave they make a smoke fire, and smoke themselves, so that they may not carry home any disease." So, according to A. C. Kruyt, in the Central Celebes, "persons coming from a village in which there is illness, are obliged by the priestess to pass beneath a basket containing rice and bananas, to destroy the contamination which adheres to them." Again, in South Africa, the men accompanying A. Merensky, when in a place where smallpox is prevalent say to him, "If one of us should get this disease, none of us can go home again. For fear of our bringing this disease with us, they will forbid us to set foot in the country." H. A. Junod says of the Bantus, "They are quite alive to the physical contagion in eruptive maladies, especially smallpox. . . . But the diseases in which contagion is especially dreaded are *phthisis* and *leprosy*. . . . Here their conception of infection is confused. It seems at times to be a bodily contagion; for instance, a consumptive person must always eat his portion from the common pot *after the others* and, if there is then any of it left, it is thrown away. But most of the taboos that relate to these two dreaded diseases seem to reveal another conception of contamination. The uncleanness of phthisis resembles that of death, and of the lochial discharges, and it is treated in the same way. Thus, grave-diggers are not allowed to eat with their fingers until they have completed their purificatory rites. They must make use of special spoons, or else they will become *consumptives.* . . . So too, the woman in childbed . . . must have a special wooden spoon . . . for if she touched the food, *it would make her phthisical*." Lévy-Bruhl, however, concludes that "Junod is right in saying that, despite appearances, the ba-Ronga do not think that phthisical infection is the result of mere physical contact. As he bids us note, it is a question of an 'impurity' comparable with that which comes from death or from the blood lost by a woman in childbed. The taboos are protections against the evil influences emanating from the corpse, or from this blood, or from consumptives, or lepers, etc." The essentially animistic conceptions involved are illustrated by the highly elaborate quarantine procedures imposed by the Ao Nagas in India in the family of one who has died—not from contagious disease, but by violence.

Similar medleys of religious taboo and empirical isolation are described by Sticker among the ancient Egyptians, the Chinese (who, for many centuries, have rigidly isolated lepers), the Hindus, the Assyro-Babylonians and, particularly, the Persians. According to this author, the idea of contagion by contact was already present among "the priests of the Hamitic Egyptians who ordained Moses. The daily baths, the regular washing before and after meals, the careful clipping and removal of hair, the cutting of the nails and the foreskin, the monthly purification of the digestive channels by cathartics, the frequent withdrawal of humor by means of blood-letting and cupping instruments, the strict choice of food, the linen garments and paper shoes, the differentiation between holy and unholy, clean and unclean animals which the Egyptian priestly law prescribed, all of these duties may have been conceived as purely ceremonial practices in late times; they arose out of the requirements of life in a prosperous country which brought its leaders into steady contact with a population of black aborigines and the surging of streaming hordes of immoral slaves and with their filthy impurities and diseases; a land which gave birth to endless plagues of vermin which multiplied themselves in annual waves, which swarmed out of air, water, earth and food, and could only be overcome by consistent opposition."

Recognition of the relation of human plague to diseases of rodents suggests an implication of contagion. In the Bhagavata Parana, one of the early Hindu scriptures, men are warned to leave their homes when a rat falls from the roof, jumps drunkenly about the floor, and falls dead, "for then be sure the plague is at hand." So, in I Samuel 6, golden images of "your mice that mar the land" are offered to God as a trespass offering to ward off the plague. Susruta (fifth century A.D.) describes malarial fever and relates it to mosquitoes.

It is among the Iranians that sanitary-religious isolation practices reached their height. Here, as Sticker says, "the stranger, the outcast, the despiser of religion is expelled; in far distant ages the weakly, aged, the useless infant, the helpless invalid and the loathsome were also expelled. To the aborigines of the Iranians a marked, a spotted person is loathsome; . . . This spot or mark is doubtless a bodily affliction or at least a bodily stain. . . . We know nothing more definite about what the leprous spot was among the old Iranians. In the median period it was in no sense our leprosy. Those who were expelled at the time were infected by a white desquamation, which is as little indicative of leprosy as the turning gray of the hair. Each spot was regarded as a divine punishment and as a sign of a curse; it struck the follower of the Avesta who sinned grievously against the holy law. . . . If a citizen has leprosy or white leprosy, cutaneous scale or a white spot he cannot walk about in the city or have intercourse with other Persians; it is said that he who sinned against the sun has this spot, every stranger, whoever, who is infected by it they expel from the country; many chase away the white pigeons for the same reason. . . . The custom of expulsion for those who have white spots is a sacramental ceremony in the Median period, no quarantine in our sense, but an expulsion in the most general sense with such a purely spiritual motive as the *interdictio aquae et ignis* among the Romans and the papal ban in the Middle Ages among the Christians."

Yet in all these religious practices there was perhaps an underlying basis of empirical sanitary experience. Indeed, Sticker says that the most ancient Iranian regulations "make it plain that the conception of the danger of contagion from the corpse was originally derived from experiences."

In the Hebrew Scriptures, we find the same combination of religious taboo and sanitary precaution, but with an enormous difference in relative emphasis. The Persian writings impress one as mysticism with a trace of science—the Hebrew Testament, as science with a trace of mysticism. Sticker concludes that this difference "goes through the entire Semitic and Aryan history, at least as long as the separate nations of these branches remain separated and thus remain free from reciprocal influences as well as from the mixture with black and yellow nations and their dark superstition and frightful spirit-worship."

Garrison is quite correct when he states that "The ancient Hebrews were, in fact, the founders of prophylaxis, and the high priests were true medical police."

In this connection, the program for the control of "leprosy" in Chapters xiii-xv of the Book of Leviticus is of primary importance. This was almost certainly not our leprosy. Sticker thinks the term may probably have included syphilis and gonorrhea; but, whatever the disease may have been, the precautions for its control were developed on highly scientific lines. The individual who shows signs of "the plague" is to be brought to the priests who examine him with minute care as to the character of lesions in the skin and the changes of color of hair in the affected areas. If the diagnosis of leprosy be made, the patient is declared unclean. If it remains doubtful, he is isolated for seven days and reexamined; if the lesion has not progressed he is again isolated and reexamined after another week. Apparently, a certain stage of the infection was recognized as so far advanced as to be no longer contagious. "Then the priest shall consider; and behold, if the leprosy have covered all his flesh, he shall pronounce him clean that hath the plague: it is all turned white: he is clean. But when raw flesh appeareth in him, he shall be unclean" (xiii, 13-14).

"And the leper in whom the plague is, his clothes shall be rent and his head bare, and he shall put a covering upon his upper lip, and shall cry, unclean, unclean. All the days wherein the plague shall be in him he shall be defiled; he is unclean: he shall dwell alone; without the camp shall his habitation be" (xiii, 45-46).

If the plague be in any garment, the priest shall examine that garment after seven days to see if the plague be spread in the garment (as a greenish or reddish discoloration). If so "He shall therefore burn that garment, whether warp or woof, in woolen or in linen, or anything of skin, wherein the plague is; for it is a fretting leprosy; it shall be burnt in the fire" (xiii, 52).

Chapter xiv outlines the procedure for release from quarantine—"This shall be the law of the leper in the day of his cleansing." The priest goes out of the camp to the place where the leper is and examines him to see if the lesions are healed. After a ceremony involving the sacrifice of one bird (atonement) and the liberation of another (transference), the convalescent "shall wash his clothes, and shave off all his hair, and wash himself in water, that he may be clean; and after that he shall come into the camp, and shall tarry abroad out of his tent seven days. But it shall be on the seventh day, that he shall shave all his hair off his head and his beard and his eyebrows, even all his hair he shall shave off; and he shall wash his clothes, also he shall wash his flesh in water, and he shall be clean" (xiv, 8-9).

Later on in the same chapter are directions for dealing with infection in a dwelling. The infection manifests itself in "hollow strakes, greenish or reddish" in the walls. If these "strakes" have spread after the house has been closed for seven days, the discolored stones must be removed and cast away. If the disease shall break out again after the house has been scraped and plastered, it must be destroyed; and the clothes of all who have slept or eaten in the house must be washed. Chapter xv deals with a "running issue" out of the flesh (perhaps gonorrhea) and provides elaborate precautions for cleansing of the infected person, of his bed, clothing, saddle seats, utensils and of anyone who has touched fomites infected by him.

Again in the Book of Numbers, the children of Israel are commanded "that they put out of the camp every leper, and every one that hath an issue, and whosoever is defiled by the dead" (v, 2). Later passages in this book are less concrete and more reminiscent of Persian taboos. "He that toucheth the dead body of any man shall be unclean seven days" (xix, 11). "This is the law, when a man dieth in a tent; all that come into the tent, and all that is in the tent, shall be unclean seven days. And every open vessel, which hath no covering hard upon it, is unclean" (xix, 14-15).

In the Book of Deuteronomy it is decreed that "If there be among you any man, that is not clean by reason of uncleanness that chanceth him by night, then shall he go abroad out of the camp, he shall not come within the camp. But it shall be, when evening cometh on, he shall wash himself with water; and when the sun is down, he shall come into the camp again" (xxiii, 10-11). Most remarkable are the succeeding passages with respect to the disposal of excreta—the first known contributions to military sanitation. "Thou shalt have a place also without the camp, whither thou shalt go forth abroad; and thou shalt have a paddle upon thy weapon; and it shall be, when thou wilt ease thyself abroad, thou shalt dig therewith, and shalt turn back and cover that which cometh from thee" (xxiii, 12-13).

In later Talmudic writings there is much additional evidence of public health practices among the Hebrew peoples. Garrison says that "Diphtheria was so much feared by the Hebrews that the first case located in a community was immediately heralded by a warning blast of the shofar, although the instrument was ordinarily sounded only after the occurrence of the third case of an infectious disease." There is much emphasis on washing the hands before and after meals in the Talmud (Cohen). According to the Midrasch, the Jews while in Palestine drank water only from cisterns and springs; after the episode of the Tower of Babel they drank the water of the Euphrates and many of them died as a result (Preuss).

Too much stress need not be laid on taboos with regard to strange women which are of doubtful sanitary significance or on the long lists of unclean beasts in Leviticus 11 and Deuteronomy 14. It may be that the flesh of swine was not eaten for scientific reasons but the major part of these regulations seem to be of a mystical nature. The system for controlling "leprosy," however, involving differential diagnosis, isolation, quarantine and disinfection, remains the most brilliant application of rational epidemiology of ancient times and was a controlling influence in public health practice down to modern days.

Our next source of inspiration with regard to the concept of contagion comes from the non-medical writers—the historians and poets—of Greece and Rome. Sticker cites the following instances from legendary sources. In Elis Hercules led the rivers Alpheus and Pereus through the manure-laden stables of the King Augeas. He freed the scene of the Olympian games in Elis from the fever-generating swarms of flies. Agamemnon had the army of the Achaians wash off their spots in the sea before Troy, which wiped out all impurity. Odysseus banished the evil corpse vapors of the one hundred and eight slain suitors and their servants by wood fires and the steam of brimstone from house and hall and chambers. The killing of the suitors and the purification took place on Apollo's annual festival. The attempts of Empedocles come within historical times, the attempts to divert the disease-bringing and crop-failure-bearing south wind from the plain at Akragas by closing up a mountain cleft, so that the city became healthy. He led the clean water of the Hypsa river through a stagnant decaying swamp at Silenus in Sikelia and thereby rescued the city from annual wholesale deaths.

Passing from legend to documentary evidence, we find by far the most remarkable contemporaneous analysis of this problem—either medical or non-medical—in Book II of Thucydides' history of the Peloponnesian Wars. This is a description of an epidemic which cannot be identified with any known disease today but which raged in Mediterranean countries for a period of three years, working terrible damage. In certain places, one-fourth of the population was destroyed. Thucydides, himself, was not only an eye-witness but a sufferer.

The malady is said to have begun "south of Egypt in Aethiopia; hence it descended into Egypt and Libya and, after spreading over the greater part of the Persian empire, suddenly fell upon Athens" (in 430 B.C.). It was most severe in the most populous places. The Athenians first attributed it to poisoning of the wells by the Peloponnesians but, as the disease spread to other areas, this idea was abandoned. The historian is very cautious with regard to etiology. He says of the epidemic, "As to its probable origin or the causes which might or could have produced such a disturbance of nature, every man, whether a physician or not, will give his own opinion. But I shall describe its actual course."

Yet Thucydides was quite clear about one vital point—the contagiousness of the disease. He says, "Appalling too was the rapidity with which men caught the infection; dying like sheep if they attended on one another; and this was the principal cause of mortality. When they were afraid to visit one another, the sufferers died in their solitude, so that many houses were empty because there had been no one left to take care of the sick; or if they ventured they perished, especially those who aspired to heroism. For they went to see their friends without thought of themselves and were ashamed to leave them, even at a time when the very relations of the dying were at last growing weary and ceased to make lamentations, overwhelmed by the vastness of the calamity. But whatever instances there may have been of such devotion, more often the sick and dying were tended by the pitying care of those who had recovered, because they knew the course of the disease and were themselves free from apprehensions. For no one was ever attacked a second time, or not with a fatal result."

Furthermore, Thucydides even maintains that the contagion of the disease affected animals as well as men. "There was one circumstance in particular which distinguished it from ordinary diseases. The birds and animals which feed on human flesh, although so many bodies were lying unburied, either never came near them, or died if they touched them."

It is interesting to note that Thucydides advances the idea of transmutation of one disease into another which was to hamper epidemiological thinking up to the days of Sydenham and beyond. He says, "if anybody was already ill of any other disease it was absorbed in this";

and, "None of the ordinary sicknesses attacked any one while it lasted or, if they did, they ended in the plague."

For several centuries, this classic account of the plague stood alone—so far as surviving records are concerned. In the first century B.C., however, we find many Roman writers echoing the pioneer analysis of Thucydides. Most important of these, perhaps, is Lucretius, who concludes his most famous poem with a description of the Athenian plague of 430 B.C. In discussing its nature, the poet demands "What is its cause?" and he answers—working out his atomic theory of the universe—that "just as there are seeds (*semina*) of things helpful to our life, so, for sure, others fly about that cause disease and death."

A contemporary of Lucretius, Diodorus Siculus in the "Library of History" describes a "plague" among the Carthaginians at Syracuse in 397 B.C. and says, "This god-sent calamity was increased by the crowding of tens of thousands into the same place, by the fact that the time of year was very conducive to disease and, in addition by the extraordinary heats prevailing that summer." It seems that the place, too, had something to do with the intensity of the trouble; for when the Athenians had earlier occupied the same camp, many of them had perished from disease, the place being marshy and low-lying. At first, before sunrise, owing to the coldness of the air from the marshes, shiverings were produced in the body while the heat of midday naturally had "stifling effect upon such a crowd gathered together in a confined space"; and later "everybody who came much about the sufferers fell a victim to the disease."

Ovid in "The Metamorphoses" (Book VII) gives a famous description of a plague at Aegina which is often said to be based on Thucydides but which contains much fanciful embroidery. It attributes the epidemic primarily to "the anger of the vengeful Juno" and contains reference to meteorological phenomena—"the heaven encompassed the earth with thick darkness"—and hot south winds (the epidemic constitution of the atmosphere). There are, however, several references to infection, as in the following passage: "The cruel malady breaks out upon even those who administer remedies; and their own arts become an injury to their owners. The nearer at hand any one is, and the more faithfully he attends on the sick, the sooner does he come in for his share of the fatality." Yet that he was thinking rather of miasms than of contagion in the modern sense is made clear by these lines: "A faintness seizes all animals; both in the woods, in the fields, and in the roads, loathsome carcasses lie strewed. The air is corrupted with the smell of them. I am relating strange events. The dogs, and the ravenous birds, and the hoary wolves, touch them not; falling away, they rot, and by their exhalations produce harmful effects, and spread the contagion far and wide." He adds still another complication when he adds, "It is known for a fact that the infection came even into fountains and lakes, and that many thousands of serpents were wandering over the uncultivated fields, and were tainting the rivers with their venom." It may be good poetry but pretty bad epidemiology which combines the wrath of the gods, the south winds, the doctrine of miasms, a vague concept of contagion, and the venom of serpents, in one glorious medley. Most of these etiological factors, it will be noted, are also found in the passage cited from Diodorus.

Virgil describes anthrax in sheep and indicates a knowledge of the spread of contagion from herd to herd.

Another interesting line of thought among classical writers may be mentioned here, since, though not directly related to contagion, it links up the concept of miasms with that of particulate causes of diseases. This is the frequent discussion of the relation of malaria to marshy areas, often with reference to insects and animalculae. The most important passages of this kind are to be found in Varro. He says, in one place, "If the farm is unhealthy by reason of the plight of the land itself, or of the water supply, or is exposed to the miasma which breeds in some localities, or if the farm is too hot on account of the climate, or is exposed to mischievous winds, these discomforts can be mitigated by one who knows what to do and is willing to spend some money. What is of the greatest importance in this respect is the situation of the farm buildings, their plan and convenience, and what is the aspect of their doors and gates and windows. During the great plague, Hippocrates the physician saved not merely one farm but many cities because he knew this. But why should I summon him as a witness: for when the army and the fleet lay at Corcyra and all the houses were crowded with the sick and dying, did not our Varro here contrive to open new windows to the healthy North wind and close those which gave entrance to the infected breezes of the South, to change doors and to do other such things, and so succeed in restoring his comrades safe and sound to their native land?"

Again, "when you plan to build, try your best to locate the steading at the foot of a wooded hill where the pastures are rich, and turn it so as to catch the healthiest prevailing breeze. The best situation is facing the east so to secure shade in summer and sun in winter. But if you must build on the bank of a river, take care that you do not let the steading face the river, for it will be very cold in winter and unhealthy in summer. Like precautions must be taken against swampy places for the same reasons and particularly because as they dry, swamps breed certain animalculae which cannot be seen with the eyes and which we breathe through the nose and mouth into the body where they cause grave maladies."

In a still later passage, "Take care to avoid having the steading face the direction from which disagreeable winds blow, yet you should not build in a hollow. High ground is the best location for a steading: for by ventilation all noxious gases are dissipated, and the steading is healthier if exposed to the sun all day: with the further advantage that any insects which may be bred in or brought upon the premises are either blown away or quickly perish where there is no damp. Sudden rains and overflowed streams are dangerous to those who have their steadings in low or hollow places, and they are more at the hazard of the ruthless hand of the robber because he is able to take advantage of those who are unprepared. Against either of these risks the higher places are safer."

Other writers on architecture, such as Vitruvius, and Columella give similar attention to the orientation, position and drainage of buildings. Considering this dread of the neighborhood of marshes on the part of these practical sanitarians, and in view of modern knowledge of the mosquito-borne character of malaria, it is entertaining to find the mosquito net (*conopeum*) ridiculed by the poets Horace, Juvenal, and Propertius.

Through all this period, then, the historians and the poets were suggesting that epidemic disease was actually spread by contagion and were hinting at a relation of certain maladies to particulate agents of infection and insect carriers. It is a curious and interesting fact that among medical writers, while these concepts did appear, they were far less prominent. It has been pointed out in a previous chapter that in the Pseudo-Aristotle, phthisis and ophthalmia are recognized as contagious but the fevers are specifically stated to be non-infectious.

Galen recognizes that rabies is caused by the bite of a mad dog; and, as we have seen, adds plague and skin diseases to the two contagious maladies mentioned in the Pseudo-Aristotle. The most important passage bearing on this question has been cited in Chapter IV.

In summary, it may be said that, among many primitive tribes, as well as in the highly-developed sacerdotal practices of such peoples as the Persians, we find suggestive fragments of isolation practice embedded in a matrix of religious taboo. In the Old Testament, on the other hand, is the first clean-cut conception of contagion and—built upon this conception—a definite and well-conceived program of differential diagnosis, isolation, quarantine and disinfection. The passages cited from the Book of Leviticus are as objective and precise as a sanitary code of the present day and almost as free from any element of supernaturalism.

In the writings of the historians of ancient Greece and Rome, we find again a clear recognition of the fact that epidemics are spread by direct contact between the sick and the well, first and most fully expounded by Thucydides. Some writers, notably Lucretius and Varro, go further and identify the infection with "seeds" which "fly about and cause disease and death," or "animalculae which cannot be seen with the eyes and which we breathe through the nose and mouth"—an interesting poetic forecast of the germ theory of disease.

Galen, as representative of the medicine of classical times, recognizes plague, tuberculosis, ophthalmia and skin diseases as contagious. It is important, however, to note that in medical, as contrasted with lay writing, miasmatic and constitutional factors are the only ones which are strongly emphasized. To the Greek and Roman physicians, contagion—though recognized as operating in certain diseases—was relegated to a minor role. This difference of emphasis between medical and non-medical thought was to persist for many centuries and to trace and to explain this difference will be one of our tasks in later chapters.

As we pass from the classical to the earlier centuries of the Christian Era, we find the contagiousness of leprosy playing a major role, no doubt on the basis of the Old Testament teaching. The spread of this disease by contagion was mentioned by Archigenes in the second century and by Aretaeus of Cappodocia in the third, the breath being assumed as the vehicle of transmission.

The first historic pandemic of bubonic plague, in the sixth century, furnished another powerful stimulus to the concept of contagion. Evagrius of Antioch, who was himself a victim of the disease in 540, "considered the disease to be contagious and to be acquired in various ways, such as sharing beds, by actual contact, by visiting infected houses, or even by casual meetings in the market-place."

The most important extant account of this "Plague of Justinian"—that of Procopius of Caesarea—however, takes the opposite view. In his *History of the Wars* (Book II, Chapters XXII and XXIII), the symptoms of the disease and the course of the epidemic are described with remarkable vividness and accuracy. It is noted that it proceeded in definite sequence from one locality to another "always moving forward and travelling at times favorable to it." "This disease always took its start from the coast and from there went up into the interior." Yet the concept of contagion is specifically denied. In speaking of the sufferings of those attending on the sick, he says, "everybody pitied them no less than the sufferers, not because they were threatened by the pestilence in going near it (for neither physicians nor other persons were found to contract this malady through contact with the sick or with the dead, for many who were constantly engaged either in burying or in attending those in no way connected with them held out in the performance of this service beyond all expectation, while with many others the disease came on without warning and they died straightway); but they pitied them because of the great hardships which they were undergoing."

Nor does the theory of an epidemic constitution enter into Procopius's analysis. He reverts without reserve to the Old Testament concept of the wrath of God.

"During these times," he says, "there was a pestilence, by which the whole human race came near to being annihilated. Now in the case of all other scourges sent from Heaven some explanation of a cause might be given by daring men, such as the many theories propounded by those who are clever in these matters; for they love to conjure up causes which are absolutely incomprehensible to man, and to fabricate outlandish theories of natural philosophy, knowing well that they are saying nothing sound, but considering it sufficient for them, if they completely deceive by their argument some of those whom they meet and persuade them to their view. But for this calamity it is quite impossible either to express in words or to conceive in thought any explanation, except indeed to refer it to God. For it did not come in a part of the world nor upon certain men, nor did it confine itself to any season of the year, so that from such circumstances it might be possible to find subtle explanations of a cause, but it embraced the entire world, and blighted the lives of all men, though differing from one another in the most marked degree, respecting neither sex nor age."

In such a passage as this, we see the clear sunshine of classical reason fading into the dim twilight of religious fatalism. The Dark Ages have set in.

CHAPTER VI

THE GREAT TEACHER

"A more frightful teacher than the plague, which swept over humanity with special fury in the middle of the fourteenth century, it is difficult to imagine."
—DIEPGEN

LYNN THORNDIKE in the general field of science, and Karl Sud-hoff and his pupils in the special area of medicine, have vigorously emphasized the achievements of the medieval mind; but their evidence is not too convincing. Throughout the history of human thought, magic and science have intermingled. In the Classical Period, however, the leading thinkers show us a prevailing trend of science contaminated by occasional remnants of superstition; in the Middle Ages, the corresponding picture is one of superstition, shot through with gleams of science. The spirit of Hermes Trismegistus was for centuries more powerful than that of Aristotle. The Philosopher's Stone and the Elixir of Life dominated men's imagination, rather than the immutable laws of an orderly, objective universe.

The particular field of human knowledge which we are here considering furnishes, however, one notable exception to the general rule. Diepgen is correct when he says: "But in one essential point the Middle Ages developed far beyond antiquity, in the full recognition of infection as a cause of disease. The recognition of this progress is bound up with the works of Sudhoff and Sticker. Certainly, even in ancient times, the communicability of certain diseases and the dangers proceeding from certain patients were known; that is shown by the description of the pest of Thucydides, the reference to the communicability of inflammation of conjunctiva in Plato, the opinions of Galen about the danger of intercourse with those afflicted by the pest and people who suffer from eye infections, itches and consumption, the opinions of Aretaeus of Cappadocia (third century) in regard to infection by leprosy, which, as in the case of the pest, is caused by the breath, an opinion which agrees with the ideas of Archigenes in the second century. But otherwise the whole Greek literature is dominated by the idea of one great universal cause of epidemical disease which causes many people to become ill at the same time, by what the Hippocratic writings term miasma. In any case the idea of infection has not attained any sort of universal application in Greek medicine. The revolution does not come until medieval times."

As suggested in the quotation at the head of the present chapter, the Black Death was the great teacher in this field. A preliminary course was, however, offered by leprosy and, at the end of the fifteenth century, a post-graduate course by syphilis.

It was fortunate, perhaps, that the first widespread epidemic which threatened Europe (after the plague of Justinian) should have been leprosy. Whether this disease was actually Biblical leprosy is more than doubtful. It bore the same name, however; and this fact made it easier to carry over into the thinking of a world dominated by the Bible the contagionistic viewpoint of the Old Testament. Indeed, this whole movement was of clerical, not of medical, origin. The theory came from the Book of Leviticus and the actual practices from the East.

Leprosy is said to have been brought by Pompey's army from Egypt to Italy and to have reached Gaul as early as the second century. In the fourth century, the great Bishop Basil of Caesarea included isolation wards for lepers in his unique hospital establishment. It was in the sixth century, however, that Western Europe first felt itself seriously menaced by the spread of the disease from Egypt. As Sudhoff says "Enlightened princes of the church, moved by the increasing misery of the people, on the strength of the sacerdotal code of the Old Testament, undertook the task of interfering; the Shepherdess of the medieval peoples knew her duty." In the year 583, the free association of lepers with sound persons was restricted by the Council of Lyons, a procedure continued and elaborated by later Church councils. In the year 644, an edict of the Lombard King, Rothari, provided for the isolation of lepers. In the same century, Gregory of Tours describes a leper house in Paris. Leper houses were established at Metz, Verdun and Maestricht as early as the seventh century.

It was as a result of the Crusades, however, that leprosy really assumed epidemic proportions, brought back by the armies returning from Jerusalem. Outside that city, the Crusaders found leper hospitals in operation, took them over for various sorts of contagious diseases, and founded the order of Knights of Saint Lazarus of Jerusalem to nurse the sick between 1099 and 1113. The "lazarettos," named from the order, spread rapidly over Western Europe. The leprosy decretals of the third Lateran Council in 1179 dealt with the disease in great detail; and Matthew Paris estimates that there were ultimately some 19,000 lazarettos in Europe, used chiefly for leprosy but also for various other contagious diseases and even for epilepsy and insanity. Louis VIII left money for 2,000 leper houses in his will in 1225. In England, the first leper house was founded in 1096, the last in 1472.

The regulations governing the isolation of lepers were minute and precise. They were required to wear a special costume, to limit their walks to certain roads, to give warning of their approach by sounding a clapper, and to forbear communicating with healthy persons and drinking from or bathing in any running stream. Heine, paraphrasing an old chronicle, says of the wretched victims of this disease, "living corpses, they wandered to and fro, muffled from head to foot; a hood drawn over the face, and carrying in the hand a bell, the Lazarus-bell, as it was called, through which they were to give timely warning of their approach." The momentous decision whether a given individual suffered from leprosy or not was decided by special commissions according to regulations which went into the most minute details. In doubtful cases the patient was often sent far away in order to obtain the judgment of an especially competent commission.

When a decree of isolation was actually pronounced, the priest, according to one contemporary document, (Trouillard) blessed the robe, a pair of gloves and a clapper and presented them to the unfortunate victim with an admonition such as the following:

"I forbid you ever to enter into church, abbey, fair, mill or market or into the company of others.

"I forbid you to go out without your habit.

"I forbid you to wash your hands or anything about you at the stream or fountain, or to drink there; and if you need water to drink take it from your barrel in your cup.

"I forbid you to touch anything that you bargain for, or buy, until it is yours.

"I forbid you to go into any tavern; and if you want wine, whether you buy it or men give it you, have it put in your barrel.

"If you go on the roads and meet another person who speaks to you, I forbid you to answer till you place yourself against the wind.

"I forbid you to touch children or to give them anything.

"I forbid you to eat or drink from any vessel but your own.

"I forbid you to drink or eat in company, unless with lepers."

The awful finality of the exclusion from human society is dramatically emphasized by a twelfth century document describing the religious Ceremonial for Excluding a Leper (Loisne):

"When a leper has been judged in court by true deposition and for just cause.

"First the court assigns a day to the priest to perform and say the service. On that day the leper must be clad according to his station, very simply. He must have on his head a white shroud, falling low behind, and a grave cloth over [his garments], and carry in both his hands a little wooden cross; and so move from his house, accompanied by the church cross and by his friends mourning over him until he has taken his place at the leper hospital, and no further. And when he has come to the entrance the priest and clergy shall meet him and sprinkle holy water over him and take him by the hand and bring him into the [lepers'] cemetery and sing *Libera me Domine*.

"When they have come to the church, the priest shall begin the Vigils and the Commedaces, and when these are finished, the priest shall pray for him and say the Requiem Mass as for a dead man, with lights and candles. The leper, attired in his shroud and grave cloth, with his little wooden cross, shall kneel and lean on a low stool, his head bowed toward the altar—there where they are accustomed to place the bodies of the dead.

"And when the service is finished the priest shall go to the leper, and read what is read to the dead, and then give him the holy water. Then the priest takes him by the hand, and when they are come to the cemetery, the priest makes him kneel, and throws earth over him three times."

If we turn from the empirical practices of church and state to the theories of physicians and philosophers, we find on the other hand no significant contribution to epidemiological theory for eight hundred years after Galen. It is, of course, possible that such contributions may have existed and been lost; but this is not probable. The content of medieval thought was meager, and was worn threadbare by the repetition of copyists. If any lost works had contained jewels of thought they would almost certainly have been preserved by later commentators. The work of Beda "On the Nature of Things" in the early eighth century tells us that disease is caused by an atmosphere which is too dry or too hot or too rainy—such abnormal weather conditions being omens or signs of the just punishment of human sins. This was almost certainly the prevailing doctrine, based on the Greek doctrine of the four basic elements and on religious faith.

It was only about A.D. 900 that the infiltration of Arabian knowledge began and that Europeans once more resumed the use of their intellectual faculties. For the intervening centuries, it is to the East that we must look for any gleams of light on scientific problems. Both among the Jews and the Arabs we find a far more rational attitude than that of Christian Europe.

In the Talmud, Rabbi Akiba, when asked to explain why sick people are sometimes cured in a heathen temple replied, "Mere coincidence—human ills come to an end one day or another, and it is a mere coincidence that the sick people entered the heathen temple just at a moment when their disease was on the point of leaving them. Do you expect the Lord to change the course of nature for the sole purpose of preventing fools from falling into errors and superstitions?"

Moses Maimonides in the twelfth century displays a similar scientific attitude. He considers belief in demons (though not in angels) as idle and fallacious and condemns "all those practices which contrary to natural science are said to produce utility by special and occult virtues and properties ... such forsooth as proceed not from a natural cause but a magical operation and which rely upon the constellations to such a degree as to involve worship and veneration of them."

He classifies vicious magic processes as: one, employing the properties of plants, animals and metals; second, determining the times when these works should be performed; third, employing gesticulations, actions, and cries of the human operator.

But he accepts any procedure—even if apparently occult—that is actually demonstrated by experience.

"For whatever is proved by experience to be true, although no natural cause may be apparent, its use is permitted, because it acts as a medicine."

Among the Arabs this rational approach (combined with knowledge of the Greek classics) was applied to medicine with significant results. So far as contagion was concerned, these Arabian physicians suffered from a special handicap. The early Mohammedan writings recognized the fact of contagion. They warned the owner of healthy animals not to approach sick animals and the person in a country free from plague not to travel to a land where the disease was present. If already in an infected place, however, it was sinful to leave it, since disease was sent as a punishment for sin, and death in such circumstances (like death in battle) ensured future reward for the faithful. Yet even this paralysis of reason by religious fatalism was overcome by later writers.

It is the great Persians, Rhazes and Avicenna, who carry us furthest along the road and their doctrines—particularly those of Avicenna—mark some advance over those of their master, Galen.

Rhazes, however eminent as a diagnostician and clinician—giving admirable descriptions of smallpox and measles—was not distinguished as an epidemiologist. His explanation of the cause of smallpox is a highly ingenious one but exclusively humoral in nature and related to a supposed normal physiological change from the hot, moist blood of children to the cold, dry blood of adult life. "The blood of infants and children may be compared to must, in which the coction leading to perfect ripeness has not yet begun, nor the movement toward fermentation taken place; the blood of young men may be compared to must, which has already fermented and made a hissing noise, and has thrown out abundant vapors, and its superfluous parts, like wine which is now still and quiet and arrived at its full strength; and as to the blood of old men, it may be compared to wine which has now lost its strength and is beginning to grow vapid and sour."

"Now the Small-pox arises when the blood putrefies and ferments, so that the superfluous vapors are thrown out of it, and it is changed from the blood of infants, which is like must, into the blood of young men, which is like wine perfectly ripened; and the Small-pox itself may be compared to the fermentation and the hissing noise which take place in must at that time. And this is the reason why children, especially males, rarely escape being seized with this disease, because it is impossible to prevent the blood's changing from this state into its second state, just as it is impossible to prevent must (whose nature it is to make a hissing noise and to ferment) from changing into the state which happens to it after its making a hissing noise and its fermentation."

Smallpox happens in young men only to those whose normal fermentative change has been delayed; and "as for old men, the Small-pox seldom happens to them, except in pestilential, putrid, and malignant constitutions of the air, in which this disease is chiefly prevalent. For a putrid air, which has an undue proportion of heat and moisture and also an inflamed air, promotes the eruption of this disease." Thus, even where corruption of the air is mentioned, it is tied to the Procrustean bed of humoralism.

"Occult dispositions of the air, which necessarily cause these diseases and predispose bodies to them" are mentioned casually; but, throughout, Rhazes' thinking is so dominated by the dogma of "heat" and "moisture" that he can really see nothing else. Prophylaxis against smallpox is to be attained by blood-letting and use of "cooling" foods.

Avicenna (Ibn Sînā, 980-1037) on the other hand, presents a serious and well-thought-out body of epidemiological theory. This "prince of physicians," court physician to several caliphs and famous *bon vivant*, has, like Galen, been depreciated as a mere compiler; but in neither case is the criticism justified. Avicenna's Canon of Medicine has been said to be the "most popular treatise on medicine ever penned"; and, in view of its great influence on medieval thinkers, its treatment of epidemiological theory is of major importance.

In the first book of the Canon, he discusses the Transmission of Disease from Person to Person; and classifies such transmission under three main heads:

"229. A. Transmission by infection. (1) From one house to an adjoining one. Here belong lepra, scabies, variola, pestilential fever, septic inflammatory swellings and ulcers; (2) from a house in the wind-track to another; (3) where one person gazes closely at another (e.g. ophthalmia); (4) fancy: e.g. when a person's teeth chatter when he thinks of something sour; (5) such diseases as phthisis, impetigo, leprosy.

"B. Hereditary transmission. Vitiligo alba; premature baldness; gout; phthisis; lepra.

"C. Racial transmission. The sweating sickness of Angelica; elephantiasis in Alexandria; aurigo in Apulia; endemic goiter and many the like."

The air is, of course, the chief vehicle by which disease is transmitted; and the way in which it is corrupted is described in some detail:

"308. Air may be changed in (1) substance, (2) qualities. The substance may become depraved apart from any increase or decrease in some of the intrinsic qualities. Such an air is termed 'pestilential.' One must remember that putrefactive processes can occur in the atmosphere just as they do in stagnant water."

"311. Air generally becomes pestilential from putrefactive changes towards the end of summer and during autumn."

In Book IV, Part I, Section 4, this subject is further elaborated. It is explained that air becomes putrid from "bad vapors which, after being mixed with it, render the whole of bad quality. And, at one time and another, that is the cause of those winds which bring to a good place bad fumes from stinking places where there are deep valleys and bodies dried up after battle, the killed previously not having been buried nor covered. Possibly there may also be a cause near to the place of origin. And, occasionally, in the interior of the soil, decay occurs for reasons unknown, making water and air harmful." Some fevers (*febris cholerica*) are associated with dry air; but the "pestilential fevers" are caused by turbid and humid air.

Finally, in addition to these terrestrial factors, there are slight and obscure references to the underlying influence of celestial conditions. "The principle behind all these changes is a celestial figure making necessary what we do not know to be approaching. There may be people who distinguish as to the proportionality of causes; it is necessary for you to know how far primary causes are to be found in distant celestial figures and in near conditions of the earth."

Yet Avicenna, like Galen, was essentially a practical man. He did not devote much attention to the stars. He was much more interested in telling his readers (Book 1, 368) that "Bad water may be purified by sublimation and distillation. If that is not feasible, boiling will suffice, for boiled water, as the learned know, is less likely to cause inflammation." It is of interest to note that Avicenna cites as a sign of pestilence that mice and subterranean animals flee to the surface of the earth and behave as if intoxicated.

In this Canon of Avicenna are to be found most of the germs of European medieval thought in regard to epidemiology, as it developed with the cult of Arabian learning during the next few centuries. In medicine, as in other branches of human thought, a marked change became manifest at this period. The Regimen of the School of Salernum has scarcely a trace of magic in it and almost no metaphysical science, except perhaps the specification of lunar days for blood-letting. In the field of epidemiology, the only item of importance is the couplet:

> "Let air you breath be sunny, clear and light,
> Free from disease or cesspools' fetid blight."

Albertus Magnus in the thirteenth century again exhibits a sound scientific spirit. He tells us that "natural science is not simply receiving what one is told, but the investigation of causes in natural phenomena." He accepts magic as primarily the work of demons; but thinks that magical wonders are really the product of natural forces, accelerated or modified by demonic influence. In our special field he says, that "a conjunction of Jupiter and Mars with others aiding in the sign of Gemini" causes "pestilential winds and corruption of the air resulting in a plague by which a multitude of men and beasts suddenly perish."

Arnold of Villanova and Peter of Abano carried forward the development of an objective viewpoint; and Bernard Gordon, who taught at Montpellier between 1285 and 1307 made an important contribution to epidemiology in his famous list of the eight diseases which were contagious. These were acute fever, phthisis, epilepsy, scabies, erysipelas, anthrax, trachoma and leprosy. If we assume that acute fever and phthisis correspond to the similar terms used by Galen, that trachoma is his disease of the eyes and erysipelas and scabies were included under his skin diseases, we have anthrax, epilepsy and leprosy in addition. The list agrees with that of Avicenna in including pestilential fever, scabies, leprosy, phthisis, ophthalmia (trachoma) and skin diseases; but omits variola, septic inflammations and ulcers. Commenting on Gordon's list, Garrison notes its persistence in an ordinance of the city of Basel (1350), in the Pest Regimen of Hans Wincker (1450) and in the *Tractatulus de regimine sanitatis* of Siegmund Abich of Prag (1484). Gordon's epidemiological theory is merely a rehash of Avicenna, mentioning celestial forces causing corruption of air and water.

The concept of contagion seems, until 1348, to have been much less prominent in European than in Arabian thought. According to Eager, Guglielmo Varignara, professor of medicine at Bologna in 1302, not only denied the contagious nature of measles and smallpox (which Gilbert of England had nearly a century before described as contagious) but even declared that the buboes of plague could not transmit infection.

It was the Black Death which at last taught the communicability of disease beyond any peradventure.

This epidemic of bubonic (and in places pneumonic) plague was perhaps the greatest single calamity ever visited upon the human race. Introduced to Constantinople from Asia in the spring of 1347, it raged in that city for a year. It spread quickly through Greece and the Mediterranean islands, reached Sicily in October and had passed on to Naples and Genoa, to Marseilles and to Dalmatia before the end of the year. Early in 1348 it had established itself in southern France, Italy and Spain. By June, it was in Paris, by fall in England and Ireland. Germany and the Netherlands succumbed a little later, and by 1350 all Europe from Russia to Scandinavia (including such dependencies as Iceland and Greenland, according to Campbell) was in the grip of the plague. Guy de Chauliac, the greatest physician of his age, at that time court physician to Clement VI at Avignon, says of this epidemic: "I call it great, because it covered the whole world, or lacked little of doing so. For it began in the East, and thus casting its darts against the world, passed through our region toward the West. It was so great that it left scarcely a fourth part of the people. And I say that it was such that its like has never been heard tell of before; of the pestilences in the past that we read of, none was so great as this. For those covered only one region, this the whole world; these could be treated in some way, this in none."

Later students vary in their estimates of the mortality directly due to the plague. Hecker, the most conservative, places the figure at one-fourth of the population of Europe; Krafft-Ebing, at three-fourths. Seebohm and Gasquet estimate that one-half the population of England perished. In individual localities, the figure must have been even higher. A Belgian cleric, writing from Avignon on April 17, 1348, says that half the inhabitants of that city are dead and four-fifths of the population of Marseilles.

The social dislocation which resulted from the Black Death was, in some ways, even more serious than the immediate mortality. The poet, Guillaume de Machaut, describes the situation as an eye-witness: "For lack of men you saw many a fair and fine heritage lying unploughed. No one could have his fields tilled, his wheat sowed, his vines trimmed without paying triple wages, so many were dead; and it happened that in the fields the dumb animals lay all bewildered, and went among the wheat and vines wherever they would; they had neither lord nor shepherd nor man to go with them. No one claimed them, nor demanded his own. Many heritages were left without lords. The living dared not stay at all at the manors where death had been, whether in winter or in summer; and if anyone did so he put himself in peril of death."

The power of the church and of the law was shattered. The monasteries and the universities were robbed of their leadership. Commerce was destroyed. The sect of the Flagellants and the victims of the Dancing Mania spread over Europe, and among the more intelligent there developed an obsessive cult of death. This was the end of the Middle Ages—and cleared the way for the new European civilization which was to be built upon the ruins of the old. Campbell quotes A. L. Maycock as saying that "the year 1348 marks the nearest approach to a definite break in the continuity of history that has ever occurred"; and Gasquet names this catastrophe as marking "the real close of the medieval period and the beginning of the modern age."

It was natural that such a cataclysm should stir up among the ignorant all sorts of blind resentments. The Belgian cleric tells his correspondent that "Some wretched men have been caught with a certain dust; and whether justly or unjustly God only knows, they are accused of the crime of poisoning the waters." Guy de Chauliac says, "In some places they believed that the Jews had poisoned the world, and so they killed them. In some other places they believed it was the poor cripples, and they drove them away. In other places that it was the nobles; and so they feared to go ábroad. Finally, it went so far that they set guards at the villages; and let no one enter who was not well known. And if they found powders or salves on any man, fearing that they were poisons, they made him swallow them."

In the fourteenth century, however, these were delusions of the vulgar, not, as in the twentieth, part of the official philosophy of great nations. Both Pope Clement VI and King Casimir of Poland took vigorous steps to protect and succor the Jews. The literate, both medical and lay, sought for rational explanations of these calamities. On the medical side, such explanations were put forth in a great number of plague tractates explaining to the public the causes of the epidemic and the symptoms and treatment of the disease. These tractates offer, perhaps, the first large-scale example of popular instruction in the field of public health. They have been exhaustively studied in recent years by Sudhoff, who reviews 141 such tractates from Germany, 77 from Italy, 21 from France, 9 from Spain, 9 from England and 7 from Switzerland. Sudhoff's material covers a period of several hundred years following the Black Death; and Campbell bases her analysis of the subject on sixteen contemporary treatises written between 1348 and 1350. The most important of these early documents are the letter of Jacme d'Agramont to the city fathers of Lerida, dated April 24, 1348, the *Consilia contra pestilentiam* of Gentile da Foligno (who died of the plague in 1348); the *Compendium de epidemia* of the Faculty of Medicine of Paris (prepared on the request of Philip of Valois, the earliest surviving record of the august body which prepared it); the *Morbi in posterum vitandi Descriptia & Remedia* of Ibn Khātimah of Almeria; the *Tractatus de epidemia*, written by "a physician of Montpellier"; a *Very Useful Inquiry into the Horrible Sickness* by Ibn al-Khatîb of

Andalusia; and *Concerning the Judgment of the Sun at the Banquet of Saturn* by Simon of Covino.

The writer has had the privilege of consulting an unpublished translation from the Catalan of the first of the documents cited (that of Jehan Jacme) made by Dr. Arnold C. Klebs of Nyon, Switzerland, for which courtesy he wishes to express his deep gratitude to Dr. Klebs. This letter is of very special interest, since it is the first of all known plague tractates, written apparently before the plague had actually reached Lerida but was present "in certain parts and regions near to ours" as a means of teaching his fellow-townsmen how to protect themselves against it.

Other early plague tractates consulted are those of Johannes Jacobi, of Amplonianus and of Magister Bartholomaüs of Brügge. The tract of Jacobi is identical with that ascribed to Knut, Bishop of Vesteras and Dr. Klebs, and other authorities have suggested that Johannes Jacobi and Jehan Jacme may have been the same person. The texts of the two documents, however, are quite different. The comments of Guy de Chauliac are, of course, of primary importance; and, of lay commentaries of the period, we have the letter of the Belgian cleric at Avignon, and the poem, *La jugement du roi de Navarre*, by Guillaume de Machaut, to which reference has been made above.

Later in the fourteenth century there appeared many significant documents of a similar type, of which the following have been consulted: a letter from Magister Henricus de Bremis (probably identical with that of Henricus de Ribeniz of Prag); the Advice of Pietro da Tussignano (1398); the *Regimen bonum in Epidimia* of Johannes de Tornamira (circa 1400); the pest tractate of Heinrich Steinhöwel of Ulm and the *Consiglio* of Marsilio Ficino—the last two dating from the fifteenth century.

On these eighteen representative documents, which are, on the whole, remarkably consistent in their interpretation, (although relative emphasis on various factors differs widely) the following analysis of the fourteenth century approach to epidemiology has been based.

The first conclusion which emerges from such an analysis is the universal acceptance of the fact of contagion. Not all the documents mention contagion; but none challenge it. As Michon says, "Was the plague contagious? All the authors of the time, medical and non-medical, are unanimously in accord on this point."

Contagion is not stressed by Jacme, and this is natural since he had not yet actually experienced the great plague but wrote of it as an approaching menace only. Yet he does mention as one reason for its prevalence in a particular locality, "frequentation of those sick of the pestilential malady, because from them it is transferred to others just as fire spreads. And so it spreads until God in his pity gives us his grace.

"And if one asks me which are the maladies that can be transferred from one to the other I say that these are also leprosy, scabies, phthisis, running eyes, pestilential fever, smallpox, measles and mange. And in general all maladies that come from pestilential air."

In another place, he mentions the danger of "associating with a patient who has the pestilential malady. It has been said by persons worthy of belief that when the masters fall ill the servants also get the malady, as also the physician and the confessor."

Gentile da Foligno recognizes that the plague "proceeds not only from one man to another but also from one community to another." He notes that traces of the pestilence remain in a locality for a long time and compares its action to that of a ferment. He warns against contact with the sick or entrance into an infected house. After discussing treatment, he concludes, "Finally I conclude that to flee, as I have said, is best in this particular pestilence; for this illness is the most poisonous of poisons, and by its spread and blight it infects all."

The Medical Faculty of Paris reports that "It is specially to be observed that the well be put at a distance from all ill-smelling infected persons; for the sick of this sort are contagious. For the corrupted and poisoned air, breathed out by these sick, infects those present. That is why all or most people in the same house die, and especially those related to the sick, or connected with them." The Physician of Montpellier is equally emphatic in regard to contagion although he considers the eye as the chief source of danger. Yet he is quite naturalistic in this view which he justifies as follows: "For anyone familiar with the theories of Euclid on mirrors such contagion has nothing marvellous about it; for one can call a phenomenon marvellous only when one does not understand its principle and the natural cause which produces it."

The doctrine of contagion is most clearly stated, perhaps, by the two Mohammedan physicians. Ibn Khātimah, according to Campbell's translation, says, "That the evil spreads is evident from observation and experience, it having not yet happened that a well man remained long with a sick one without being attacked by the disease. Almost as harmful as the air breathed out by the sick, if not entirely so, are the fumes from their bodies, pieces of clothing, beds and linen on which the sick lay, if they are used again. The author has observed that the inhabitants of a portion of Almeria, where the clothing and bed linen of the sick were sold, died almost without exception, while dealers in other markets under the same conditions fared as other people. He also observed that cities which forbade the entry of people from stricken places remained spared as long as possible; most of the smitten living in strongholds about Almeria, date the entrance of the disease from the arrival of someone from a pestilential place." Yet he feels compelled to make his gesture to ecclesiastical authority by concluding piously that the spread of the disease "is a law which God has placed in the nature of the thing. God is first of all and above all the one who works. With this we refute the sort of generation which the erring maintain and refer to as infection."

Ibn al-Khatîb scorns any such genuflection. If he is asked how he can grant infection when religious law proscribes it, he replies "The existence of infection stands firm through experience, research, mental perception, autopsy and authentic knowledge of fact, and these are the materials of proof." In another place, he says, "when we speak of the corruption of the special air, we mean, for instance, the air of the house which is attacked, and then the air of the city, while the plague is established there, while the air of the neighboring territory remains unaltered; and we exclude the corruption of the air in general, since that next it remains sound."

Simon de Covino, a doctor of Paris who probably witnessed the course of the disease at Montpellier, wrote an account of his experiences in poetic form in 1350. He says:

"It has been proved that when it once entered a house scarcely one of those who dwelt in it escaped. . . . It happened also that priests, those sacred physicians of souls, were seized by the plague whilst administering spiritual aid; and often by a single touch, or a single breath of the plague-stricken, they perished even before the sick person they had come to assist." Clothes were regarded as infected and also furniture.

Guy de Chauliac, describes both the pneumonic and bubonic forms of the disease and says: "The contagion was so great (especially when there was blood-spitting) that not only by remaining [with the sick], but even by looking [at them] people seemed to take it; so much so, that many died without any to serve them, and were buried without priests to pray over their graves.

"A father did not visit his son, nor the son his father. Charity was dead! The mortality was so great that it left hardly a fourth part of the population. Even the doctors did not dare to visit the sick from fear of infection, and when they did visit them they attempted nothing to heal them, and thus, almost all those who were taken ill died, except toward the end of the epidemic, when some few recovered.

"As for me, to avoid infamy, I did not dare to absent myself, but still was I in continual fear."

Guillaume de Machaut says "Few dared venture into the open air or approach near to any to talk to them. For the breath of the corrupted in turn corrupted those who were well." Amplonianus is one of the many writers who stresses the use of vinegar for washing the hands and washing out the mouth and nose on leaving the sickroom as a prophylactic against contagion. Magister Bartholomaüs makes the same recommendation and notes that patients near death are the most contagious. Magister Henricus warns against visiting the sick during the plague and against visiting baths, churches, social gatherings and damp places. Pietro da Tussignano recognizes contagion and recommends elaborate procedures for purifying the air. In an extraordinarily interesting passage, he says, "those surviving after an epidemic may infect newcomers; just as does unleavened bread which is surrounded by meal: as one arranges the meal for fermentation, so in this case the pestilential air affects human bodies; therefore, one should not return to those places in which the epidemic has been." Heinrich Steinhöwel says that, to escape the plague, one should "fly quickly and fly far" from the infected place; and, if that is impossible, purify the house by sunlight, fumigation and the lavish use of vinegar.

Finally, Boccaccio in the Introduction to the Decameron (Kelly's translation) says: "What gave the more virulence to this plague, was that, by being communicated from the sick to the hale, it spread daily, like fire when it comes in contact with large masses of combustibles. Nor was it caught only by conversing with, or coming near the sick, but even by touching their clothes, or anything that they had before touched."

The plague, then, was clearly contagious. But what was the nature of the communicable element? Here, again, there is almost complete unity of opinion. No writer hints at a *contagium animatum*, nor even at a particulate solid particle of any kind. It was a chemical property of the air which all these commentators visualized—as was to be the case for many centuries to come.

Jehan Jacme, in the earliest of the plague tracts, is particularly clear and circumstantial on this point. Normal health, he says, and protection against poisons, noxious beasts and pestilences depend on temperate, clean and clear air. (In the air of certain isles of Ireland, no poisonous beasts can live.) Changes in the quality or substance of the air (putrefaction) causes disease (as in Avicenna). It is of special interest, however, to note that Jacme apparently recognizes a specificity in such atmospheric alterations which many later medical writers ignored. He says, "and that to a diversity of putrefactions there correspond a diversity of properties is easily proved as we see that by putrefaction of phlegm outside of the veins a fever arises called 'quotidian,' with the property of beginning every day, and by putrefaction of bile another fever arises which is named 'tertian' with the property of beginning every other day. And through the putrefaction of black bile arises the 'quartan' with the property of beginning every fourth day. And when I say *outside the veins* it is because all the above said humors can putrefy, inside the veins in which case a continuous fever is produced." Later, he continues, "Therefore, if in the air through all these various alterations as well in its qualities as in its substance diverse properties can develop and from diverse properties follow diverse consequences, no man can wonder when the air sometimes becomes the cause of sudden deaths among people, or of the occurrence of diverse pestilential fevers or tumors or apostematas in the axilla or the inguinal region or that in other places reigns the smallpox or worms or other maladies, most perilous and mortal. And such times can be called times of epidemic or of pestilence." Thus, "pestilence is alteration *contra natura* of the air in its qualities and in its substance." Alteration of the waters may cause death of fishes; but alteration of the air affects men, birds, beasts and plants that live in the air. Since plants grown in corrupted air themselves become corrupt "where people live on corn brought from afar, they must ascertain with care from what region it came. Thus they must ask for certificates [of origin] from the grocery if they suspect that they [foods] come from regions and ports in which such a pestilence reigns." Here is an extraordinarily interesting link between the concepts of contagion and of atmospheric miasms. Still another such link appears in a passage where Jacme describes the passage of an epidemic from one area to another. "Because all plagues begin in one region. But then sometimes it moves to others by one of three reasons. First, by contiguity, because one air corrupts easily another air which touches it, and one sees manifestly that this is so by the experience in a similar case, viz. when a tree has rotten apples only the ones near to them rot also. One sees also that when such a tree has apples partly rotten, the rot soon is conveyed to the whole tree and all the apples. Second, by transport of foods, meal and meat from a pestilential region to another, so that those who eat them fall ill of similar maladies and worse ones, the same as those from where they came. Thirdly, winds that carry and move corrupt and pestilential air from one to another region."

As to the question why pestilence becomes universal "for a whole region or for several," Jacme suggests four factors: the wrath of God, corruption of dead bodies, of waters and of vapors formed in the interior of the earth, unnatural hot and humid winds and the conjunction of stars and planets. Its prevalence in a particular locality, he attributes to contagion, proximity of swamps, lack of purifying sunshine due to a shut-in position among hills or to an excess of trees (the shade of the walnut and fig being particularly harmful), to excretal and other decomposing filth, and to excessive indulgence in foods, particularly fruits.

Jacme stresses the harmful influence of hot and humid southerly winds or of any weather which is unusually hot or cold. He also mentions putrefaction of dead bodies as a cause of the corruption of the atmosphere and illustrates by the analogy that "from decayed bodies arise flies and poisonous worms in great quantity"; also humid vapors formed in the interior of the earth such as those which "at times make the earth shake"; also "malicious and dangerous" vapors from certain putrefactions in water. "The odor of the leaves of decaying cabbage has the property of corrupting the air."

Gentile da Foligno is also quite clear about corruption of the atmosphere being the major issue. He says, very acutely, in commenting on the influence of the stars (which we shall discuss later) "Which of the aforesaid causes it is, however, is of no great moment. It must be believed that whatever may be the case in regard to the aforesaid causes, the immediate and particular cause is a certain poisonous material which is generated about the heart and lungs. Its impression is not from the excess in degree of primary qualities, but through properties of poisonousness; whence poisonous vapors having been communicated by means of the air breathed out and in, great extension and transition of this plague takes place, not only from man to man, but from country to country. And, as has been intimated before, it is no great matter in these causes whether it is a constellation or an earthly or aquarian figure, if only we may know how to resist it, and that a stand must be made against it to destroy it lest it destroy us. As for those wishing to extinguish a fire burning a house, it is enough to know that it is a fire, that it may not destroy us, whether it be produced by fire or by motion; and for those wishing to resist the poisonous bite of a dry asp, it is enough to know that the asp was biting, whether it was generated by coition or from putrefaction" (Campbell).

The Medical Faculty of Paris, as we have seen, refers to "corrupted and poisoned air breathed out by the sick"; and in another paragraph we read that "the present epidemic or pest comes directly from air corrupted in its substance. For air which is pure and clear in its nature, does not decay or become corrupt unless it is mixed with evil vapors." Ibn Khātimah stresses this factor with particular emphasis and analyzes in great detail the metaphysical possibilities of "partial" or "total" alteration of the normal properties of the atmosphere. The possibilities of "total" change, he illustrates by the condition which may exist in old store-houses and wells where lights go out and animals die. This is the sort of deadly alteration which he considers to be manifest in severe epidemics, where thousands of people die in a few days. Ibn al-Khatîb considers "corruption of air" the proximate cause of the epidemic. Guillaume de Machaut describes the air during an epidemic as "no longer fresh and pure, but dirty and vile, black and obscure," so that it becomes entirely corrupted. Pietro da Tussignano says that "a disease is a change made in the air" and follows Ibn Khātimah in discussing partial and total corruption of the atmosphere. Marsilio Ficino defines pestilential fever as "a poisonous vapor hostile to life, created in the air," hostile "not because of its elementary quality but because of a specific property."

The next problem, of course, is "How does the air become corrupted so as to spread infection?" Here again, there is little conflict of opinion, though considerable variation in emphasis. So far as terrestrial phenomena are concerned, the Hippocratic and Galenic conceptions of organic decay and abnormal weather conditions are dominant. Gentile da Foligno refers to the opening of wells and caverns shut up

too long, to emanations from lakes or ponds, to evil-smelling putrefactions of dead bodies of men or animals. The Paris Compendium
refers to decaying matter piled up in the interior of the earth, such as
causes earthquakes and to south winds carrying vapors from swamps,
lakes, deep valleys and unburied corpses. Ibn Khātimah lists putrid
fumes of decaying matter, such as manure, stagnant bodies of water,
low swampy fields, rotting plants and vegetables, unburied corpses on
battlefields and plague-stricken cattle; but he also stresses abnormal
seasons and weather conditions.

Johannes Jacobi mentions particularly the air of "a seat or privy next
to a room or of any particular thing which corrupteth the air in its
substance and quality" and, again, that pestilence sometimes "cometh
of dead carrion or corruption of standing water in ditches or sloughs
and other corrupt places." Magister Henricus mentions (after astrological factors) "corruption of the air because of decay," and "fetid
exhalations," as the second and third causes of atmospheric deterioration. Pietro da Tussignano gives a somewhat individual list of causes
of corrupt vapors; "they have been lifted up from the corrupt earth: so
it is when caves are found or enclosures of air: or when some things are
placed in water: like the rope of hemp: and similar things: or such as
dead bodies which are not buried: or trees of evil nature: such as the
nut: the fig-tree: and similar things." Johannes de Tornamira says,
"In times of epidemic, you must first of all avoid corrupted air which
may come from marshy, muddy and fetid places, from stagnant water
and ditches, from burial places, from stables of draught animals—avoid
completely such places. Furthermore, beware of fog and fetid air and,
as far as possible, select clear and pure air." Heinrich Steinhöwel warns
against miasms of decaying bodies, heat and unseasonal weather.

There remains, however, another problem to be solved. Granted that
the plague is a contagious corruption of the air, beginning with some
form of decay of non-living materials and later spreading from man
to man, why did this corruption assume such appalling proportions in
1348? This is still the unknown "x factor" in epidemiology. We do not
really know why influenza became pandemic in 1918 any more than
the authors of the plague tractates knew why plague became pandemic
in 1348. We guess that a variation occurred in the virulence of a living
germ; this is only an assumption, backed by no concrete evidence. It
is the most plausible assumption in the twentieth century; but could

not have been postulated in the fourteenth. Our predecessors, working —as they inevitably did—on the basis of a theory of atmospheric corruption (of a chemical, not a biologic nature) and dealing with an effect which was world-wide and not local, naturally resorted to the celestial universe for an explanation. So we find the physician of the time turning to a malign conjunction of the stars as the ultimate cause of the phenomenon which they were seeking to explain.

Jacme's references to astrological influence are brief and highly naturalistic (on the basis of the humoral theory). He stresses the effects of "hot" or "cold" planets as they approach the sun upon the "hotness" or "coldness" of the air; and in another place illustrates the more specific power of certain planets by the attractive force of a magnet. Gentile da Foligno quotes Avicenna in support of the view that remote causes, or heavenly figures, impress themselves upon the near or earthly figures in such a way as to render the air putrid and produce a pestilence and refers to the conjunction of Saturn and Mars as particularly threatening. His primary interest, however, as we have seen was in the actual corruption of the air. The Arab writers also touch lightly on celestial influences, and Ibn al-Khatîb specifically states that astronomical factors lie outside the scope of medical interest.

It was the Paris Faculty which worked out the astrological influence in detail and with major emphasis and deeply impressed this theory upon European medical thought. Its Compendium is altogether positive about the whole matter. On March 20, 1345, at one o'clock in the afternoon, occurred a conjunction of Mars, Jupiter and Saturn in the sign of Aquarius which, with other conjunctions and eclipses was the whole cause of the trouble. Following the teaching of Albert of Cologne, these authors explain in detail how Jupiter, a warm and humid planet, drew up evil vapors from earth and water and how Mars, a malevolent planet generating choler and wars, was from October 6, 1347, to May 1348 in the constellation of the Lion together with the head of the Dragon. Mars, being on the wane, was particularly active in drawing up vapors and, since its evil aspect was turned toward Jupiter, a disposition or quality hostile to human life was engendered. "It is a property of Jupiter to engender strong winds which, with a generally prevailing southerly direction, brought an excess of heat and humidity. In our own region, the humidity was even more excessive than the heat. This was the ultimate and general cause of the present epidemic."

It must be noted that the authors of this theory were dealing not with a magical but with what they conceived as an objective natural process. It is significant to note how the famous "practitioner of Montpellier" explains that the "reason why the epidemic rages in two distant towns and not in places between them is on account of the aspects and rays of the planets which strike these places, like the glance of the eyes upon an object; as when Saturn looks upon Mars with malignant aspect, or Mars with malignant aspect upon humane Jupiter, then the rays of those planets kill where they strike."

Apparently, all later fourteenth century writers accepted the general theory of the Paris Faculty as to the ultimate primary cause of the epidemic. Thus Pietro da Tussignano says, "The reasons [for disease] are twofold. The first is universal and remote; it is a disposition coming from the forms and images of the sky. . . . And the dispositions contaminate the waters and thus they produce putrefying contaminations in the inmost parts of the earth and that especially happens about the time of the eclipse of the sun and moon and at the conjunction of the planets. Especially about Saturn and Mars with the fixed stars." And, so Marsilio Ficino, "Poisonous vapor forms itself in the air during the plague epidemics, more generally during the evil conjunctions of stars, particularly Mars and Saturn."

These astrological ideas are, of course, to be found among the physicians of Greece and Rome (note Hippocrates' references to the Dog-Star); but they played a much more prominent part in the fourteenth century than in the first. It may reasonably be maintained, however, that this is no discredit to the physicians of 1348. It is evidence that they did not ignore the crucial problem, "Why did disease become pandemic at a certain moment?" They met this question squarely and answered it in the most plausible manner made possible by the knowledge of the times.

Aside from contagion, miasms and planetary influence, many of the fourteenth century commentators include a fourth set of factors relating to the occurrence of remarkable terrestrial phenomena. As I interpret the texts, however, these were incidents secondary to celestial and atmospheric influences rather than direct causes. They are often referred to as "signs" of an epidemic constitution.

Jehan Jacme says, on this point, "by the putrefaction of the earth is generated a multitude of living things, each one of divers kind and divers property such as serpents and lizards, mice and leeches [?]. And by the putrefaction of the air are generated flies and mosquitoes and locusts, each one of divers kinds and divers properties. And by the putrefaction of the water are generated toads and serpents and eels. But in the element of fire no putrefaction whatever can take place because of its heat and dryness." Among the "signs" of pestilence, Jacme mentions comets and various other appearances of flashing or flaming in the air [falling stars ?], planetary conjunctions, harmful winds and weather, occurrence of plagues of frogs, snakes, worms, etc., bad crops and the prevalence of other diseases than the major pestilence. He does not make as clear a distinction between "causes" and "signs" as do some later writers. Indeed, he says of fire from heaven that "this sign of the pestilence is not only a sign but the cause itself which gives rise to pestilence. But everything that presents to our understanding that which may become, can be called a sign."

The Paris Faculty, in discussing the influence of "decaying matter piled up in the interior of the earth," suggests that such matter may cause earthquakes as well as corruption of the air. Its Compendium lists among the portents and signs of epidemic disease, unseasonable weather; exhalations and flashes such as the dragon and the flying stars; yellowish sky and reddish air on account of burning fumes; thunder storms and violent southerly winds; a multitude of dead fish and animals; trees covered with dust; and a multitude of frogs and reptiles. A tractate entitled "Is it From Divine Wrath," reviewed by Campbell, considers the epidemic as primarily due to corruption of the air caused by an earthquake which occurred in 1347; but this is an unusual position. Simon de Covino repeats the Paris references to lightning and falling stars, mist and clouds, and deadly south winds. Ibn Khātimah notes the withering of plants, their leaves appearing as if covered with dust, the rotting of fruits before they are ripe and rotting fish piled up opposite the plague-stricken Turkish coast as signs of an epidemic constitution.

Johannes Jacobi states the case rather fully, clearly distinguishing between "tokens" and "causes" of the epidemic. The "tokens" are as follows:

"Seven things ought to be noted in the same. The first is, when in a summer's day the weather often times changeth—as in the morning it appeareth to rain—afterwards it appeareth cloudy and at last windy in the south.

"The second token is when in summer the days appear all dark and like to rain and yet it raineth not and if many days so continue there is dread of a great pestilence.

"The third token is when there is a great multitude of flies upon the earth, then it is a sign that the air is venomous and infected.

"The fourth token is when the stars seem oftentimes to fall; then it is a token that the air is infected with much venomous vapor.

"The fifth token is when a blazing star is seen in the element—then there should happen soon after to be great manslaughter in battle.

"The sixth token is when there is great thunder and lightning, namely out of the south.

"The seventh token is when great winds come out of the south which are foul and unclean."

Jacme is one of the very few medical authorities to stress Divine Wrath as a factor in epidemics. He quotes Exodus 6-11, Deuteronomy 28, II Kings 24. He also mentions malign human influence: "From another cause may come the plague and pestilence, that is from bad people, children of the devil, who with diverse medicines and poisons corrupt the foodstuffs with evil skill and malevolent industry. But properly speaking such mortality is not the pestilence of which we speak here."

It is a somewhat remarkable fact that other medical writers of the time (except Ibn Khātimah) make no reference—or only the most perfunctory reference—to the conception of disease as a punishment for sin. Their explanation is throughout naturalistic. With the lay commentators it is different. Guillaume de Machaut tells us that "When God saw from his mansion the corruption of the world which was everywhere so great, it is no marvel that He desired to take cruel vengeance on that great disorder. At once, without longer tarrying, to take justice and vengeance, He made Death go forth from her cage, full of folly and of rage, without bit, without bridle, without rein, without faith, without love, without measure, so full of pride and so arrogant, so gluttonous and so famished, that she could not satisfy herself with anything that she devoured. And she ran throughout the world, against all whom she met."

So, Boccaccio, in speculating on the fundamental origin of the plague, says diplomatically that it may have been due to "the influence of the planets, or that it was sent from God, as a just punishment for our sins."

Many of the medical authorities emphasize the importance of individual predisposition, to explain the fact that not all persons in an infected house are stricken down. Jacme thinks the individuals in special danger are "those that have a body full of humors, especially corrupt and putrid humors. And also those who the whole year long rejoice in eating and drinking much. And those who have frequent intercourse with women. And those who have the porosities of their bodies naturally or artificially open, as those who bathe frequently. Naturally, those who are oversensitive to hot or cold. And those who without much reason sweat. And those whose bodies are hairy, because abundance of hair denotes wide porosities of the body."

The Paris Faculty considers that those whose bodies are replete with humors are most susceptible; Ibn Khātimah specifies more specifically young and corpulent persons, particularly young women (whose temperament is hot and moist); Ibn al-Khatîb, women and children; Simon de Covino, on the other hand, points to the frail and poorly nourished as particularly susceptible. Johannes Jacobi considers that bodies having open pores "as men which abuse themselves with women or bathe very frequently or men that are heated with labor or great anger" are more liable to infection than bodies "having the pores stopped with many humors." The humoral theory, as usual, led its devotees to fantastic extremes.

For practical prevention—aside from avoidance of sick persons and infected localities, which we have discussed above, our authors have various suggestions.

Jacme's prophylactic regimen for protection against the plague is extensive, occupying nearly half of his tractate. He is far more voluminous and far more self-confident than later authorities who had had actual experience with the epidemic. If the air is pestilential because of heat one should keep cool in the mountains or underground or by sprinkling water on the floor or evaporating it from large bowls or from drenched linen sheets. One should wear light clothes (but carefully avoid chilling) and eat "cold" foods. Opposite precautions must be taken when "the air is pestilential because of excessive cold."

"If air is pestilential because of putrefaction and corruption of its substance, one must consider whether its corruption or putrefaction was sent for our good, or for our sins, or whether it came from the infection of the earth, or of the water, or of allied things, or whether it came from higher or superior causes such as by the influence of conjunctions or opposition of planets." If sent by divine power, there is nothing to do but repent and pray. "When God wisheth not, Saints cannot." If putrefaction comes from the earth, one should seek high places, if from the skies, low and underground places (and keep the windows tightly shut). Fumigation of the house with rosemary, cypress, myrtle, incense, myrrh and other substances is recommended and "it is most beneficial to sprinkle the floor of the room with rosewater and vinegar."

Violent exercise is harmful. Eating and drinking must be temperate and meat of humid flesh and slimy fishes avoided. Theriac and the marvellous antidote of Mithridates, and other drugs are recommended and, of course, purging and bleeding.

Finally, Jacme stresses the importance of good mental hygiene. "To prove the great efficacy and the great virtue of our imagination on our body and on our work," he quotes from Genesis the success of Jacob in producing the ring-straked lambs and kids and continues as follows: "Another proof of this proposition can be made and induced by the following experiment: When somebody stands on a square board on the flat floor he needs in no direction something to hold on to so as not to fall off, but when this same board is placed in a high and perilous position, he would dislike very much to stand upon this said board. Evidently the difference is due wholly to the imagination. Because in the first case he is not afraid and in the other he is afraid. Thus it is evidently very dangerous and perilous in such times to imagine death and to have fear. Therefore nothing must make us discouraged or despair, such fear only does great damage and no good whatsoever."

Jacme sets one excellent example to other writers on plague (as well as to much later health propagandists) by his emphasis on the importance of sanitation. He says, "To prevent pestilence in a town one must prevent with energy that entrails and refuse of beasts or dead beasts be thrown out near the town. Nor should manure heaps be placed inside the town. Nor must it be allowed that behind the town in the public, neither in day time or night time, any excrements be discharged or thrown, nor must there be kept behind the town skins to be tanned, nor should cattle or other beasts be killed or butchered. Because from all these great infection of the air occurs. And this precaution is valid for Paris, for Avignon and for Lerida." If such precautions had been general, the rodent carriers of plague would certainly have been substantially reduced in numbers.

Most of the other writers are less confident and less detailed. Most of them follow the Hippocratic tradition in stressing avoidance of dangerous winds. The Paris Faculty warns against a habitation near marshy, miry and fetid places, evil standing water and ditches. Windows should open toward the north, and those facing south should be kept closed, at least till the sun has risen or a fire been lighted. In general, windows should be glazed or covered with waxed cloth to keep out all but the pure north air at midday. Ibn Khātimah emphasizes much the same things and considers that cities on a southern exposure toward the sea are particularly dangerous because the rays of sun and stars are reflected from the water mirror so as to make those cities hotter and more moist.

Many of the writers recommend the purification of the air by fumigation. The Paris Compendium specifies the fragrant fumes of juniper and ash, grape, rosemary, young oak and thorn. The burning of aromatics, wood of aloes, amber and musk for the rich, cypress, laurel, mastic and costus, for the poor, is helpful. In summer, sprinkling the house with vinegar and rosewater, and inhaling the odors of flowers is recommended (Ibn Khātimah). The "amber apple" is specially valuable, to be smelt as a prophylactic; but it is costly and various cheaper substitutes are suggested for the poor. The boiling of water is stressed by many of our authors.

From the standpoint of personal hygiene, all medical authorities emphasize the importance of the temperate life. Pietro da Tussignano refers specifically to the Non-naturals of Galen. His list of the Non-naturals, however, differs from many early Galenic texts in including food and omitting sexual moderation and the control of the passions and affections of the mind. Many of the tractates contain elaborate specifications as to safe and dangerous foods, into which it is difficult to read any possible scientific significance. Most of them consider bathing—particularly, hot bathing—as hazardous because it opens the pores of the skin and thus predisposes to infection. It is possible that the spread of the disease in public bath-houses may have furnished some basis for such a conception. Sexual intercourse is considered dangerous, particularly by the Christian writers.

Antidotes of various sorts were recommended as prophylactics, pills of aloes, myrrh and saffron by the Paris Faculty, figs, filberts and rue before breakfast, a powder of black pepper and cummin (the practitioner of Montpellier), and the four traditional antidotes against poison —theriac, mithridate, vol Armeniac and terra sigilata, powdered emerald, etc. Purging and bleeding were suggested as general prophylactics. Ibn Khātimah is particularly emphatic on venesection. He has seen as much as eight pounds of blood drawn at one time and he says, "After people learned this and saw its effects, they began to have bleeding done for themselves, without medical prescription, several times a month, without consideration or fear, without feeling harm or weakness, without contracting sickness in consequence."

Many authorities, such as the Paris Faculty and Johannes Jacobi, emphasize the importance of seeking competent physicians for treatment; but Guy de Chauliac, the really great physician of his time, says, as quoted above, that when doctors did visit patients "they accomplished almost nothing and gained nothing. For all the sick died, except a few toward the end." Yet this modest and heroic healer continued to perform his hopeless and unrewarded duties until he was stricken down himself.

In the final decade of the fifteenth century a third formidable teacher, Syphilis, powerfully reenforced the teachings of Leprosy and Plague; this episode will be discussed in the next chapter. It seems clear, however, that from the experience of the Black Death, the medical leaders of 1400 had developed a clear and remarkably logical theory of epidemiology—even if their prophylaxis and therapeusis were inevitably futile. Their main conceptions of causation may be summarized as follows:

A. Such a disease as the plague was highly contagious, spreading from the sick to the well by contact (according to some authorities by the glance of the eye); and infection was associated with objects and places used or occupied by the sick.

B. The infection consisted in a corruption of the air (of what we should call a chemical nature).

C. This corruption of the air arose from decomposing organic matter, unburied bodies of the dead, marshy and putrid waters and the like; and was favored by certain meteorological conditions, such as heat, dampness and southerly winds.

D. The basic factor which made possible the generation of particularly virulent corruption (such as characterized a great and unusual pandemic) was a malign conjunction of the planets and fixed stars.

E. Such a conjunction was apt to be associated with other unusual earthly and heavenly phenomena such as unseasonable weather, earthquakes, falling stars, thunderstorms and the like; but these were "signs" of an epidemic constitution of the atmosphere rather than "causes" of such a condition.

F. Individual predisposition played a considerable part in determining which particular persons were stricken in the course of an epidemic.

No single author presents the total picture in quite so logical a form but no one of the tractates with which I am familiar is inconsistent with it. The conception as a whole was a reasonable one in view of the knowledge of the day, and marks a tremendous advance over the etiological thinking of classical times. All of the elements in it are present in Galen but they are much more fully detailed and more logically related by the fourteenth century writers and the role of contagion is far more prominent.

It is of particular interest to note that these authorities saw no antithesis among the six factors mentioned above. There was no conflict in their minds between "contagionistic" and "miasmatic" theories such as arose in later centuries. They were free from that sinister intellectual error—the assumption of one necessary and sufficient cause which excludes all others. There is, however, marked difference in emphasis on various factors. The philosophically-minded Faculty of Paris was chiefly interested in primary celestial factors; the concrete practical interest of Gentile da Foligno, Ibn Khatimah, Ibn al-Khatîb, and Guy de Chauliac was concentrated on contagion. Miasmatic factors were stressed by Jehan Jacme, da Foligno, Ibn Khātimah, Johannes Jacobi and Pietro da Tussignano. The terrestrial wonders which were to be taken as signs of the disease are particularly prominent in the Paris Compendium and in Johannes Jacobi. Yet there are no really deep differences of opinion as to major causes.

There was nothing much to be done about the stars or the earthquakes or the weather (except to keep out harmful winds by shutting south windows). The corruption of the air was dealt with, as we have seen, by fumigation, sprinkling with odoriferous substances and the like, and by sanitation (Jacme). Vital resistance was built up by attention to the Non-naturals. The chief defense was, however, avoidance of infection; and the practices of isolation and quarantine, already developed in connection with leprosy, underwent a rapid and general development.

According to Eager, "The Venetians were, it is generally admitted, the first to make provision for maritime sanitation. As far back as the year 1000 there were overseers of public health, but at first the office was not a permanent one. The incumbents were appointed to serve during the prevalence of an epidemic only. The first information we have of this kind of public office is under date of 1348, when Nicholas Veneria, Marinus Querino, and Paulus Belegna (their Christian names given in the Latin of the text) were appointed overseers of public health. These officers were authorized to spend public money for the purpose of isolating infected ships, goods, and persons at an island of the lagoon. A medical man was stationed with the sick." About 1374, Venice enacted orders forbidding entrance to the city of infected or suspected ships, travelers or freight; and in 1403, the city established the first thoroughly equipped maritime quarantine station of which we have record on the island of Santa Maria di Nazareth.

Eager says that "One of the most ancient edicts commanding the segregation of sufferers from pestilential maladies had for its authors two laymen, Sagacio and Pietro da Gazata, and is found in the Chronicles of Reggio d'Emilia. The document, dated 1374 and written in Low Latin, orders that all persons sick with pest be taken outside the city, into the open country, a camp, or the woods, there to remain until dead or cured. The parish priests are required to promptly report all cases of pest under pain of death by fire. After registering these historical facts, the chronicler adds: 'And I saw in this same year that these orders were observed in Reggio, for which cause all were grieved and terrified more than by the fear of the illness which, when God permits, cannot be averted.' "

Diepgen tells us that a quarantine station was established at Ragusa in 1377. He adds, "In Ragusa all visitors who had come from pest-suspected localities were detained for one month outside the city for purification by the sun and wind. Anyone who associated with them was isolated; the personnel which cared for their nourishment was strictly supervised. Because thirty days did not seem to suffice, forty days were introduced." In commenting on general quarantine practices, he continues, "Houses are aired out for weeks and fumigated. Beds and other furniture are placed in the sun and cleaned with water; possessions of the pest-inflicted which have only a small value are burned. Domestic animals are controlled, the keeping of dogs, cats, birds, rabbits and pigs in the city boundaries is limited or prohibited. Meetings of great masses of people are prohibited. . . . The duty of reporting gains more and more general importance. These are all beginnings in a systematic combatting of epidemics which are elaborated further in the course of the modern age and are expanded to other infections, but to the principle itself nothing essential has been added even in the most modern state regulations for epidemics."

CHAPTER VII

FRACASTORIUS

"As for my studies, they are very various. I have written a good treatise on Contagion . . . and on Critical Days, which I ascribe, not to the moon but to our humors."—LETTER FROM FRACASTORIUS TO RANNUSIO

AFTER the initial catastrophe of 1348, plague continued to rage in Europe for more than three centuries. From the painstaking chronicle of Lersch, we may glean a few examples of the long and terrible experience. In 1359 and 1360, one-third of the population in certain regions are said to have died; in 1360 and 1361, many Polish towns lost half their inhabitants; in 1361 there were 500 deaths a day in Montpellier; between 1360 and 1364 Russia suffered severely; in 1370 there were 80,000 deaths in Lubeck; in the early 'eighties many cities suffered their fourth visitation of the disease; 16,000 deaths in Florence in 1418, and 50,000 in Paris; 40,000 deaths in Constance in 1438; 40,000 in Paris in 1450, and again in 1467; 30,000 in Venice in 1477-1478; 500 deaths a day in Brussels in 1502; 18,000 in Vienna in 1542.

Ambroise Paré, the great military surgeon of his day, ranking as a medical pioneer with such contemporary leaders as Vesalius, Paracelsus and Fracastorius, wrote an important treatise on plague, based on his own experience, in 1568, which forms the Twenty-Fourth Book of his collected works. He begins with a description of the disease as "coming of the wrath of God, furious, sudden, swift, monstrous, dreadful, contagious, terrible, called by Galen a wild beast, savage, and most cruel." "It comes not only of simple corruption, but also of contagion of the infected air, past all words, and past understanding." More pious than most medical writers of the time, he devotes an entire chapter to asseverating, with many scriptural quotations, that the plague is primarily an Act of God and a punishment for sin. The disease has also, however, "human or natural causes; the infection and corruption of the air" and "the vitiation of the humors of the body, so that they are predisposed to take the plague from the air." The corruption of the air is attributed in orthodox Hippocratic fashion to abnormal weather conditions, to emanations from the bodies of dead men and animals, to exhalations from stagnant waters or from the bowels of the earth. The putrefaction of plague is, however, a highly specific one, "different from all other putrefactions. It has the power, however, to transmute other corruptions into its own likeness"; so that all boils and putrid fevers, and other diseases that come of putrefaction, are apt in time of plague to acquire this especial and most mysterious malignancy.

On the danger of contagion, however, he is quite sound. "When the times are thus constituted, we must avoid all infected places, and all association with them that are stricken, lest we be infected by the vapor and exhalation of the corrupt air." He urges magistrates and public officers to keep houses and streets clean, to remove dead animals and filth of all sorts, to supervise water and food-supplies, and to close public hot baths (not to escape infection but to avoid opening the pores of the skin). Those who are sick must be isolated and provided with medical attendance; and quarantine must be established by towns not yet attacked. "And they must hang a cloth, or some such token, from the windows of houses where any are dead of the plague. And the surgeons, and all who have to do with the patients, must carry white staves in their hands when they go through the town, that men may keep away from them." He gives detailed directions on the duties of those chosen to attend plague patients "above all things, they must remember that they are called of God to this vocation for the exercise of surgery: therefore they should go to it with a high courage free of all fear, having firm faith that God both gives and takes away our lives as and when it pleases Him." They must, however, take many precautions:—build up vital resistance (by bleeding and purging, if necessary); washing their bodies frequently with a special aromatic composition; placing a sachet of some poison over the heart "to accustom the heart to the poison of the plague and to fortify it"; wearing special non-porous clothing; avoiding too close contact with the patients and keeping in the mouth a clove or a morsel of canella or angelica root or a juniper berry to ward off infection. The last chapter of Paré's treatise contains one of the most vivid accounts ever penned of the horrors of a plague epidemic and the moral deterioration and social dislocation produced thereby. During the epidemic at Lyons, he tells us that "if the physicians, surgeons, and barbers appointed to dress the patients, were but seen in the streets, everybody ran after them throwing stones to kill them like mad dogs, bidding them go by night only, lest they should infect them that were healthy."

Nor was plague, by any means, the only menace. In 1485, England was first visited by the strange and deadly "sweating-sickness," so that in many places one-third of the population died. In 1506 it returned and, in some communities, half the people died. A third epidemic occurred in 1516-1517 and a fourth in 1529. This time it spread over all of northern Europe; but according to Lersch, it was held to be not contagious! In 1551 there was the last great epidemic of this disease.

Influenza is recorded on many occasions. In 1410-1411 there were 100,000 cases in Paris. Another epidemic occurred in 1427, another in 1510, another in 1557-1558 and another in 1580—all, however, with very low mortality. Typhus fever was always present, but had particularly wide prevalence in the ninth decade of the fifteenth century. Smallpox, measles, diphtheria, cholera and dysentery at times assumed widespread epidemic proportions.

Many fourteenth and fifteenth century writers dwelt on the contagiousness of plague. Among these may be mentioned Jacopo da Forli, Michele Savonarola and Marsilio Ficino, who has been cited in a previous chapter. They do not, however, deserve the special credit given them by Eager, for, as we have seen, nearly all the earlier plague tractates set forth the same conclusion. Savonarola stresses well carriers and Benedetti, fomites. Quarantine practice continued apace along the lines laid down in the fourteenth century. A quarantine station was established at Genoa in 1467 and at Marseilles in 1526. Venice began the fumigating of letters and the washing with vinegar of money from infected regions in 1493.

The procedure of disinfection was, in general, governed by a very definite philosophy. The contagious element of disease was supposed to be absorbed by porous substances but did not adhere to smooth solid ones or to liquids. Thus, Nicola Massa, a Venetian physician, in 1556, considers wool, hair, cotton, linen, hemp, silk, thread and all things made from these substances; skins, feathers and the like; and all merchandise, as well as sacks, baskets, boxes, casks and cords to be dangerous fomites. On the other hand, metals and objects made of them, including arms and cooking utensils, precious stones and marble; grain, flour and meal; vegetables, fruit (fresh and dried) and nuts, wine, oil and vinegar; and all drugs and aromatics, were non-infectible.

Eager has unearthed a number of interesting legal records of quarantine procedures of the time. As an example of land quarantine he

quotes instructions issued in Naples in 1557. "Citizens, usually mer-
chants, were stationed at the gates of the city to examine bulletins
of health. Corruption and lack of diligence on the part of these
persons were punishable by death. Sentinels, some on foot and some
on horseback, made a patrol about the city walls to prevent clan-
destine entrance. Bills of health to be acceptable had to be stamped
with the seal of the university of the place from which the traveler
came. They gave not only the day but the hour of departure, together
with a description of the traveler. Sanitary bulletins were also issued
to accompany merchandise, but in times of severe pest all articles
except aromatics and medicaments were considered suspicious."

Maritime quarantine in the sixteenth century is illustrated by the
precautions taken with regard to a Catalan ship arriving at Palermo
from Barcelona. "This vessel had 97 persons aboard, 18 of them passengers. Three seamen and two passengers had died of a disease suspected of being pest. The deaths occurred while the vessel was taking on
cargo in the harbor where she lay at anchor. The cargo consisted of barrels of salted fish, cases of sugar (destined for Palermo, and already dis-
embarked and in store), salted cheese, salt in bulk, a quantity of sumac,
and merchandise, including many bales of cloth from Barcelona, a port
not under suspicion. The master of the vessel was at once required to
give 20,000 scudi security not to leave the harbor until given pra-
tique. To make assurance doubly sure, the rudder was taken away
from the ship and a watch set. All persons, except the sick and a
sufficient number of seamen to guard the ship, were sent ashore to
a place known as the Borgo, where all garments were taken from
them, and they themselves exposed to the fumes of boiling pitch
and afterwards washed with vinegar. Some of the clothing was
burned and some washed, aired, and perfumed for fifty days. The
sick were sent to a lazaretto, the Cuba, a huge stone building which
still stands at Palermo as a monument of early quarantine.

"The treatment given the cargo was as follows: Barrels of salted
fish, washed outside, first with sea water and then with vinegar;
cases of sugar, salted cheese and sumac, coverings removed and
burned and the commodities without further treatment delivered to
the owners; salt, no treatment, not being considered infectible; merchandise, aired and perfumed ashore for fifty days, and the cloth
unrolled and hung from the rigging of the ship for fifty days.
The sails and cordage of the ship were taken down, submerged in

the sea for a week, and then hung from the masts, yards, and booms in the air, sun and dew, by day and night, as long as the ship remained in quarantine. Fumigation was made in the interior of the ship by boiling pitch in caldrons between decks. Fifty days were set as the period of detention, instead of forty, because the season was winter."

Finally—since all these details are so significant of the epidemiological thinking of the time—we may quote one more extract from Eager, this time describing isolation procedures pursued within a city during the course of an epidemic. The passage is from a treatise by Alessandro Massarina who was in charge of sanitary measures at Vicenza in 1577. "The first death was attributed to garments clandestinely introduced from Padua, where plague prevailed. After a necropsy establishing the diagnosis the furniture in the house was burned and every exposed person stripped, given new clothes, and removed outside the city. The house was purified by aromatic fumigations and painted with milk of lime. All infected vestments and bedding received a treatment with strong lye. The disease, however, spread, and in one year the city, with a population of 30,000, suffered 1,908 deaths from plague. As soon as the epidemic established itself the city was divided into thirty-two sections and a daily house-to-house inspection made by sixty-four trustworthy citizens, two to each precinct. All cases of sickness were reported to one of four public physicians. These physicians served for periods of fourteen days. Infected habitations received the same treatment as in the initial case, except that the furniture was not burned in all instances, but washed instead with lye and left in the sun and open air for thirty days. All garments were put in running water for two days. Persons exposed or under suspicion went to the Campo di Marte, outside the city walls, where wooden houses had been built. A river separated the isolation camp from the lazaretto, where the sick were lodged and where physicians and nurses were in attendance. Suspects developing plague in the isolation camp were taken across the river to the lazaretto, and convalescents from the latter place were transferred to the former. Those who kept well in the Campo di Marte for twenty-two days returned to their disinfected homes in the city, there to remain under observation for an additional twenty-two days. Convalescents from the lazaretto passed twenty-two days in the isolation camp, and were afterwards confined to their houses in the city for another twenty-two days. At the height of the epidemic all the houses in the city were closed for forty days, and none but the guards were allowed in the streets. At this time 5,000 persons were fed from public funds, and there were about 400 persons in the lazaretto and 500 on the Campo di Marte."

Through the courtesy of Dr. John F. Fulton I have recently had the opportunity of studying a pamphlet entitled "Certain Necessary Directions, as well for the Cure of the Plague, as for preventing the Infection, etc." published by Robert Barker, in London in 1636. This collection of documents, intended for the information of magistrates and prepared at the command of King Charles I under date of April 22, 1636, gives an excellent picture of seventeenth century administrative procedure; and, though dating from a later period, may be cited as a continuation of plague quarantine practice. It includes, first of all, a circular prepared by the College of Physicians which emphasizes the following major points: the appointment of doctors, apothecaries and chirurgeons for the special care of plague patients; the quarantine of persons and goods coming from infected places; the strict control of corrupt flesh or fish, or nuisances and of domestic animals; the isolation of the sick and the closing of infected houses for forty days; the control of spread to other areas by regulation of flight of inhabitants from an infected town; "the correcting of the infectious aire" by building fires in the streets and shooting off cannon and by burning fumigants in houses and by the individual use of perfumes; the building up of resistance by adequate diet and tonics and by purging and bleeding. Many drugs are listed for general and local treatment of cases of the disease. This report of the College of Physicians is followed by a reprinting of Orders in Council issued in 1603. These orders provide for a formal conference of the justices of any county in which plague occurs for the development of an organized plan for the control of the epidemic and the care of the sick, and for the raising of the monies needed for these purposes. All the essentials outlined by the College of Physicians are provided for. In the field of quarantine, infected houses (in closely settled areas) must be closed for six weeks after the cessation of sickness. In rural areas where the inhabitants must come out to care for their cattle, they are required to "weare some mark in their uppermost garments, or beare white rods in their hands" as a warning. Watchmen shall be appointed to see that the regulations are carried out and other persons to deliver necessary supplies to the quarantined houses, and these persons must themselves bear a characteristic mark or carry a white rod. Ministers, curates and churchwardens must report cases of disease in their parishes. Clothes, bedding, and other materials used by the infected must be burned or aired by a locally approved method. A most interesting provision runs as follows: "If there be any person Ecclesiastical or Lay, that shall hold and publish any opinions (as in some places report is made) that it is a vain thing to forbeare to resort to the Infected, or that it is not charitable to forbid the same, pretending that no person shall die but at their time prefixed, such persons shall be not onely reprehended, but by order of the Bishop if they be Ecclesiastical shall be forbidden to preach, and being Lay, shall be also enjoyned to forbeare to utter such dangerous opinions upon pain of imprisonment."

There follows a typical set of local orders issued by the Lord Mayor and Aldermen for the execution of these procedures in London. Next, a Royal Proclamation "for quickning the Lawes made for the reliefe of the poore, and the suppressing punishing and setling of the sturdy Rogues and Vagabonds," who may play a part in the spreading of contagion. Elizabethan laws "for the reliefe of the poore," "for the necessary reliefe of Souldiers and Mariners," and "for punishment of Rogues, Vagabonds and Sturdy Beggers," with a Jacobean annex to the latter, in view of the possible bearing of this legislation on relief and police problems arising in connection with plague control, are cited. Next, we have a Jacobean Act specially framed "for the charitable reliefe and ordering of persons infected with the Plague." This provides for county assistance to local areas unable to meet the costs involved and prescribes heavy penalties for those who defy quarantine regulations. Finally, the volume closes with the records of two Star Chamber proceedings dealing with the control of insanitary tenements which are of the greatest interest from the standpoint of the housing movement. Truly, a remarkably complete compendium of information for the health administrator of 1636!

The sanitary practices of this period were still mainly directed against plague; but, at the close of the fifteenth century, a new pestilence had already served as the third of the great teachers in the field of epidemiology. This was syphilis, a malady which—on account of its chronic character—finds little place in the standard histories of epidemics, but which must have wrought more damage than any one of them, except the plague itself.

The prevailing concept of the time was that this disease was quite new to Europe, and was introduced from the New World by the sailors of Columbus on their return from the fateful voyage of 1492. This view was attacked by Sudhoff on the ground of the prior existence in Europe of maladies resembling syphilis which were treated by the use of mercurials. In recent years, however, the older view has received new support. There has been rediscovered a lost work by the Spanish physician, de Isla, in which he describes the treatment for syphilis of several members of Columbus's crew on their return from Haiti in 1493; and, most important of all, skulls and long bones have been found in pre-Columbian graves of American aborigines bearing apparent evidence of syphilitic infection. The view of an origin in Asia or in southern or eastern Europe is still maintained by certain competent authorities; but, to the writer, the case for a Columbian source seems still the stronger.

Whether syphilis was actually introduced from the New World in 1493 or not, it is certain that toward the end of the fifteenth century it began to spread throughout the continent of Europe as an epidemic of tremendous deadliness. First generally noted by historians among the Spanish troops sent by Ferdinand and Isabella to the aid of Alphonso of Naples, it quickly spread to the troops of Charles VIII of France when they occupied Naples in 1495. The disease was apparently already present in Spain and in France (where one of Columbus's ships had touched); but the mercenaries from many nations who made up the French army played an important role in the spread of the disease. It reached Germany and Switzerland in 1495, Holland and England in 1496, and Vasco da Gama is supposed to have carried the infection round the Cape in 1497 causing an outbreak in India in 1498 which in turn spread eastward, reaching Canton in 1505. As is usual in pandemics, each nation cast the blame on the preceding victim. To Turks, syphilis was the disease of the Christians, to the English it was the French Pox, to the French the Neapolitan disease, to the Italians the Spanish disease. At least eleven printed documents referring to syphilis are extant for the two years 1495 and 1496, while no earlier references are known which can certainly be associated with it. In the words of J. Johnston Abraham: "As the disease was new to Europe, it fell upon nations totally unprepared. There was no acquired immunity, and it raged therefore with a ferocity now seldom seen. Frequently the victims were prostrated with acute fever, severe headache, intense osteoscopic pains and delirium. Death was not an uncommon sequela."

It was a tremendously vivid and vital world which the new plague was attacking—a world enormously different from that which the Black Death had assailed in 1348. This was the day of Ferdinand and Isabella and of Cesare Borgia. In 1498 Savonarola preached his last sermon in Florence, and Machiavelli was sent by the signory on his mission to Caterina Sforza—that hard-bitten countess who, when rebels besieging her castle held her children captive and threatened to slaughter them, defied the besiegers to do their worst with that gorgeous phrase, "I can make more children," so typical of the essential spirit of the Italian Renaissance. The paintings of Raphael and the sculptures of Michelangelo were delighting the eye of the artist and the first half-century's output of the printing press was intoxicating the imagination of the scholar. Leonardo was experimenting with his flying machine and prophesying that "The human bird shall take his first flight, filling the world with amazement, all writings with his fame, and bringing glory to the nest whence he sprang."

In medicine, too, the spirit of the Renaissance was at work; and the menace of syphilis challenged the powers of some of the ablest minds of any age. A dozen medical tracts on the subject appeared between 1497 and 1501 of which that of Leonicenus was an outstanding example. The general symptoms of the disease and its relation to venery were clearly recognized (Leonicenus called it "the love disease"). The treatment by the use of mercury suggested by the Arabian practice of treating other skin diseases with mercurial ointments, was introduced in 1496.

In the sixteenth century there were two great leaders in medicine, whose names remain supremely illustrious today—Fracastorius and Paracelsus; and both made their important contributions to syphilology. Paracelsus (1493-1541) spent his life in traveling from one end of Europe to the other, attacking his predecessors and quarreling with his contemporaries—the first medical teacher who dared to lecture in the vernacular and to challenge the sacred Galenical theories of ancient medicine. Paracelsus was sometimes a mystic and sometimes an empiricist—always a wanderer and a rebel. As a mystic he belonged to the Middle Ages, but as an empiricist he was of the Renaissance. He hoped to free medicine from its worst errors "not by following that which those of old taught, but by our own observation of nature, confirmed by extensive practice and long experience. . . . If I want to prove anything, I shall not try to do it by quoting authorities, but by experiment and by reasoning thereon."

Both his experiments and his mysticism led Paracelsus to lay great stress upon the pharmacological value of the metallic salts, particularly those of lead, mercury, iron, antimony, copper and sulphur and, in particular, he wrote several influential tracts defending the mercurial treat-ment of syphilis. In the field of epidemiological theory, the contributions of Paracelsus were not of major significance. In one passage, he distinguishes four kinds of plague, due, respectively, to earth, air, fire and water (in the historic tradition exemplified by the hot and cold plagues of Jehan Jacme). In another place he lists five causes of disease (*entia*): cosmic agencies (*ens astrorum*); pathologic poisons (*ens venene*), including auto-intoxications and contagia; natural causes (*ens naturale*) or predisposition to disease from organic defects; psychic causes (*ens spirituale*) and divine intervention (*ens deale*). This is a highly suggestive general etiology; but not practically helpful with regard to the cause of epidemic disease.

On the whole, the mystic in Paracelsus dominated the scientist. Yet with all his faults he rendered a great service to European thought as an iconoclast. No medical writer did more to break the shackles of classical dogma; but it was perhaps fortunate that the vagaries of his psychopathic personality prevented him from imposing his own metaphysics in place of the theories which he did so much to overthrow.

There could be no more striking contrast than that between this stormy iconoclast from north of the Alps and the orderly scholar and polished humanist, Fracastorius. With him, too, we pass from the world of legendary names associated with scattered literary fragments to a human being with known history and clearly envisaged personality.

Hieronymus Fracastorius (in the Latin form, used in his medical works—often called Fracastoro in Italian, Fracastor in English or French) was born at Verona in 1478 (not 1483 as often stated in older books of reference). He studied at Padua, where he was a contemporary of Copernicus and Erasmus and an intimate of Girolamo della Torre, professor of medicine, and his three sons. In 1500 he married and in 1501 was appointed lecturer in logic at the University. In 1508 he was driven out by the German invasion (under the auspices of the League of Cambrai) and took refuge, first in Verona and later in his villa at Incaffi on the Lake of Garda. In 1516 he returned to Verona where he lived and practiced for some twenty years. In 1530, he published his poem on syphilis and by 1534 he had retired from the active practice of medicine and devoted himself to his literary labors. In 1538 he published an important astronomical treatise, *Homocentrica*, and in 1546 came his greatest work, on *Contagion*. Throughout most of his life he was closely associated with the ecclesiastical leaders of Italy and enjoyed the patronage of Gilberti, Bishop of Verona, of Cardinal Bembo, Cardinal Farnese, and of Pope Paul III. He made his one appearance on the stage of world history in 1547 when—as one of the two official physicians to the Council of Trent—he certified to the presence of an epidemic of typhus fever in the city and caused the transfer of the Council to Bologna. This was a change greatly desired by Pope Paul and the position taken by Fracastorius was criticized by the adherents of Emperor Charles V as vehemently as it was praised by the Papal party. Six years later, in 1553, Fracastorius died in his villa at Incaffi, from cerebral apoplexy.

Fracastorius is described by the editor of his collected works (1555) as "of short stature, but stockily built; his shoulders were broad and he wore a becoming and well-groomed beard; his long black hair framed a round face, his eyes were brown." A number of contemporary pictures exist which reveal a fine high brow, a straight aquiline nose, a rather cold, stern eye and the "well-groomed beard"—the very essence of a serious, dignified, taciturn scholar.

Besides the three major works mentioned above, Fracastorius wrote a number of other treatises, on the temperature of wines, on the rise of the Nile, on critical days, on sympathies and antipathies, on poetry, on the mind and on the soul. He was astronomer, geographer, botanist and mathematician, as well as physician and philosopher. He understood the true nature of sedimentary rocks, anticipated the principle of Mercator's projection, and described a primitive telescope.

The poem on syphilis was an enormous literary success. Cardinal Bembo called its author the equal of Lucretius and Virgil, which was clearly extravagant; but when at his death he was commonly described as "the Virgil of his time" his admirers were not perhaps far from the truth. Competent humanists now consider him at least the equal of any of his contemporary poets. A monument was erected to him in the

Piazza dei Signori in Verona and a bronze medallion on the Porta San Benedetto in Padua.

From our standpoint, only the works on syphilis and on contagion need be considered. The first of these was not only a chef-d'oeuvre of Renaissance Latin but easily the most important of sixteenth century contributions to medical knowledge in this field. The poem is in three books. The first deals with the origin of the disease and must be reviewed in some detail. The second discusses treatment, emphasizing the use of mercury. These two books were completed in 1525 and sent to Cardinal Bembo, to whom the work was to be dedicated. The Cardinal urged the omission of certain passages from Book II dealing with mercury and the inclusion of a discussion of the new drug, guaiac, then coming into use. The use of excessive doses of mercury had brought this remedy into disrepute. Fracastorius could not bring himself to any elisions in Book II but he did add (before publication in 1530) a Third Book singing the praises of guaiac, in which the Shepherd, Syphilus, from whose name that of the poem and the disease was derived, enters the picture. It is of interest to note that guaiacum was not removed from the British Pharmacopeia until 1932.

The two vitally important points in an understanding of the etiology of syphilis were a recognition of the specific identity of the disease and of the ways in which contagion spread from one person to another. Both these points were clearly understood by most medical authorities in the first half of the sixteenth century. Fernel (1506-1588) in his treatise on *Medicine* in 1554 treats gonorrhea and syphilis as distinct diseases. Yet even in Fracastorius's lifetime, the contrary view was espoused by Paracelsus and later was adopted by Paré and Sydenham. Over two hundred years later the great John Hunter (1728-1793) in his *Textbook on the Venereal Disease* (1786) denied the existence of hereditary syphilis and the possibility of extragenital infection (in the course of nature). Furthermore, in order to prove that syphilis was the same disease as gonorrhea he inoculated himself with pus from a gonorrheal case and (presumably dealing with a mixed infection) succeeded in infecting himself with syphilis. In the early nineteenth century, a still more tragic episode occurred in Paris where F. J. V. Broussais (1772-1838) denied the existence of a syphilitic virus, and an unfortunate pupil inoculated himself in the arm with the discharge from a syphilitic sore and when generalized syphilis resulted committed suicide. Clearly, in three hundred years, retrogression rather than progress had marked the attitude of medicine toward the basic facts of etiology. From Fernel down, many writers had made correct surmises, but real proof— such as must have convinced leaders like Hunter and Broussais—was clearly lacking. It was not till 1838 that Philippe Ricord (1799-1889) in his treatise on venereal infections finally established the separate identity of gonorrhea and syphilis and gave the fundamental classification of the latter disease in its primary, secondary and tertiary stages.

In the early years of the sixteenth century, however, the extreme severity of epidemic syphilis made its individuality very clear. As to its mode of transmission, however, it is a curious fact that nowhere in Fracastorius's poem is there clear recognition of its relation to sexual intercourse except perhaps one phrase in Book II which runs as follows: "Above all things fly from desire and the soft embraces of love, for nothing is more harmful than these; fair Venus herself, and tender maidens likewise, abhor this pestilence." Yet even this reference is in the form of counsel to the infected, not as a means of prophylaxis.

On the whole, the *Syphilis* poem does not add significantly to epidemiological theory, giving us little more than a poetical version of the same theories advanced by medical writers from Avicenna down through the period of the plague tracts. It is true that Fracastorius refers to syphilis as a "contagion"; but so do earlier writers refer to the plague. It is true also that he describes the causative agents as "*semina*," a word which Wynne-Finch translates sometimes as "seeds" and once as "germs." Indeed the very first line of the poem sets forth as its aim the elucidation of the question, "What various chances in Life, what seeds conveyed this strange disease." Yet, as we have seen in earlier chapters, the same word was used by classical writers without any conception of a *contagium animatum*; and it will be pointed out in a later paragraph that it is quite improbable that Fracastorius employed it in any modern sense.

Indeed near the beginning of Book I he gives us a magnificent description of the process of contagion, as we now understand it, only to discard it in favor of the traditional miasmatic-astrological theories. He says,

"What causes after so many ages brought forth for us this unaccustomed disease? Was it borne by the Western Sea, and so came to our world at the time when a chosen band set sail from the shores of Spain, and dared to attack the foam and the unknown waters of the wandering ocean and search out lands lying in a new world? For there, they say, that sickness held sway with everlasting ruin through all the cities, and wandered hither and thither by endless fault of heaven, sparing but few. Must we then think that by means of traffic this contagion was carried to reach us—a contagion which, small in the beginning, but soon gaining strength and matter to feed on by degrees, spread itself throughout all lands? Just as oftentimes when by chance a spark from a torch which a shepherd has carelessly left in the cornfield falls among the stubble, it is small indeed at first, and moves with lingering pace. But before long, increasing little by little as it goes, it raises itself aloft and lays waste the conquered fields, the harvest and the neighbouring woods, its flames surging up to the sky. Then Jove's wood where none can walk crackles and thunders afar, and the wide heavens around and the plains give back the glow."

This view, however, he then rejects; and for the same reasons which proved a stumbling-block in the way of acceptance of a complete theory of contagion for three centuries to come. First, the occurrence of the disease in persons not known to have been exposed: "For certainly it is not fair to deem that the disease is foreign to us and borne across the ocean; since in the first place, we can show many who of their own accord, without contact with any other, have contracted this same malady." Second, the rapid spread of the epidemic: "Besides, a single contagion would not have been able to reach so many lands at once in so short a time." Therefore, "Since these things be so, doubtless this pestilence has a more deep-seated beginning; its course, unless I am mistaken, is more mysterious and grave, its origin more profound."

It seems clear that Fracastorius is not denying the immediate fact of contagion, which he was to develop so brilliantly in his later book. Like the authors of the plague tractates, he was seeking for some underlying cause, imminent throughout a wide area at a given time; and, like them, he could find such a cause only in the atmosphere. "And when you consider that the seeds of so great a disease cannot lie either in the bosom of the earth or in the sea you are bound to decide after deliberation that the source and seat of the evil must exist in the air itself; the air which is diffused round all the earth, which insinuates itself everywhere throughout our bodies, and has continually inflicted this plague on the race of living beings. The air, indeed, is the Father of all things and the Author of their being. Often, too, it brings grievous maladies to mortals; born in many ways, it starts corruption in the tender body, easily receiving the taint and passing it on."

The cause of this corruption of the circumambient air is astrological. Just as the summer sun produces the heat of summer, and as the moon controls the tides, just as a conjunction of Mars and Saturn caused the Great Plague of two centuries before, so has a similar conjunction produced the plague of syphilis.

The exact process involved is obscure. "Was it that, when so many stars came into conjunction with the blazing sun, the fiery energy drew many vapors from sea and land; and that these, mingled with thin air and seized by the new taint, conveyed a corruption too fine to be seen? Or did some other thing sent down from the upper air infect far and wide the realms of the sky?" Of one thing, however, Fracastorius is certain—the specificity of the corruptions engendered by particular astrological and atmospheric conditions. Sometimes the corruption produced affected plants only, sometimes goats, sometimes men; "and although grapes are softer than apples, one does not infect the other; but grape taints grape." The infection of syphilis had probably been produced before and would be produced again; but it was a perfectly distinct entity. Here, at least, Fracastorius was in advance of the vague pythogenic theories of the nineteenth century.

It was *Syphilis* which made the European reputation of Fracastorius in the sixteenth century, and it is by the chance that his name for the disease was accepted that he is chiefly known in medicine today. The essay on *Contagion*, published twenty-one years after the completion of the first two books of *Syphilis* is, however, his real title to enduring fame. From a scientific standpoint, it is an infinitely greater achievement.

The full title of this work in the admirable English translation by Mrs. Wilmer Cave Wright is "Contagion and Contagious Diseases and Their Treatment"; and it is from this volume by Mrs. Wright that quotations are made in succeeding pages. In the introductory dedication to Cardinal Alexander Farnese the author sets himself a difficult and challenging task. He is unsatisfied with the vague conclusion of earlier writers that contagious diseases were due to certain "occult properties." "None of these authorities," he continues, "attempted to say: what is in general the nature of contagions; by what principle they infect; how they are generated; why some of them leave fomes, and some propagate themselves even from a distance; why some diseases are contagious, though they are milder and more gentle, while others, though much more acute and more virulent, are not at all contagious; how contagion differs from poisons; and many other questions of the same sort."

This task Fracastorius approaches in a spirit of practical empiricism which was rare and refreshing in a day when men devoted so large a part of their energies to debate about ultimate and essential metaphysical principles. He says, "Now there are three classes of causes; those that are very general and very remote from things; those that are nearer and more special; and finally those that are very near and very special. In obscure and difficult matters, to arrive at the special and nearest causes is surely the affair of God or of the divine; to rest content with the most general causes is a sign of a lazy and boorish mind; but to investigate the intermediate causes, and to try to arrive at the special, so far as a human being may, is surely the task of a philosopher." Here is the true humility and the real opportunity of science.

Book I of the treatise deals with contagion and Chapter I gives a tentative definition of the subject to be considered. Contagion, the author says, is "a certain precisely similar corruption which develops in the substance of a combination, passes from one thing to another, and is originally caused by infection of the imperceptible particles." We note that the infection in this case must be "precisely similar in both the carrier and receiver of the contagion"; reproducible specificity is the test. Further, the contagion affects the "imperceptible particles," not the object as a whole, as fire would do.

Chapter II gives Fracastorius's fundamental classification of three different types of contagion—those which infect by direct contact only, those which may also spread by fomes, and those which may infect at a distance. Those spread at a distance may also be carried by fomes and those spread by fomes are also transferred by direct contact. Our sixteenth century authority was too clear-headed to hold the idea current in the nineteenth century that such a disease as typhoid fever could be "infectious" but not "contagious."

Chapter III treats of the spread by contact only and illustrates the phenomenon by analogy with "that which occurs in fruits, as when grape infects grape, or apple infects apple." He analyzes this phenomenon in terms of the classical theory of four properties (hot, cold, moist, dry) and concludes that, in such a case, "hot, moist particles—moist either independently or in combination—that evaporate from the first fruit, are the principle and germ of the putrefaction that occurs in the second fruit." The imperceptible particles concerned, Fracastorius calls germs (*seminaria* or "seedbeds") of contagion, a somewhat stronger term than the famous allusion of Lucretius to "*semina*" which "fly about bringing disease and death."

Garrison, in commenting on this work, says that Fracastorius "seems by some remarkable power of divination or clairvoyance, to have seen morbid processes in terms of bacteriology more than a hundred years before Kircher, Leeuwenhoek and the other men who worked with magnifying glass or microscope. . . . Thus Fracastorius seems to have had a clear notion (or prevision) of the causation of disease by micro-organisms, and he appears to have seen these organisms as made up of those gelatinous or 'dispersed' systems which modern physical chemists call colloidal states of substance."

I yield to none in admiration of Fracastorius; but this is to read into his treatise results of modern science of which he had no conception. When Fracastorius used the word "germs" (*seminaria*) there is the clearest evidence from the text that he had no conception whatever of a living micro-organism. The word, which Wright translates sometimes as "germ" and sometimes as "seed" meant what the latter translation means to us, or what the word "germ" means to us when we speak of the "germ of an idea." It is made clear throughout the text that the concept involved is a chemical, not a biological one—exactly the concept we employ when we speak of bacteriophagy as "transmissible lysis." It is precisely the glory of Fracastorius that, by close observation and clear thinking, he worked out a clear and essentially accurate analysis of the way in which living "germs" operate, without ever suspecting that they were living.

In Chapter IV, our author considers the second class of contagions, those which infect by fomes as well as direct contact. The essential difference (manifest, as we know today, by the contrast between measles and smallpox on the one hand and typhoid and cholera on the other) is the power of the "germ" to persist for a longer period in the environment. Fracastorius maintains that he has seen phthisis and plague thus persist in fomes for two or three years. He illustrates this phenomenon aptly by the persistence of odors in clothes, or of soot on a smoky wall. The power to spread by fomes is attributed to the ability of these particular kinds of germs to penetrate porous substances (associated with fineness and volatility) and to their capacity for survival (associated with viscosity). Hence, the importance of porosity in determining medieval disinfection practices. "It follows," he says, "that iron, stone and bodies of that sort which are cold and not porous, are not adapted to become fomes whereas wool, rags, and many kinds of wood are well-adapted."

Chapter v opens the subject of contagions which may also be transmitted at a distance. "There is a kind of ophthalmia with which the sufferer infects everyone who looks at him." Furthermore pestiferous fevers, phthisis, and indeed "the majority of the diseases we are investigating," fall in this class, infecting those who live with the sufferer without actual contact. This mode of transmission is compared to the action of gaseous poisons and with the power of "the animal called catablepha" (a sort of basilisk which could kill by its glance at a distance of a mile).

Several chapters are devoted to analysis of this sort of action in a way which indicates that the author was a little worried, subconsciously, about the phenomena involved. In Chapter vi he makes it clear that no "occult" properties can be in question, on account of the specificity of the effects involved. In Chapter vii, he illustrates the process by running of the eyes caused by the smell of onions or garlic and sneezing induced by pepper (with other less happy examples); and he compares the spread of contagion to the diffusion of smoke through a room. The ability of the "germs" to survive exposure to the air, in the course of such a process, is due to their highly viscous nature. They cannot, however, "endure violent alteration. Hence the germs of all contagions are consumed by fire, and are broken up by very cold water also."

An interesting discussion follows as to the method by which the seeds of infection penetrate the body. This may be by passage through the breath and blood-vessels or by a process similar to evaporation. But "One method of penetration is by propagation and, so to speak, progeny. For the original germs which have adhered to the neighboring humors with which they are analogous, generate and propagate other germs precisely like themselves, and these in turn propagate others, until the whole mass and bulk of humors is infected by them." This passage is highly suggestive but the alternative process of evaporation and the introduction of the phrase "so to speak" make it apparent that Fracastorius is thinking in terms of something like what we call transmissible lysis and not in terms of living organisms. The final conclusion of this chapter is that contagions transmitted at a distance differ from others only in the more viscous and more resistant nature of their particles.

Chapter viii emphasizes the highly important concept of the specificity of contagions, some affecting trees and crops, some certain animal species, some children, some women, some old men—as a result of analogy between the infecting agent and the infected object.

In Chapter IX, Fracastorius discusses the question whether every contagion is a kind of putrefaction and concludes that such is the case. Putrefactions are of various sorts and need not be always characterized by foul odors. If they are simple and merely characterized by evaporation of moisture and release of innate heat you have ordinary putrefactive decomposition. In other putrefactions, however, there "occurs simultaneously some generation, whether of some animal form or of something else which has a single and definite form" (such as vinegar). But, "all contagions consist in some form of putrefaction." In diseases not spread by direct contact only, contagion may be defined as "a precisely similar putrefaction which passes from one thing to another; its germs have great activity; they are made up of a strong and viscous combination; and they have not only a material but also a spiritual antipathy to the animal organism."

Chapter x deals with the question why some diseases are contagious while others—though more inflammatory and dangerous—are not; and concludes that the power of contagion is due to the more moist and viscous quality of the particles, in the former case. Chapter XI analyzes the difference between contagions and poisons and explains that the latter do not reproduce themselves (one person who has been poisoned does not poison another) because their particles are hot and dry.

Chapter XII is of special importance for our discussion since it deals with the origin of the seeds of contagion. These seeds may "arise originally in ourselves, not only in the case of scabies, achores and phthisis, but also in the case of fevers that are called pestiferous," as a result of "obstructions, plethora and malignity of the humors"; once so generated they may—in a second person—"propagate and engender what is similar to themselves."

The "principles and germs of contagion" may also, however, arise in the external world. "For we often observe them roving about and affecting many people, and one calls them Epidemics. Of these some are common to many communities or districts, but are not contagious and are merely called 'common.'[1] But others again are contagious, that is when once they are engendered in an individual, without any general disposition of the atmosphere, they transfer the contagion to another, and these are called not merely 'common,' but contagious as well. Of this sort are

---

[1] Later known as "endemic."

pestilences such as that plague about which Thucydides writes, which roved all over Greece, and like those which in our time have appeared in Italy and are called by some *'lenticulae'* and by others *'puncticulae.'* "[2]

Of those contagions which thus come from without "the air is the most potent cause, though they may also come from water, marshes and other sources."

Fracastorius next proceeds to an analysis of the role of the heavenly bodies in relation to epidemics. He accepts the fact that "astrologers often predict that certain diseases and epidemics will arise; for example, it is well known that they predicted syphilis (or the French Sickness, as it is called) long before it had made its appearance." He concludes, however, that "Certainly, since nothing that touches us very nearly can be sent down to earth from the sky, unless it be something spiritual like 'luminousness,' or something else of the same sort, if we look back to what was said above about the activities of spiritual things, we shall see that no contagions *per se* can be produced by the sky; but there is no reason why certain contagions should not be produced by it, by accident,[3] and they might even be predicted by astrologers. For since they know the phenomena most frequently produced by the heavenly bodies *per se*, they can also foresee what phenomena are most frequently connected with them, by accident. Now the heavenly bodies may of themselves become heated, and this increase of heat results in the rise of a great mass of vapors from the waters and the earth; these vapors presently may produce various and diverse kinds of corruption, some new, some familiar to us, some unusually severe, according to the different constitutions of these heavenly bodies. Astrologers and learned men observe these conditions, and can foretell the effects that they usually produce. Now these effects, though they occur by accident, under the influence of the stars, are nevertheless very often accompanied by the phenomena that occur *per se*; and there is no reason why certain phenomena should not arise from the heavenly bodies by accident, and that very often."

In this chapter, too, the question is raised "whether we can immunize ourselves against pestilences as one can against poisons," a question to be considered in Book III.

Finally, Chapter XIII of Book I discusses the "signs" of contagion

---

[2] Typhus.

[3] It is of course obvious that "accident" is used to mean a secondary indirect result, not a chance happening (as in our common speech).

which we have discussed in connection with the early plague tracts. These do not warrant definite prognostications, but are merely "signs of probability." Conjunctions of the planets, excessive dampness, great heat, falling stars, comets, earthquakes, etc. "indicate that putrefaction is occurring around the earth" and that there are present vapors of an "unctuous and viscous kind." South winds, abnormal mists, a dust-laden atmosphere, are similar indications, as are the breeding of vast numbers of insects, particularly locusts, or the presence of corpses of men slain in battle. "One should not only fear, but flee, when objects placed in the open air, such as provisions, linen and the like, contract a kind of decay and mildew."

The last two books of *Contagion*—though they contain many acute clinical observations—may for our present purposes, be passed over very briefly, citing only those incidental passages which further illuminate Fracastorius's theories of contagion.

Book II deals with the characteristics of the specific fevers recognized by the author. The poxes and measles are first discussed, and it is of interest to note that both are considered universal and benign. Apparently, alastrim must have been the prevailing form of smallpox in that day. Exposure and record of previous attack are listed among the questions to be considered in making a diagnosis.

Chapters III, IV and V discuss the pestilent fevers as some length. Fracastorius develops a long but courteous argument against the views of Galen and of Montanus, his own distinguished contemporary, as to the essential nature of these diseases. He says that "countless persons who are perfectly healthy and whose humors have suffered no depravity, nevertheless catch that contagion from merely associating with the plague-stricken or from his clothes." Therefore, the peculiar character of such fevers is not related to the humors affected but primarily to the specific nature of the diseases. "The principles of contagions *per se* are the germs themselves."

Pestilent fevers may be of external origin, due to germs arising in the air or the earth. "I say germs, not simple vapors for, as I have said above, there is a great difference between germs and vapors." Or, on the other hand, the germs may be produced within the body by internal putrefaction. In any case, their contagiousness "is the most important indication."

In Chapter V he discusses the English sweating sickness. "It is not only contagious from one person to another; it also roves from one town to another, and has been observed to travel not only through the island of Britain, which is almost the only place where it ever appears, but also to her neighbor, Belgium." The special predilection of this disease for Britain is attributed to some local quality of the air.

Chapter VI deals with typhus, a disease in which contagion spreads only by direct contact. In 1528, there was an epidemic due to general corruption of the atmosphere; but the disease had become sporadic due to the fact that the germs have become less keen and strong.

Chapter IX on contagious phthisis again emphasizes the two forms of the disease, one arising within the body and the other contagious. "For it may happen that a man who has never suffered from catarrh, who has no ruptured blood-vessels, has never been afflicted with an ulcer in the chest, never had pleurisy, in short has never had serious illness, but is in excellent health, nevertheless contracts the disease either from association with or living with a sufferer from phthisis, or from fomes; for it is really astonishing with what tenacity and for how long a time that virus is preserved in fomes. In fact it has often been observed that the clothes which a phthisical person has worn have conveyed the contagion even after the lapse of two years. Furthermore, the rooms, beds, and floors where a sufferer from phthisis has died, also become fomes. We must therefore conclude that in that sort of fomes are left behind the very germs of contagion that evaporate from the putrefaction produced in phthisis." This chapter also contains interesting original observations of Fracastorius on lung pathology; and some reference to hereditary predisposition.

In Chapter X, on rabies, the mode of infection and the prolonged incubation period are well described.

Chapters XI and XII deal with syphilis. Here, Fracastorius clearly recognizes the venereal nature of the disease; but also insists that it may arise spontaneously within the body, or be transmitted to infants in mother's milk or, rarely, by fomes. "In certain individuals it would arise without any contagion having been contracted from another person; in other cases, and these were the majority, it was contracted by contagion, but not from every kind of contact, nor readily, but only when two bodies in close contact with each other become extremely heated. Now this happened in sexual intercourse especially, and it was by that means that the great majority of persons were infected." He still maintains, as in *Syphilis* that a general corruption of the air (predicted by astrologers from the conjunction of Mars, Saturn and Jupiter) was the cause of the severe epidemic at the turn of the century. During the last twenty years (prior to 1546) there had been a steady tendency for the disease to become milder and more chronic. The primary atmospheric cause having disappeared, the germs—once sharp and viscous—have, he says, become drier and more earthy. The disease is in its old age and will ultimately cease to propagate itself and disappear—to return at some future date when the necessary peculiar constitution of the atmosphere should again arise. Epidemiologists of our own time have advanced ambitious theories in regard to cyclical variations in microbic virulence on much more slender grounds of evidence than those available to Fracastorius.

Chapters xiv and xv include a discussion of leprosy, scabies, and various cutaneous infections, highly confused by uncertain terminology and dubious humoral theories. The author finally concludes that those infections of the skin which are contagious include "the plague bubo;[4] those exanthemata which we call fersae and variolae; certain ulcerated strumae; some forms of lichen; scabies, elephantia, achores, alopecia, syphilis, mentagra, and any others there may be in which foul putrefaction develops."

Book iii deals with the "Treatment of the Contagia." Here the point of special interest is Fracastorius's continuing emphasis on specific treatment of individual diseases. It is not enough to treat symptoms. In each case, one must "destroy the germs of that contagion by the means that I shall now prescribe. For once the germs are killed (*interempta*), the disease will progress no further." The following ideals set forth are admirable, even if they must have been difficult of attainment in the sixteenth century. "He who wishes to treat contagions must pay attention to the following points. First let him observe what sort of contagion it is, whether it is one of those that come to us from without, and if so whether it has been contracted from the air or from another person; or whether it is one of those which develop originally in us; whether it infects by direct contact only, or also by fomes, or infects also at a distance. Then let him consider whether it is acute or sluggish; in what humor it is seated and what is its analogy (selective property); also how far it has progressed, whether it is in the initial stage, or has progressed far; also, what parts of the body are mainly attacked, whether it is wholly internal, or wholly external, or everywhere; whether it has taken hold of the solid parts, or is only roving over the periphery; whether it

---

[4] The inclusion of the plague bubo as a skin infection is curious in view of the fact that plague has previously been clearly recognized as a true pestiferous fever.

is traveling quickly and widely, or slowly, and in narrow limits. In a word, all the differential symptoms of contagions must be closely observed."

In Chapter II he develops the methods available in order that the germs "may be blotted out and, so to speak, slain, expelled, or broken and altered or driven back." The Latin word *"enecari"* suggests a concept of a living entity but it is modified by the term "so to speak," which indicates that the phrase is not to be read literally. The methods of destroying the germs are chilling (cold drinks or cold bathing), heating, drying (by use of salt for instance), evacuation, blood-letting and the use of antipathetic substances. It is interesting to note that both extreme heat and extreme cold are being used to control infection in the body today; and Fracastorius's discussion of antipathetic substances would serve as an excellent description of serum therapy: "Just as poisons and germs of contagions have an antipathy toward the soul and the natural heat, so there are certain other things which, like some antidotes, have an antipathy towards poisons and the germs themselves and repel them, and perhaps in some other way blunt their force as well."

In Chapter III, we pass from methods of destroying the seeds of infection to those designed to check the putrefactive changes which those seeds have set in motion. The power of a small amount of substance to effect profound changes is happily illustrated by the coagulation of milk by rennet and the preservation of wine by addition of alum. The actual drugs suggested for these admirable purposes are, of course, more or less fantastic, involving a very long list of vegetable and mineral substances, including powdered emerald (in regard to which Fracastorius is sceptical) and the horn of the unicorn.

Fracastorius's conservatism in regard to bleeding and purging is highly commendable. In mild diseases, such as measles and smallpox, one should not hinder nature by such treatment but assist her healing processes through rest and proper diet.

Chapter VII deals with the treatment of true pestilent fevers[5] and contains extensive recommendations on what we should call isolation and quarantine. "This contagion often has its source in the air; often travels from one person to another; is often contracted from fomes; and some-

---

[5] It is difficult to understand what distinction—if any—Fracastorius drew between "pestilent" and "pestiferous" fevers or what he meant by "true" pestilent fevers. Smallpox, measles, typhus, syphilis and the sweating sickness stand out clearly. Probably "true pestilent fever" was primarily the plague.

times arises originally in ourselves." "Where the plague is due to some taint in the air, though this happens seldom, there is no remedy more salutary than flight, as the proverb says, and the search for healthier air. But if that is not possible, for one cannot always abandon cities, furniture, houses and loved ones, then at least purify the air by the means that have been mentioned above. 'You will do well to set alight the broad fields of stubble, and burn down virgin woods and sacred groves.'

"Also observe carefully whether the contagion is being conveyed into your district from some other district. Then shut the windows on that side, and live on the other side of the house. Beware of every kind of fomes, such as wood, clothes, and every object that has been handled by the plague-stricken. Those governments act most wisely which provide by custom and law that all furniture in an infected house must be burned, and the heirs compensated from the public funds." A case is cited where "one coat made of skins caused the death of no fewer than twenty-five German soldiers for when one died another put it on, and at his death another, and so on, until they took warning from so many deaths and burned the coat."

Passing now to the care of the patient, those windows looking toward the north should be opened and flowers and sweet-smelling chilly fruits placed in the sickroom. Fumigation should be performed with vaporized rose-water, camphor and cloves. To avoid infection, "it is wiser not to visit any sick person, if possible, to flee from all crowds, and to remain at home; keep the house clean and well-ventilated; and avoid becoming heated, lest, by opening the pores of the skin, you contract the contagion. That the air which you breathe may be purer, always keep in your mouth either juniper berries or gentian root or galanga root or cassia bark or macer, or the seed of a citron. Also keep touching your nostrils with a small sponge soaked in vinegar and rose-water. Wear very clean clothes, made if possible, not of wool but silk, and change them very often."

Chapter x, on syphilis, follows much the lines of Fracastorius's earlier poem. The number of drugs cited as of possible value is staggering; but guaiac is still to the fore. Mercury may be desirable in more serious cases and the symptoms of mercurialism, due to excessive doses, are described. It is interesting to note that a sweating process was the last and most drastic resource. There is strong emphasis on general personal and mental hygiene.

The actual therapeutic procedures of the sixteenth century were confused and largely fantastic. Diagnosis had, however, made astonishing progress; and the general scientific approach was logical and clear and bold. From the standpoint of the etiology of the communicable diseases, the success of the author in building up a rational theory of contagion—without the aid of the microscope and the culture tube—was really astounding. If we apply this theory to the virus diseases, rather than to the bacterial infections, it is essentially correct today.

Let us summarize the main points in Fracastorius's etiology and see how far they correspond with modern knowledge. The essentials of his theory were as follows:

1. A wide variety of diseases are caused by transmissible, self-propagating entities ("germs"). These are conceived, not as living organisms, but as chemical substances, susceptible to evaporation and atmospheric diffusion. This is a difference which seemed fundamental a quarter of a century ago but appears less significant today, since the crystallization of viruses has so effectively broken down the barrier between the living and the non-living.

2. Each disease is specific and has its specific "germ." This emphasis on specificity is of primary importance; its neglect by later authorities is responsible for much of the medical confusion of succeeding centuries.

3. The "germ" propagates itself in the tissues of the infected host and causes disease by setting up chemical, putrefactive changes in those tissues.

4. The "germs" of different diseases vary in power of persistence in the environment and in invasiveness. The "germs" of a particular disease may exhibit cyclical changes in these properties leading to more epidemic or more sporadic prevalence and to greater or less severity.

5. The "germs" may originally arise either within the body or in the external world. Whether this is true or not, who can say? Pathogenes presumably first appeared as variations from some saprophytic form.

6. The "germs" are spread from person to person by direct contact, by fomes and by transmission at a distance, the latter two types of transmission depending on special properties of the "germs" involved.

7. Under unusual conditions, such as produce widespread pandemics, the general atmosphere becomes infected; and this special condition is associated with—though not directly caused by—abnormal astrological conditions and atmospheric and terrestrial phenomena. This is the one

important point on which we differ from Fracastorius, but, as pointed out in an earlier chapter, we are still only able to conjecture as to the causes of pandemicity.

8. In order that a "germ" may produce infection, it must find a corresponding "analogy" in the tissues of the host. Here is, of course, a logical, though vague, explanation of vital resistance.

9. Treatment of the diseases in question must follow three main lines: destruction of the "germs" by such processes as heat and cold (both in actual use today) or their evacuation from the body; checking of the putrefactive processes caused by the "germs"; and neutralization of the action of the "germs" by the use of antipathetic substances. The latter process obviously suggests immuno-therapy; but there is no conception that the desirable antipathetic substances can be produced by the active agency of the host-tissues themselves.

Altogether, this analysis was a truly marvellous triumph of close observation and clear reasoning. It is the first really philosophical statement of the contagionistic theory of disease—a mountain peak in the history of etiology perhaps unequalled by any other writer between Hippocrates and Pasteur.

CHAPTER VIII

THE CONCEPTION OF A CONTAGIUM ANIMATUM

"The fourth sort of little animals, which drifted among the three sorts aforesaid, were incredibly small."—LEEUWENHOEK

IN THE sixteenth century, as we have seen, Fracastorius developed a remarkably complete and adequate theory of contagion, in which the only major deviation from modern conceptions was the lack of recognition of the biological nature of the contagious element. In the seventeenth century, three independent investigators presented evidence which—if it had been appraised at its true value—was sufficient to fill this gap in epidemiological thinking. Even though recent researches show us that the distinction between living and non-living matter is a theoretically tenuous one, the practical impact upon theories of contagion of a recognition of this fact should have been of major importance in an understanding of the *modus operandi* of contagion.

The seventeenth century—like the sixteenth—was again a brilliant period of human history. At the turn of the century, Cervantes was fifty-three years of age and Shakespeare thirty-six; Milton was born in 1608, Molière in 1622. Velasquez first saw the light in 1599, Rembrandt in 1607. Francis Bacon was thirty-nine years old in 1600, Galileo thirty-six, and Descartes a child of four; Kepler was born in 1571, Newton in 1642. The philosophers, Locke and Spinoza, were both children of 1632, and Leibnitz of 1646.

In the field of medicine, Vesalius and Paré were gone but Harvey and Sydenham were to take their place. Harvey graduated at Padua in 1602 and published his epoch-making *De Motu Cordis* in 1628. Sanctorius by his *Ars de Statica Medicina* in 1614 shared with Harvey the honor of initiating the science of modern experimental physiology. Sydenham was born in 1624.

By 1550, sweating sickness, leprosy and epidemic chorea had practically disappeared. Typhus fever (as in the "Black Assizes" at Oxford in 1577) and typhoid fever continued a high prevalence, and smallpox epidemics were numerous. Plague and syphilis were perhaps the major scourges of the seventeenth century, although the latter had ceased to be actively epidemic. The statement of Garrison that the actual mortality from epidemic diseases was "as great as in the Middle Ages" is probably an overstatement; but plague, at least, continued as a constant menace. The Great Plague of London occurred in 1665 and within the next two decades Vienna and Prague suffered from epidemics of equal severity. It was in a study of this disease, essentially a seventeenth century plague tract, that the German-born Jesuit priest, Athanasius Kircher, made his important contribution to epidemiological theory.

Kircher was born in 1602 at Geisa, near Fulda, where he was educated at the Jesuit College. He entered the Society of Jesus in 1618, studied classical and oriental languages, mathematics and physics, and was appointed professor of philosophy, mathematics, and oriental languages at Würzburg about 1630. In 1631, he was driven out by the disturbances of the Thirty Years War and took refuge at Avignon, where he turned his attention from magnetism to Egyptology. In 1635 he settled in Rome, where for eight years he taught mathematics in the Collegio Romano. He enjoyed the patronage of Pope Urban VIII, and Cardinal Barberini and Emperor Ferdinand III also aided in the publication of his monumental work on the Coptic language (1643). At about the latter date, he retired from the college to devote himself to researches in archeology and science. The plague tract which we shall discuss in detail was published in 1658; and Kircher apparently lived the quiet life of a scholar in Rome until his death in 1680.

Kircher has been somewhat unfortunate in his biographers. The *Encyclopaedia Britannica* calls him "a man of wide and varied learning, but singularly devoid of judgment and critical discernment." The author who discusses him in the *Allgemeine Deutsche Biographie* says, "Of all these folios and quartos on optics and acoustics, on mathematics, on magnetism, on the heavens, the earth and the world beneath, on plague and on prodigies of nature, there is not one, in the opinion of competent experts, which includes any real contribution to knowledge." Dobell says, "To me the *Scrutinium Pestis* appears as a farrago of nonsensical speculation by a man possessed of neither scientific acumen nor medical instinct." Even Torrey in his recent review of Kircher's work says, "He contributed no well authenticated observation to microbiology or the history of infectious disease. He established no useful generalization. He made no stimulating suggestions for research. In his own times, he belonged to the past."

Whether such criticism may or may not be justified with regard to Kircher's philology and physics, it is certainly unwarranted with respect to his *Scrutinium Physico-Medicum Contagiosae Luis, quae Pestis dicitur* (1658). This treatise has earned for its author an honored place in the history of medical science. It is of major importance in the development of epidemiological thinking.

Kircher begins Section I of his treatise (On Origin Causes and Behavior of Plague) by a chapter on plague as the scourge and arrow of God sent for the punishment of the sins of men. This is quite in the vein of Ambroise Paré, but is less surprising in an essay by a Jesuit priest dedicated to Pope Alexander VII than in one written by an army surgeon. Having paid his respects to ecclesiastical authority, he proceeds in Chapter II to define plague as a widespread disease affecting several regions, very deadly and highly contagious—distinguishing it from sporadic diseases such as dysentery, smallpox, the various fevers on the one hand and from locally-limited endemic diseases such as Egyptian elephantiasis and Alpine goiter on the other. In Chapter III, the author considers the "natural" rather than the "divine" causes of plague, and gives the usual list of the various modes by which plague may be generated by putrefaction. The list includes marshes and decaying mud, dead bodies of men and animals, and decomposing vegetable matter. Under hot and moist conditions, the general atmosphere may precipitate those contagious putrefactions called *seminaria*, which in the living produce inevitable disease and which propagate in the bodies of the dead their deadly progeny (Chapter IV). Contagious corruption is not merely an alteration in the four basic elements but rather the addition of alien foreign deleterious properties. These may be spread by direct contact, by fomites and by action at a distance (as in Fracastorius). The influence of the stars is mentioned as a "remote cause" or contributory factor (Chapter V). Chapter VI discusses contributory causes within the human body itself, such as improper diet or starvation. The first part of Chapter VII deals with the ways in which the "corpuscular" effluvia enter the body and cause disease.

So far, except for the emphasis on the "corpuscular" nature of the contagious element, we are on familiar ground. All that has gone before fits into the traditional epidemiological theories of the seventeenth—and indeed of the fourteenth—century. In a later paragraph of Chapter VII, however, Kircher makes his real contribution. In discussing the effluvia from bodies of men dead of the plague as a cause of contagion, he says that this contagion which invades the body propagates like a creeping thing through all its members. Associated with this putrefaction are the true latent germs (*seminaria*) of plague which internally cause progressive putrefaction and externally produce corruption of the air. "To whatever degree, corpuscles of this sort may be normally non-living, yet under the influence of ambient heat and in proportion to the degree of the infectious decomposition, produce an offspring of innumerable imperceptible worms, so that the more corpuscles are present in the effluvia, the greater will be the number of little worms generated. When this occurs they may be considered no longer as evidences of life but as actual living effluvia [*animata effluvia*]."

This conclusion, which the author assumes may be considered startling by his readers, Kircher then proceeds to support by records of his own original observations made with a "very delicate" microscope.

He first quotes Aristotle, Pliny and other authorities in support of the general principle that all putrefying substances generate worms "by their essential nature"; and then proceeds to discuss six "experiments" of his own. (1) Particles of meat exposed to moonlight and kept for several days, exhibit under the microscope many diverse kinds of small worms; (2) When "creeping things" (*serpentem*) are macerated in rain water and kept for several days, multitudes of new creeping things are generated; (3) on the leaves of the sage plant tiny moving animals may be seen with the microscope; (4) in decaying wood, one may observe a great development of organisms ("little worms") of which some show horns, some bear wings, others are many-legged, some have eyes like black dots with a proboscis between; (5) in an infusion of pulverized soil in water, exposed to the sun's heat in summer, the sediment at the bottom develops a great number of very minute worms, producing finally winged forms (*Cyniphes*) which fly about and attack men and animals; (6) a final "experiment" deals with generation of living things from dead bodies but is chiefly a discussion of general principles without specific original observations.

In Chapter VIII Kircher proceeds to a more general statement of his thesis that the cause of contagion is the generation from the decaying bodies of those dead of the plague of corpuscles, which may be either living or non-living. Such insensible particles may infect bread, wood or other porous substances and may be breathed in with the air or transmitted by the fingers or other forms of contact. He supports this thesis by citations from Cardanus, Agricola and other writers as to the prevalence of great numbers of worms at times of plague and by references to Cornelius, Gemma and August Hauptmann who have noted the presence of worms and other living things in the tissues of cadavers.

Chapter ix discusses the different forms of "plague," and Chapter x, "artificial" plague produced by diabolical arts. Finally, Section i closes with a long chapter on the influence of the constellations and on the various "signs" of a plague epidemic. The astrological section follows conventional lines and the signs are treated under six headings as follows: signs of plague sent by God; signs in the form of generation of great numbers of insects or of disease in plants and animals; signs in the form of abnormal conditions of the sky or air; signs relating to the presence of contagion in the air; signs of the mitigation of the plague; and signs of its complete disappearance. Under the fourth of these headings, Kircher suggests that the presence of contagion in the air can be detected by certain practical tests; such as exposing bread on the roof of a house to see whether it becomes fly-blown and poisonous for dogs or hens who eat it.

Section ii of the *Scrutinium* deals with various additional problems concerning plague, and Section iii with practical prophylactic and therapeutic measures. The first chapter of Section ii copes rather effectively with the view which Kircher attributes to Van Helmont (and by inference to Paracelsus also) that plague is generated by the force of the human imagination and against it he maintains stoutly that the "seeds" of plague must always be present as the essential cause, though imagination and fear may heighten susceptibility. In Chapter ii, he contends that the poison of plague cannot be generated in the normal human body and reviews the various sorts of external putrefaction from which it may arise. Chapter iv is particularly important for it discusses in detail the various ways in which the contagion of plague is spread. Kircher adopts the three modes of transmission of Fracastorius with a certain slight difference and without citation of that authority. His three modes are by direct contact, by transmission through the air, and by fomites at a distance. The characterization of infection by fomites, rather than atmospheric infection as operating "at a distance" seems an improvement over the analysis of Fracastorius. The author states, "It has been demonstrated that plague is, in general, a living thing; and that those, for instance, who are sick of the plague, being severely infected, suffer putrefaction in a high degree so that they are in a state favorable to the generation of worms of all sorts. The little worms propagated are particles so small, so slender and so subtle as to elude all our senses, being revealed only by a very powerful microscope. These particles reproduce themselves so actively that their numbers are beyond computation. Thus conceived and generated in corruption, they are readily given through all the openings and pores of the body, together with the breath and the sweat. When they are stirred by even the faintest breath of air, they take on a lively motion like atoms [particles of dust] when a ray of sunlight is projected into a dark place. They scatter now in this direction, now in that, and they adhere very tenaciously to anything with which they come in contact and insinuate themselves into its deepest pores."

"I was led to this belief," he says, "by the fact that the putrid blood of fever patients one or two hours after taking it I have found so full of worms that I was dumbfounded, and from that moment I was convinced that the human body [suffering from plague] whether living or dead teems with worms. It calls to mind the words of Job: 'I have said to corruption, thou art my father; to the worm, thou art my mother and my sister.'" He continues: "The same thing was observed more than once by the distinguished and learned Roman physician, Julius Placentius, in the dissection of *bubones*, which he undertook at my instance as Superintendent of the Hospital, namely, that they were filled with an innumerable brood of minutest worms. This will seem beyond belief to many medical men. But they should know that many things lie hid in Nature, unknown alike to the ancients and to men of modern times, which the acumen of our time has disclosed through the help of the eye armed [with the microscope] and, as the saying is, has demonstrated *ad oculum*."

Kircher then discusses twelve different specific modes by which contagion may be spread, which may be summarized as follows: (1) by direct contact; (2) fomites, such as "linen, bread, clothing, skins, hides, tapestry, sleeping couches, benches, tables, utensils of all sorts, even cochlearia, knives, orbes, drinking cups, shoes, girdles"; (3) by various animals such as cats, dogs, fowls and pigeons and by flies which have fed on the sick or the dead acting as passive carriers; (4) by substances such as wine, oil, butter, fats and metals of all sorts ("there is no substance which is not subject to contagion"—although enclosure of wine or other liquids in tight vessels protects them against the entrance of the germs); (5) by animals of various sorts acting not as passive carriers but as themselves victims of the disease—a phenomenon which Kircher denies; (6) by sight, sound and smell, all of which are accepted as modes of transmission; (7) by such things as letters and merchandise which may carry infection to distant places; (8) by physicians in attendance on

ince "the virulent corpuscles which have been breathed out
ed by manual contact will adhere in the innermost recesses
s so that contagion may readily be communicated to those not
.nfected with the disease"; (9) by carriage by the wind; (10') by
s. .ntercourse; (11) by fomites in which contagion may persist for
many years; (12) through the air to a distance which Kircher estimates
at not more than five or six feet, since he believes that contagion does
not persist in the air, as it does in fomites.

Section III of the *Scrutinium* deals with prophylaxis and therapeusis
of the plague and does not concern us in the present discussion.

The microscopes available to Kircher could not have permitted him
to see bacteria, perhaps not even protozoa. His "worms" were probably
really worms or, in some cases, insect larvae. The structures observed by
him in infected tissue are conjectured by many commentators to have
been rouleaux of red blood-corpuscles.

Nor was he the first to advance the theory of living organisms as the
agents of communicable disease. Absolute priority in scientific discovery
is very rare. Singer in his scarce, privately-printed treatise on *The Development of the Doctrine of Contagium Vivum* lists many precursors
from the ancient Greeks down. Cardanus in 1557 suggested that
the seeds of disease are truly living and reproduce their kind after the
manner of minute living animals. Victor de Bonagentibus in 1556 compared the generation and conveyance of fevers to the putrefactive processes which produce "worms" in corpses. Gabriel Fallopius in 1564
applied a similar analogy specifically to syphilis and phthisis.

In the seventeenth century, the revival of the atomic theory by Descartes and the increasing use of primitive microscopes greatly stimulated
speculation along these lines. Alexander Benedictus in 1608 gives accounts of minute "lumbrici" in cheese, on the teeth, in lungs, kidneys
and skin. "He appears to have been quite familiar with living creatures
as a cause of disease and he certainly knew of the organism of scabies."
August Hauptmann in 1650 maintained that fevers were caused by
minute animalcules of the nature and form either of worms or of their
eggs.

Nevertheless, it is clear that the *Scrutinium Pestis* was the first really
effective presentation of the theory that living organisms were the primary cause of disease. The thesis is detailed and logical, on a wholly
different plane from such casual inferences as are implied by Varro's
reference to "animalculae" or indeed to the brief allusions of the six-

teenth and seventeenth century writers cited above. The *Scrutinium* is notable for the inclusion of notes on actual "experiments" which, if not experiments in our sense of the term, were at least first-hand direct observations—an innovation of no mean importance in that day. Finally, the claim to have seen under the microscope the actual germs of plague, even though it was unjustified, greatly strengthened the influence of Kircher's work. As Singer points out, his views "immediately attracted wide attention in every country in Europe." Christian Lange in Germany was perhaps his most ardent disciple, but in England, Holland and Sweden, as well as in Germany and Italy, the ideas of Kircher were echoed by many observers in the second half of the seventeenth century. The judgment of Garrison that Kircher was "undoubtedly the first to state in explicit terms the doctrine of a *contagium animatum* as the cause of infectious disease," is essentially justified.

My colleague, Professor G. L. Hendrickson, who has been good enough to check my translation of Kircher's salient passages and to read the manuscript of this chapter, permits me to quote the following comments:

"I venture to suggest that your account of Kircher should be offset by a remark or two on his incredible credulity and superstition. His central truth (or basic theory) is so overlaid with pretentious nonsense, such as Fracastoro for example would have laughed at, that it is little wonder many modern students have been loath to grant him any significance at all.

"Perhaps, also, something might be said about the probable steps which led him to the formation of his doctrine. He was a careful reader of Lucretius and understood his atomic theory very well. He was, therefore, like Fracastoro, familiar with the idea and the terminology of 'seeds of disease,' as atomic, minute, invisible, carried by the air, and thus a source of contagion. But now with the microscope, which was fascinating all the scientists of his time (especially at Rome), he saw that there were living organisms invisible to the naked eye. The problem of the transmission and spread of plague-contagion was a present and pressing one because of the epidemic in progress in Naples and in lesser degree even in Rome. By putting together, then, the Lucretian doctrine of seeds of disease and his own and others' microscopic observations it was possible to arrive at the conclusion which he enunciates, of an effluvium animatum as the explanation of contagion. . . .

"It does not matter much what Kircher saw; it was sufficient that he saw organisms below the threshold of unaided vision, and made the inference of still more minute manifestations of life beyond what he saw (cf. Lucr. 4, 115). That was enough to bridge the gap from 'atoms to organisms.'

"Apart from Kircher's doctrine of effluvia animata as a source of contagion, he makes a number of other incidental observations which may be set down to his credit, to offset a vast amount of credulity and superstition.

"First of all he professes faith in experiment as the only sure guide to knowledge. At the end of one of his tests to discover whether or not air is infected, he says (p. 105): 'I might add other signs of the presence of infected air gathered from many sources, but it has seemed best to me to set down here only those which have been verified and proven by experiment. Others which are the product only of opinion and remain unsupported by experiment I pass over.' This is good sense, but it would be more impressive if his experiments were more accurately described and controlled. The only one of his experiments which has a suggestion of real significance is no. 5 on p. 46, which describes the exposure of water in an open vessel, with the addition of a little dust, to the summer sun. It is not perfectly clear whether he thinks of the ensuing growth of worms (which become flying insects) as spontaneous generation from earth, water and heat, or that an effluvium animatum has introduced life into the water. This latter view is apparently entertained in another place, where he describes a similar experiment of clear water in an open vessel, which becomes infected by minute particles of dust in the air, and produces worms. He uses this as an analogy for infection of water or any liquid by contagious effluvia (p. 146-7). This experiment is not unlike the more careful observations of Leeuwenhoek, or even of Tyndall two centuries later."

Among the pregnant incidental suggestions in the *Scrutinium* are the recognition of insects, particularly flies, as carriers of plague infection, either intrinsically (by biting) or extrinsically (by external carriage); and the assertion that in periods of contagious effluvia, water, wine, honey and other liquids may be protected against infection by storing them in tightly closed vessels.

The major defect in Kircher's epidemiological theory was his dominant (though not consistent) conception that the living germs of disease were spontaneously generated by the decomposition of organic matter. Just ten years after the publication of the *Scrutinium*, there appeared in Italy another contribution of first-rate importance which laid the basis for correction of this erroneous assumption.

Francesco Redi (1620-1698) resembled Kircher in the wide range of his interests. Born at Arezzo, he graduated at Pisa in medicine and philosophy in 1647. He became successful in his primary profession, serving as physician to Ferdinand II and Cosmo III in Florence, and in his medical writings advocated observation as opposed to theory and emphasized hygiene rather than therapeutics. As a poet, he gained fame, the dithyrambs of his *Bacco in Toscano* being widely acclaimed. He was also a philologist and a naturalist; and it is his *Experiments on the Generation of Insects* (1668) which involved his major contribution to science.

At this period, the doctrine that living things—not merely insects but even fishes, reptiles and mammals—were spontaneously generated by organic decomposition was generally accepted. Van Helmont (1577-1644), for example, gives a famous recipe for the spontaneous production of young mice by setting away in a warm place a jar of grain containing a dirty shirt. Redi attacked this problem by direct experimentation. Huxley in his essay on *Biogenesis and Abiogenesis* gives a summary of Redi's reasoning and of the results of his experiments, as follows: "Here are dead animals, or pieces of meat, says he; I expose them to the air in hot weather, and in a few days they swarm with maggots. You tell me that these are generated in the dead flesh; but if I put similar bodies, while quite fresh, into a jar, and tie some fine gauze over the top of the jar, not a maggot makes its appearance, while the dead substances, nevertheless, putrefy just in the same way as before. It is obvious, therefore, that the maggots are not generated by the corruption of the meat; and that the cause of their formation must be a something which is kept away by gauze. But gauze will not keep away aeriform bodies, or fluids. This something must, therefore, exist in the form of solid particles too big to get through the gauze. Nor is one long left in doubt what these solid particles are; for the blow-flies, attracted by the odor of the meat, swarm round the vessel, and, urged by a powerful but in this case misleading instinct, lay eggs out of which maggots are immediately hatched, upon the gauze. The conclusion, therefore, is unavoidable; the maggots are not generated by the meat, but the eggs which give rise to them are brought through the air by the flies."

This beautifully simple demonstration, and others of like kind, led

Redi to the conclusion that, in all cases where living matter was apparently produced from dead matter, the real explanation was that the seeds (*semenza*) of the animals or plants concerned had been introduced from outside. Here was a clear and full-fledged doctrine of biogenesis; and Redi's evidence was so convincing that this doctrine gained rapid and general acceptance.

It is, of course, obvious that Redi's conclusions were concerned primarily with insects and need not necessarily apply to more primitive forms of life. In the eighteenth century, they were to be specifically challenged for the new world of "infusorial animalculae" by Buffon and Needham; but the Abbé Spallanzani (1729-1799) confuted these critics, in a brilliant series of experiments, and demonstrated for the germs of putrefaction what Redi had shown for fly maggots. Only in the nineteenth century, however, was the doctrine of abiogenesis to be definitely overthrown by Schulze and Schwann, Schroeder and von Dusch and, finally, Pasteur.

The third major contribution of the seventeenth century to the basic data available for a theory of contagion was made by the Dutchman, Antony van Leeuwenhoek. Here was no brilliant virtuoso, but a patient, indefatigable, critical observer in one narrow area of science. Kircher and Redi were typical Renaissance figures. Leeuwenhoek was a precursor of the laboratory investigator of today; and, in spite of his lack of superficial brilliance, much the greater man of the three.

Antony van Leeuwenhoek was born at Delft in 1632, the year of the birth of Locke, Spinoza, Vermeer and Sir Christopher Wren. Holland at that time was at the height of its glory "in the very front rank in the civilized world, as the home of letters, science and art" and "undoubtedly the most learned state in Europe." That Leeuwenhoek should contribute to the brilliance of his country, however, seemed improbable. He was the son of a basket-maker and at sixteen was apprenticed to a draper in Amsterdam, with no opportunities for formal education. About 1654, he returned to Delft which, with its shaded walks and canals, was described by a contemporary visitor as "a fair and populous city, very clean, well-built, and very pleasant." Here Leeuwenhoek married in the year of his return and set up his own business as a draper. He must have made rapid progress in the esteem of his fellow-townsmen, for in 1660 he was appointed "Chamberlain of the Council-Chamber of the Worshipful Sheriffs of Delft" and in 1679 he was appointed to the office of Wine Gauger. Both these posts, according to Dobell, were rather profitable sinecures, the actual duties being performed by others. Leeuwenhoek was also a qualified surveyor and on the death of his friend, Vermeer (in 1675) he was appointed administrator of the family estate.

The external side of Leeuwenhoek's life was, then, that of any solid tradesman and respected burgher. His business success or his profitable public posts, or both, made it possible for him to indulge in continuous and intensive studies of nature, in the course of which he perfected magnifying glasses of then unheard-of power and used them in a series of studies which have gained for this self-trained amateur a high place in the history of biology.

These studies must have been going forward for some time before they saw the light; but Leeuwenhoek made his first public contribution to the Royal Society of London in 1673, when he was forty-one years old. This communication was a letter sent to London with a covering endorsement in which his sponsor, Reinier de Graaf, says that the author had during the year past "devised microscopes which far surpass those which we have hitherto seen"; and the communication was also supported by Constantjn Huygens. It was the first of several hundred letters written by Leeuwenhoek during a period of fifty years on subjects chemical, physical, botanical, zoological, physiological and medical. It is these letters which constitute his title to fame, for he never published a book or a scientific memoir. It is of interest to note—as evidence of the superior civilization of the seventeenth as compared with the twentieth century—that these letters contrived to pass from Delft to London and to be published by the Royal Society, even while England and Holland were at war.

Leeuwenhoek received his first great honor when he was elected a member of the Royal Society in 1680 His discovery of a new world of life in the water and the earth and the fluids of the living body attracted wide attention, and he was universally accepted as the greatest microscopist of his time. His unique magnifiers, his simple, straightforward and acute power of observation, earned instant respect; and, although his explanations of the phenomena he observed were often fantastic, he always made a clear and honest distinction between his observations and his speculations. His simple home at Delft was visited by many of the greatest figures in Europe; and on their visits to Delft he was commanded to display his wonders to

Peter the Great of Russia and to reigning sovereigns of England and Germany.

In 1716, when Leeuwenhoek was in his eighty-fourth year, the University of Louvain honored him by sending him a medal specially designed in honor of his researches and accompanied by a Latin poem of praise. This was acknowledged in a letter containing the following delightful passage: "Notwithstanding my praises be therein sung very high, yet the poet's cleverness deserveth still higher praise for screwing them up to such a pretty pitch: and when I think on the flatteries expressed in your letter, and in the poem, I don't only blush, but my eyes filled with tears too, many a time: especially because my work, which I've done for many a long year, was not pursued in order to gain the praise I now enjoy, but chiefly from a craving after knowledge, which I notice resides in me more than in most other men. And therewithal, whenever I found out anything remarkable, I have thought it my duty to put down my discovery on paper, so that all ingenious people might be informed thereof."

Leeuwenhoek continued to put down his discoveries on paper to the end. His last letter to the Royal Society was dated in May, 1723; and he died in August, at the ripe age of ninety-one years.

The work of this extraordinary investigator was entirely based on his skill in microscopy. Robert Hooke, the botanist, in discussing "The Fate of Microscopes" in 1692, says that these instruments "are now reduced to a single Votary, which is Mr. Leeuwenhoek; besides whom I hear of none that make any other Use of that Instrument, but for Diversion and Pastime." Compound microscopes had been constructed in Holland and Italy in the first decade of the seventeenth century; but Leeuwenhoek's instrument was quite independent, being only a single-lens magnifier of unusual power. He left nearly 250 of his instruments of which about 8 are still in existence and from these, and from descriptions left by early writers, we have a clear idea of their construction. The lens was a small double convex glass mounted in a hole between two silver plates riveted together. The object to be examined was mounted on a silver point on the side of the plate away from the observer, this point being movable in three planes by screws which brought it into the required focus. Professor Harting of Utrecht found that some of Leeuwenhoek's lenses had a magnifying power of 270 diameters. Apparently, however, some very special technique involved in his procedure, was never revealed. He said in his famous letter to the Royal

Society, under date of October 9, 1676, "My method for seeing the very smallest animalcules and minute eels, I do not impart to others; nor how to see very many animalcules at one time. That I keep for myself alone." Cohen has recently reported ingenious experiments with a copy of a Leeuwenhoek lens which suggest that utilization of the inherent optical properties of the spherical drop of fluid under observation, or of air bubbles contained in that fluid, would produce the results which the Dutch microscopist obtained.

Clifford Dobell in his *Antony van Leeuwenhoek and his "Little Animals"* has given us an exhaustive and illuminating picture of Leeuwenhoek's contributions to protozoology and bacteriology, only the high points of which need be briefly reviewed here.

Letter No. 6, written on September 7, 1674, describes, incidentally, the first observation of protozoa in lake water. Letter 18 (October 9, 1676), however, is the classic document in which not only protozoa, but bacteria as well, were clearly and unmistakably described. The first sections of this long communication report several more or less clearly recognizable genera of protozoa, and in later sections Leeuwenhoek proceeds to a description of an infusion of pepper, originally made up in the hope of finding "the cause of the hotness or power whereby pepper affects the tongue." After discussing three types of protozoa present, the writer says, "The fourth sort of little animals, which drifted among the three sorts aforesaid, were incredibly small; nay, so small, in my sight, that I judged that even if 100 of these very wee animals lay stretched out one against another, they could not reach to the length of a grain of coarse sand; and if this be true, then ten hundred thousand of these living creatures could scarce equal the bulk of a coarse sandgrain. I discovered yet a fifth sort, which had about the thickness of the last-said animalcules, but which were near twice as long."

In a still later paragraph of the same letter, spirilla, as well as bacteria and bacilli, were described in pepper-water. This epoch-making discovery of the bacteria was confirmed by Robert Hooke in a communication to the Royal Society in 1678 and also by Christiaan Huygens in a manuscript report, which remained unpublished until a few years ago.

Letter 23 (1678) contains another good description of bacteria in pepper-water which "would oft-times shoot so swiftly forward with the hindmost part of their body, that you might think you saw a pike darting through the water" and of spirilla in the same medium.

Number 39 (1683) is the most important of all these letters, to the bacteriologist. It deals with the matter obtained from between the teeth. Leeuwenhoek says, in explanation: " 'Tis my wont of a morning to rub my teeth with salt, and then swill my mouth out with water; and often, after eating to clean my back teeth with a toothpick, as well as rubbing them hard with a cloth: wherefor my teeth, back and front, remain as clean and white as falleth to the lot of few men of my years, and my gums (no matter how hard the salt be that I rub them with) never start bleeding." Yet whitish matter was still present between his molars and incisors; in this matter, suspended in clean rain water, he observed and figured cocci, short rods, long thread-forms (*Leptothrix*) and spirochetes. We have here a clear picture of the characteristic flora of the mouth and the movement of each type of bacterial organism is accurately described. Leeuwenhoek concludes "(howbeit I clean my mouth like I've already said), that all the people living in our United Netherlands are not as many as the living animals that I carry in my own mouth this very day."

The observations on his own mouth were confirmed by examination of matter from the teeth of "two different womenfolk that I'm sure clean their teeth every day"; of a child eight years old; of an old man who led a very sober life but had "never washed his mouth in all his life"; of another old man who never washed his mouth in his life with water "but it gets a good swill with wine or brandy every day." In all these instances he found his little animals, with very little variation except that the temperate but dirty old man had a particularly extensive flora with spirochetes very abundant. Furthermore, Leeuwenhoek showed that, although wine vinegar promptly killed his animalculae *in vitro*, thorough rinsing of the mouth with this disinfectant was ineffective. "From this," he says, "I drew the conclusion that the vinegar, when I filled my mouth with it, didn't penetrate through all the matter that is firmly lodged between the front teeth and the grinders, and killed only those animalcules that were in the outermost parts of the white matter." Here was a well-planned and soundly interpreted experiment in oral disinfection.

Letter 75 (1692) adds new observations (with a rather poor figure) on the bacteria of the mouth and reports that the matter from between the observer's front teeth was almost free from animalculae, while that from his back teeth was swarming with them, a fact which he attributes to the sterilization of the anterior part of the mouth by the drinking each morning of coffee, "so hot that it puts me into a sweat."

Letter 96 (1695) describes bacteria in an infusion of fresh-water mussels; and Letter 110 (1697) again returns briefly to the bacteriology of the mouth.

Clearly, Dobell is justified in designating Leeuwenhoek as the "Father of Protozoology and Bacteriology." He made many other important contributions to biological science. He described the red blood corpuscles and observed the capillary circulation (confirming the work of Malpighi). He described the spermatozoa and the bone corpuscles and the cross-striation of voluntary muscle. He made significant contributions to helminthology. His primary claim to scientific renown is, however, the fact that he was the first to see either bacteria or protozoa.

Leeuwenhoek did not himself make any clear application of his discovery of the "little animals" to the causation of disease. He did, however, observe bacteria in the mouth and spirochetes as well as protozoa in the feces of men and animals (Letter 34, 1681 and Letter 38, 1683). Others, however, were not slow to realize the possible medical implications of his discoveries. Benjamin Marten in 1720, three years before Leeuwenhoek's death, assumes that tuberculosis is caused by invisible "animalculae," like those discovered by Leeuwenhoek; and it is of extraordinary interest to note that Linnaeus in the twelfth edition of his *Systema Naturae* presents in an appendix six doubtful kinds of "living molecules" in addition to *Chaos infusorium*, the single species including all forms of infusoria. These kinds of living molecules are translated by Dobell as follows: "a. The contagion of eruptive fevers? b. The cause of paroxysmal fevers? c. The moist virus of syphilis? d. Leeuwenhoek's spermatic animalcules? e. The aery mist floating in the month of blossoming? f. Münchhausen's septic agent of fermentation and putrefaction?"

Linnaeus, of course, wrote in the eighteenth century. It is clear, however, that by 1700 there was available theoretical and observational evidence which should have made possible the formulation of our modern germ-theory of disease. Kircher had advanced the concept of a *contagium animatum*—but held to the doctrine of spontaneous generation. Redi had presented convincing evidence that living things (at least those of macroscopic size) were not spontaneously produced by decomposition but introduced from outside. Leeuwenhoek had actually described and figured the protozoa and bacteria in the human mouth and intestine. If an open-minded and imaginative observer had put the work of these three pioneers together, the germ-theory of disease could have been developed in the seventeenth century instead of the nineteenth. Why medical thinkers were diverted from such a possible path into a wilderness of speculative theory, we shall discuss in succeeding chapters.

CHAPTER IX

THE ENGLISH HIPPOCRATES

"Sydenham, however, was indubitably the first real clinician of modern times, the first since Hippocrates to observe and to note the lineaments of disease and to record what he saw with unsurpassed objectivity."—RIESMAN

B Y 1700, the rational groundwork had been laid for a sound theory of contagion. Unhappily, however, there was no great clinician with the vision of Lister to see what the monograph of Kircher and the experiments of Redi and the observations of Leeuwenhoek might mean for medicine. On the contrary, medicine fell under the sway of a very different concept—that of the overwhelming importance of the epidemic constitution of the atmosphere; and this concept so confused the issue as to hold back epidemiological progress for two centuries.

The first noted seventeenth century advocate of this conception was Guillaume de Baillou (1538-1616), a French court physician whose two books on epidemic and ephemeral diseases were published posthumously in 1640. The most influential representative of the school, however, was Thomas Sydenham and we may profitably study him as its exemplar.

Extraordinarily little is really known of Sydenham's life. He was born at Winford Eagle in 1624, of a locally prominent family of Dorsetshire landowners. He was entered at Oxford in 1642 but is believed to have shortly left the University to join the Parliamentary Army. He returned to Oxford after the Civil Wars and took his M.B. in 1648. During the Protectorate his career is obscure, but he is thought to have occupied himself with politics. With the Restoration in 1660 his chances of political preferment ceased and he devoted his energies seriously to medicine in London. He became a licentiate of the College of Physicians in 1663 and took his M.D. at Cambridge only in 1676. His first publication on fevers appeared in 1666. He was a friend of Locke and of Boyle but did not make a great impression upon his compatriots. His reputation on the continent was greater than at home, and between 1684 and 1689 his works were issued in Amsterdam, Leyden and Geneva editions. He was a great sufferer from gout and died in 1689. Through Boerhaave at Leyden and his disciples at Vienna, Dublin and, later, Philadelphia,

Sydenham exerted a wide influence throughout the eighteenth century. His clinical descriptions were masterly as in the cases of chorea, dysentery, gout, malaria, measles, smallpox, syphilis and tuberculosis; and his general emphasis on bedside observation was absolutely invaluable in its influence upon medical thought.

In the author's preface to the third edition of his *Collected Works*, Sydenham outlines a broad and admirable program of research. "The improvement of physic," he says, "in my opinion depends (1) upon collecting a genuine and natural description, or history, of all diseases, as can be procured; and (2) laying down a fixed and complete method of cure." "All diseases then ought to be reduced to certain and determinate kinds, with the same exactness as we see it done by botanic writers in their treatises of plants." In writing a history of diseases, "every philosophical hypothesis which hath prepossessed the writer in its favor ought to be totally laid aside, and then the manifest and natural phenomena of diseases, however minute, must be noted with the utmost accuracy, imitating in this the great exactness of painters, who, in their pictures, copy the smallest spots or moles in the originals." In the description of a disease, special attention must be paid to the effect upon its course of the age and constitution of the patient and to the influence of the season of the year.

The greatest contribution of Sydenham was his revival of the objective and naturalistic spirit of Hippocrates and he led a wholesome reaction against the sterile philosophical disputations of the iatro-chemists and the iatro-physicists which dominated the medical thinking of the time. In one important respect, however, he perhaps made an important advance over his Grecian master. Sigerist says "Hippocrates recognized only disease, not diseases. He knew only sick individuals, only cases of illness. The patient and his malady were for him inseparably connected as a unique happening, one which would never recur. But what Sydenham saw above all in the patient—what he wrenched forth to contemplate—was the typical, the pathological process which he had observed in others before and expected to see in others again. In every patient there appeared a specific kind of illness. For him, maladies were entities, and his outlook upon illness was, therefore, ontological. Hippocrates wrote the histories of sick persons, but Sydenham wrote the history of diseases."

It is perhaps significant that the concept of entities was thus emphasized by a physician whose preoccupation was with epidemic diseases, with which the vast majority of Sydenham's contributions were concerned. Nearly half of the total volume of his writings was made up of a major treatise on the "acute diseases"; and many of his minor communications return to the same topic. These contributions must be analyzed in detail in so far as they relate to our theme.

In a collection of writings devoted so largely to epidemic diseases we might expect to find much of interest for the present volume. Indeed, Garrison says that "Sydenham's studies in the geography and meteorology of epidemic diseases and the rhythmic periodicity of their occurrence makes him with Hippocrates and Baillou one of the main founders of epidemiology."

How far such a judgment may be justified can be determined only by a somewhat detailed study of Sydenham's actual writings. We are too prone to honor (or dishonor) the great men of the past without ever reading them to see what they really said.

For this purpose, I have examined meticulously the *Collected Works*, using the Swan translation which I have preferred because its English is particularly clear and vigorous; but important passages have been checked for their meaning against the Latham translation of 1848.

Section 1, on the "acute diseases in general" begins with the definition of disease as "a vigorous effort of nature to throw off the morbific matter, and thus recover the patient. For as God has been pleased so to create mankind, that they should be fitted to receive various impressions from without, they could not, upon this account, but be liable to different disorders; which arise (1) either from such particles of the air, as having a disagreement with the juices, insinuate themselves into the body and, mixing with the blood, taint the whole frame; or (2) from different kinds of fermentations and putrefactions of humours detained too long in the body, for want of its being able to digest, and discharge them, on account of their too large bulk, or unsuitable nature." Here, at the start is a clear and important distinction between the extrinsic and intrinsic factors in disease. Plague is cited as an example of the first class, due to "morbific particles" (taken in with the air we breathe); and gout as an example of the second, or intrinsic class. The first are rapid acute diseases, characterized by fever, the second, chronic diseases. The acute diseases, Sydenham divides into "epidemic distempers," which "proceed from a latent and inexplicable alteration of the air, infecting the bodies of men" and "intercurrent or sporadic" acute diseases "arising from some peculiar indisposition of particular persons." This distinction seems to clash with the primary definition of extrinsic diseases as a whole. Apparently, Sydenham separated acute from chronic diseases on a clinical basis and then subdivided acute diseases on an etiological basis.

Chapter II of the treatise elaborates Sydenham's basic theory of the causation of epidemic diseases in detail. This theory is primarily dominated by his whole-hearted acceptance of the determining effect of season and atmosphere upon the nature of disease. Sydenham is not sure whether "certain tribes of epidemic disorders constantly follow others, in one determined series, or circle, as it were; or whether they all return indiscriminately, and without any order, according to the secret disposition of the air, and the inexplicable succession of seasons." He is quite convinced, however, that diseases occurring at various seasons are so radically different as to require diverse treatments. The effects of the atmosphere in determining disease are of a twofold kind. One influence is related to the four basic qualities of the air—"for instance, pleurisies, quinsies, and the like, which generally happen when an intense and long-continued cold is immediately succeeded by a sudden heat." The other influence is much more subtle—"There are various general constitutions of years, that owe their origin neither to heat, cold, dryness, nor moisture; but rather depend upon a certain secret and inexplicable alteration in the bowels of the earth, whence the air becomes impregnated with such kinds of *effluvia*, as subject the human body to particular distempers, so long as that kind of constitution prevails."

A generally sound distinction is drawn between two broad groups of epidemics, the *vernal* and the *autumnal*. The former, appearing as early as January, include measles and "vernal tertians"; the latter include plague, smallpox, cholera morbus, and autumnal dysenteries, tertians and quartans. The whole picture is, however, confused by Sydenham's emphasis on the epidemic constitution peculiar to a given year, which influences the character of all the epidemics of that year, impressing upon their symptoms its own peculiar characteristics. A specific epidemic (one can hardly speak of a specific disease) is the result of interplay between the physical atmospheric qualities of the season and the occult influence ruling over the year. "In whatever years these several species (of diseases) prevail at one and the same time, the symptoms wherewith they come on are alike in all."

Each new epidemic, then, is almost an entity *sui generis* for which a specific therapeusis must be devised. "Under so much darkness and ignorance, therefore, my chief care, as soon as any new fever arises, is to wait a little, and proceed very slowly, especially in the use of powerful remedies; in the meantime carefully observing its nature and procedure, and by what means the patient was either relieved or injured."

The rest of Section 1 and the whole of Sections 11-v are devoted to detailed description of the various epidemics which the author had observed in the years 1661 to 1675, and of the methods he had found useful for their treatment. Invaluable as they may be from the standpoint of clinical observation, these chapters (which include over one-third of Sydenham's total writings) add little or nothing to the theory of epidemiology outlined above. In Chapter iv of Section 1, it is of interest to note that he coins the term "commotion" to describe the pathological process involved in a fever rather than "fermentation" or "ebullition"; "For tho' the commotion of the blood in fevers does at different times resemble the fermentations and ebullitions of vegetable liquor; yet there are those who think this commotion very different from both."

In Chapter v, the vernal intermittent fevers are described in terms which make it clear that Sydenham conceives them as due fundamentally to the influence of season upon the humors of the body "For the spirits being concentrated by the winter's cold, gather strength in their recess, and in this lively state are invited out by the heat of the approaching sun, and, being mixed with the viscid juices, wherewith nature had stock'd the blood during that season, . . . are, whilst they endeavor to escape, detained, and as it were entangled, and consequently occasion this *vernal ebullition,* in the same manner as is observed to happen upon exposing bottles filled with beer to the fire, after having been long kept buried in sand, or in a cool cellar, whence the liquor begins to work, and endangers the bursting of the bottles." A similar humoral-climatic theory is elaborated to explain the autumnal intermittent fevers. The autumnal quartans are to be treated by "the bark" which, however, "more frequently checks, than cures the disease." Completion of "commotion" (for which Sydenham continually uses the condemned words, fermentation and ebullition) is essential to complete cure; therefore, "the bark" should not be administered too soon. The swelling of the abdomen in children is "a good sign." "There is no hopes of vanquishing the disease till the *abdomen* (especially that part of it near the spleen) swells and grows hard; the distemper abating in the same degree, as this symptom manifests itself."

Section II deals with the fateful plague years of 1665 and 1666. The year 1665, according to Sydenham, was marked by severe "peripneu-monies, pleurisies and quinsies" in the winter months, by a peculiar epidemic fever in late winter and early spring, and by the outbreak of the plague in mid-year. Both the malignant fever and the plague are related to the mysterious epidemic constitution of 1665. In the case of plague, however, another factor is at work. Sydenham says:

"4. But besides the constitution of the air, as a more general cause, there must be another previous circumstance to produce the plague, *viz.* the receiving the effluvia, or *seminium*, from an infected person, either immediately by contact, or mediately by pestilential matter, conveyed from some other place. And when this happens in such a constitution, as we have mentioned above, the whole air of that tract of land is quickly infected with the plague, by means of the breath of the diseased, and the steam or vapour arising from the dead bodies, so as to render the way of propagating this dreadful disease by infection entirely unnecessary: for tho' a person be most cautiously removed from the infected, yet the air, received in by breathing, will of itself be sufficient to infect him, provided his juices be disposed to receive the infection.

"5. Tho' this distemper, when it is only *sporadic*, seizes some few persons, without any regard to the season, the infection being, as it were, communicated from one to another; yet when an epidemic constitution of the air likewise prevails, it arises in the intermediate season between spring and summer; this season being the fittest to produce a disease, the essence of which chiefly consists in an inflammatory state of the juices, as we shall afterwards shew. Again, this disease has its times of increase and declension, like other kinds of natural things. It begins at the time above set down, as the year advances it spreads, and as that declines it abates, till, at length, winter introduces a state of the air contrary to it.

"6. For if the changes of the season were to have no effect on this disease, the true pestilential *seminium*, unconquerable by any alteration of the air, would be conveyed from one person to another in a continued succession; so that when once it had got into a populous city, it would rage more and more, and never cease till it had destroyed all the inhabitants. But that the contrary frequently happens, appears from the number of the dead, which rose to some thousands in one week in August, but decreased very much, and was inconsiderable toward the end of *November*. I must own, however, what some authors have likewise asserted, that the plague appears at other seasons of the year; but this seldom happens, and it is not then very violent.

"7. Mean time I much doubt if the disposition of the air, tho' it be pestilential, is of itself able to produce the *plague*; but the plague, being always in some place or other, it is conveyed by pestilential particles, or the coming of an infected person from some place where it rages into an uninfected one, and is not epidemic there, unless the constitution of the air favours it. Otherwise I cannot conceive how it should happen that when the *plague* rages violently in one town in the same climate, a neighbouring one should totally escape it, by strictly forbidding all intercourse with the infected place; an instance of which we had some few years ago, when the plague raged with extreme violence in most parts of *Italy*, and yet the Grand Duke by his vigilance and prudence entirely prevented its penetrating the borders of Tuscany."

The paragraphs cited give us Sydenham's first real mention of the factor of contagion; and his recognition of the two factors of season and contagion is entirely sound, so far as plague is concerned.

Section III deals with the epidemics of 1667-1669, which included smallpox, a "variolous fever" resembling smallpox, and dysentery. The latter, however, "so nearly resembled the then reigning variolous fever, that it should seem to be only the fever turned inwards, and fixed upon the bowels." Nowhere is there a reference to contagion.

Section IV discusses the epidemics of 1669-1672 which included cholera morbus, dysentery, continued fever, measles, anomalous small-pox and bilious colic. A passage in Chapter I of this section illustrates the intimate specificity of the relationship between constitution and disease postulated by Sydenham. He explains the lesser severity of intestinal disease in summer than in autumn by the assumption "that the then reigning constitution had not yet so perfect a tendency to a dysentery, as to be able to produce all those symptoms in every subject, which affect such as are seized with this disease; for in the following *autumn*, when the gripes returned, the *dysentery* was accompanied with every pathognomic symptom." Here, too, Sydenham launches one of his dominant theories—that one epidemic tends to expel another. Measles in 1670 and tertian fever in 1671 "prevailed so considerably as to over-power the smallpox, and prevent its spreading much in the beginning of these years." In the late summer of 1672, dysentery became mild and some smallpox occurred. In Sydenham's view, "the constitution of the air, having a less tendency to produce the dysentery rendered the smallpox powerful enough to equal it." Chapter II deals with the cholera morbus of 1669 and contains the following example of Sydenham's overwhelming emphasis, when he says, "as if there lay concealed some peculiar disposition in the air of this particular month, which is able to impregnate the blood, or ferment of the stomach, with a kind of specific alteration adapted only to this disease." Chapter III on dysenteries again indicates the conception that constitutions—not diseases in our sense—were the specific entities: "For possibly there may be as many sorts of dysenteries, as there are kinds of smallpox, and other epidemics peculiar to different constitutions, and which may therefor require a different method of cure in some particulars." Chapters IV-VII on epidemics of continued fever, measles, anomalous smallpox and bilious colic in 1670-1672 contain precisely similar passages.

Section V deals with epidemics of the years 1673 to 1675, and follows the same lines, one disease "introducing" or "passing into" or "changing into" another, always under the primary influence of the epidemic constitution, as modified by season. In Chapter V is the following more detailed explanation of the genesis of a particular constitution or "disposition." "I conceive it more probable," Sydenham says, "that a certain particular tract of air becomes replete with *effluvia* from some mineral fermentation, which infecting the air through which they pass, with such particles as prove destructive, sometimes to one kind of animals, and sometimes to another, continue to propagate the diseases peculiar to the various dispositions of the earth, till the subterraneous supplies of those *effluvia* fail." Again, he says, "that diseases have certain periods, resulting from the secret and hitherto unknown alterations happening in the bowels of the earth." In Chapter V, he states that "the malignity in epidemics, whatever its specific nature may be, consists and centers in very hot and spirituous particles, that are more or less opposite to the nature of the circulating fluids." Where, as in plague, these particles are very subtle, they can be eliminated by sweating; in other fevers they may be less subtle and so mixed with grosser humors, that sweating is of no avail. In Chapter VI, which is a recapitulation, recognition of the prevailing "disposition" is given primary weight in diagnosis. When a physician is called in to attend a continued fever, "he may easily learn, either from his own observation, or the relation of others, what other diseases besides this fever rage epidemically in those places, and of what kind they are: which being known, he will no longer be in doubt of what kind that fever is, which accompanies the other then reigning epidemic."

Section VI deals with a group of what Sydenham calls "Intercurrent Fevers," diseases which are less strikingly related to any peculiar constitution than those previously discussed. These are the diseases which later were called "endemic"; and they include scarlet fever, pleurisy, bastard peripneumony, rheumatism, erysipelatous fever and the quinsy. These diseases "generally arise from some peculiar disorder of particular bodies, whereby the blood and juices are some way vitiated, yet sometimes they proceed *mediately* from some general cause in the air, which, by its manifest qualities so disposes the human body, as to occasion certain disorders of the blood and juices, which prove the immediate causes of such *epidemic intercurrents*." This is an extremely interesting recognition of those diseases in which lowering of vital resistance plays an important role—which Dr. E. S. Godfrey has recently described as "opportunistic infections." As to their external causes, such fevers, Sydenham tells us, resemble in certain respects the "stationary fevers"—those which are chiefly determined by the epidemic constitution. "For not to mention infection, which sometimes communicates stationary fevers[1] and *surfeits*, which give rise to both stationary and intercurrent fevers, the manifest external cause of the greater part of fevers is to be sought for hence; either (1) a person hath left off his clothes too soon, or (2) imprudently exposed his body to the cold after being heated with violent exercise; whence the pores being suddenly closed, and the perspirable matter retained in the body, that would otherwise have passed thro' them, such a particular kind of fever is raised in the blood, as the then reigning general constitution, or the particular depravity of the juices, is most inclined to produce. And indeed I am of opinion, that abundance more have been destroyed by this means than by the *plague, sword*, and *famine* together; for if a physician examines his patient strictly concerning the first occasion of the disease, he will generally find it to proceed from one of these causes, provided it be of the number of those acute diseases we have treated of above. Upon this account I always advise my friends never to leave off any wearing apparel till a month before midsummer; and not to expose themselves to the cold after being heated by exercise."

In Chapter II of this section, scarlet fever is described as an autumnal disease which "seems to me to be nothing more than a moderate effervescence of the blood, occasioned by the heat of the preceding summer." In Chapter III pleurisy, which occurs in the spring, is explained by the theory that "the blood being then heated by the fresh approach of the sun, is much disposed to fermentation and immoderate commotions."

[1] This appears to be the second reference to contagion in Sydenham's voluminous works.

"Bastard peripneumony" in Chapter IV is attributed to the blood "loaden with phlegmatic humours collected in the winter" and "put into fresh motion by the approaching spring." Chapters V-VII discuss rheumatism, erysipelatous fever and the quinsy but add nothing of epidemiological significance.

Thus closes Sydenham's basic memoir on the acute diseases, which makes up about half of his *Collected Works*. It is followed by a series of letters in answer to requests for further information. The first of these, addressed to Dr. R. Brady, deals with the epidemic constitution of the period 1675 to 1680. In view of the prevalence of tertian and quotidian fevers,[2] much space is devoted to treatment with Peruvian bark. Unusual prevalence of coughs in 1679 gives occasion for the following highly mechanical explanation of their cause: "the month of October having been wetter than usual (for it seldom ceased raining) the blood, corresponding with the season, drank in abundance of crude, watery particles, by reason that perspiration was stopt upon the first coming of the cold, whence nature endeavored to expel them, by means of a cough."

Sir Henry Panam wrote to Sydenham for guidance in regard to the treatment of venereal disease since "it is enough for the patient to be punished by the Supreme Being, and not to be tormented more severely by his physician"; and a long letter on this subject follows, as Sydenham's first contribution to the subject of chronic diseases. He accepts the Columbian origin of syphilis and has a complete understanding of its transmissibility, being far ahead of many later medical authorities in this regard. Furthermore, he recognizes congenital infection (from either parent!), transmission to children by suckling or other contact, as well as by the more usual method of sexual intercourse. Symptomatic description of venereal disease is admirable, although gonorrhea is interpreted rather as a symptom or stage of the disease than as an independent entity.[3] The gonorrheal stage of the disease is to be treated chiefly by purging, the more advanced stage (syphilis) by mercurials, which owe their power entirely to their power of producing salivation.

A letter from Dr. William Cole elicits a third epistle on smallpox and hysteric diseases. The first part of this essay, dealing with smallpox, is chiefly an argument against too early confinement to bed, and contains

---

[2] It is interesting to note the high incidence of malaria in England at this period.

[3] Although he recognizes, with characteristic acuteness of observation "that though a salivation excels every other remedy in curing a *confirmed pox*, yet it is not able to conquer a *gonorrhea*, when joined therewith, for this disorder continues after the former is perfectly cured."

nothing of epidemiological interest, except the theory that an unusual severity of the disease in 1681 was due to the extreme dryness of the season. In the latter part of the memoir, he makes the interesting observation that "as fevers with their attendants constitute two-thirds of the diseases to which mankind are liable, upon comparing them with the whole tribe of chronic distempers, so hysteric disorders, or at least such as are so called, make up half the remaining third part, that is, they constitute one moiety of chronic distempers." This discussion of hysteric disorders, although beyond the scope of the present volume, is one of the most remarkable of Sydenham's writings and constitutes a highly significant contribution to mental hygiene. As illustrated by Galen earlier and Rush later, the great clinicians have always been keenly conscious of this problem. There is, in this chapter, however, one interesting casual reference in our field, in allusion to quartan fever "wherewith a person in perfect health may be seized, by residing two or three days in moist and marshy places." Horseback riding is recommended for hysteric diseases and also—less fortunately—for consumptions.

There follows a long essay on the gout and dropsy, which includes a passage of interest to us. Sydenham digresses at one point to discuss the general difference between acute and chronic diseases and has this to say of the former:

"Now, whether the inmost bowels of the earth (if the expression be allowable) undergo various alterations, so as to infect the air by the vapours thence arising, which seems very probable to me; or whether the whole atmosphere be infected by means of an alteration, resulting from a peculiar conjunction of any of the planets; certain it is, that the air sometimes abounds with such particles as injure the human body; as at another time it becomes impregnated with such particles as prove pernicious to some species of brutes. During this state of the air, as oft as we receive into the blood by breathing the poisonous corpuscles which are prejudicial to the body, and contract such epidemic diseases, as such tainted air is apt to produce, nature raises a fever, which is the ordinary instrument it employs to free the blood from any noxious matter therein contained." Chronic diseases on the other hand are "of a very different nature"; for "though a certain and unwholesome air may greatly contribute to their production, yet they do not so immediately proceed from the air, but generally from the indigestion of the humors, the common origin of all these diseases." He draws the sound conclusion that chronic disease can be controlled only by a continued program of personal hygiene.

Schedula Monitoria or an Essay on the Rise of a New Fever (possibly typhus?) contains no epidemiology except the brief repetition of an earlier statement, "that the change of a constitution depends principally on some secret and hidden alteration in the bowels of the earth, communicated to the whole atmosphere, or on some influence of the planets."

Finally, the most systematic of Sydenham's works is his *Processus Integri*; or Complete Methods of Curing Most Diseases—a Seventeenth Century Osler. Here are only two references of significance for us. In treating of venereal disease, Sydenham again emphasizes his concept that gonorrhea and syphilis are stages of the same disease, saying, "When the blood is tainted by the long continuance of a gonorrhea, or the unadvised use of astringents, the true pox appears." In the last section on consumption, he advances the following theory.

"There are several kinds of consumptions. (1) The first mostly arises from taking cold in winter; abundance of persons being seized with a cough upon the coming in of cold weather, a little before the winter solstice, which happening to such as have naturally weak lungs, these parts must needs be still more weakened by frequent fits of coughing, and become so diseased at length hereby, as to be utterly unable to assimilate their proper nourishment. Hence a copious crude phlegm is collected, which by the continual agitation of the lungs, occasioned by the vehement cough accompanying this distemper, is plentifully expectorated. The lungs being hereby supplied with purulent matter, taint the whole mass of blood therewith, whence arises a putrid fever, the fit whereof comes towards evening, and goes off towards morning with profuse and debilitating sweats. Lastly, to close the scene, a looseness succeeds, occasioned partly by corrupt humours, discharged from the mesenteric arteries into the intestines, and deposited there, and partly by the weakened tone of the viscera; and thus the patient perishes at length the following summer by a distemper occasioned by the foregoing winter. And this is the principal kind of disease.

"Moreover, as the blood in winter abounds with moist particles, and perspiration is too much check'd by the sudden contraction of the pores, these particles insinuate themselves into the lungs, thro' the ramifications of the arterial vein, or pulmonary artery, which runs thro' the whole substance of the lungs, or are discharged by the salival ducts, and deposited in the glands of the throat, whence the humor being now fallen thro' the aspera arteria upon the lungs, irritates these parts continually, like a catarrh, and the frequent and violent fits of coughing, soon cause the weakness and other symptoms above enumerated. And when the lungs lose their natural tone, tubercles ordinarily breed therein, which, upon viewing the lungs of those that perish by this distemper, generally appear filled with purulent matter."

Other, less important types of consumption are due to hot acrimonious particles influenced by overheating due to drinking too much wine and to "the translation of febrile matter to the lungs in the declension of a fever, which, being more debilitated hereby, are attacked with the symptoms just enumerated." Here is a rather keen perception of the contributory influence of chilling and acute respiratory infection, of alcoholic excess, and of debilitating fevers in lowering resistance to tuberculosis.

This is the sum of Sydenham's contribution to epidemiology; and the picture presented is simple and logically clear. This was why it had so wide an influence.

The causes of disease were threefold: (1) an internal factor, the development within the body of an abnormal composition of the humors; (2) an external factor, the influence of the known factors of climate and seasons, heat, cold, moisture and dryness; and (3) a second external factor, the mysterious epidemic constitution of the atmosphere, characteristic of a given year. Such a disease as gout was chiefly determined by the humoral factor, the regularly endemic maladies, such as the respiratory diseases of winter and the intermittent fevers, chiefly by the seasonal climatic factor, widespread unusual epidemics, like plague, by the epidemic constitution. The specific characteristics of a given disease at a given time were determined by interaction of all three.

The sharp recognition of internal and external factors in the causation of disease was a valuable contribution to epidemiology, although this was, of course, no new conception. Indeed, in most respects Sydenham followed closely the classical Hippocratic doctrines, all three of his three major factors being those which are present in "Airs, Waters and Places." In his emphasis on climate and season, however, Sydenham rendered a very special service, for this

factor, since the classical period of medicine, had been somewhat neglected. It is probably this emphasis to which Garrison refers when he
speaks of Sydenham's outstanding contribution to epidemiology.

The stress laid by "the English Hippocrates" upon epidemic constitution was less fortunate. Here, indeed, he was pre-Hippocratic, rather
than Hippocratic. In "Airs, Waters and Places," major emphasis is laid
on observable factors of physical constitution and on climate and season; and the "epidemic constitution of the atmosphere" is called in to
explain only the residual phenomenon of unusual epidemic disease
which cannot be understood in any other way. From Galen down
through the plague tracts and the sixteenth century writers, this had
been the procedure followed. "Epidemic Constitution" was the *Deus
ex machina*, called in as a last resort to account for an unexplained
residuum. With Sydenham, it becomes the central feature of the etiology
of disease. This factor, in Sydenham's own words was "secret and inexplicable," having no relation to "the manifest qualities of the air." To
introduce such an influence as a sort of "x-factor," to account for residual
phenomena is a reasonable recognition of the limits of current knowledge; but to make a factor which lies beyond the realm of observation
the major basis of one's theories is to abandon science for metaphysics.
If the cause of any phenomenon is of such a nature that it cannot be
observed, it lies outside the field of science. The theory of epidemic
constitution, developed to the degree to which Sydenham developed
it, provided an imposing verbal explanation of any phenomenon which
might occur; but such a facile answer closed the door to research and
made any real progress in epidemiology slow and difficult.

A by-product of the stress laid upon epidemic constitution was the
conception that one epidemic disease merged into, and was transformed
into, another. Logically enough, Sydenham believed that, since epidemic
constitution and season determined the character of an epidemic, a
change in these factors which was favorable to one disease must be unfavorable to another. Thus, if plague increased, smallpox must necessarily decrease. There was sound basis for this view, so far as seasonal
influences are concerned. When, however, the metaphysical concept of
epidemic constitution was prominently introduced, each particular outbreak of disease became a unique and unpredictable entity. It is true, as
Sigerist says, that Sydenham passed from the Hippocratic concept of
an individual case of illness to the conception of an epidemic entity
prevailing at a given time. Yet he hindered, rather than promoted, the

true conception of a basic *disease* entity, having fundamental common characteristics, influenced by season and by unknown factors, but nevertheless unique and identifiable at various times and in various years.

As to the vital factor of contagion, Sydenham is strangely oblivious of the contributions of Galen, of Avicenna, and of the authors of the plague tracts—not to mention Fracastorius and Kircher. Contagion is mentioned by him only three times, clearly and definitely in regard to plague and venereal disease, and incidentally in his discussion of intercurrent and stationary fevers. Nowhere, however, is this important factor stressed. It is not even mentioned in connection with smallpox and measles; and not a single suggestion is ever made as to the danger of infection or any precautions suggested in the nature of isolation or quarantine. Such an omission is peculiarly significant in view of the marked developments of practice along such lines, from the thirteenth century onward. It must have been devastating in its effect on later medical thinking which was so greatly influenced by Sydenham's works.

Nothing can dim the glory of Sydenham's achievements as a clinician. His keen observation and exact recording of case histories had an incalculable influence for good upon the future of medicine. Even in the field of epidemiology, his stress upon seasonal influences was valuable and important; and his concept of an epidemic-entity perhaps led on toward the conception of a true disease-entity. On the other hand, his almost complete neglect of contagion as a practical factor in the spread of epidemic disease and his major stress upon the metaphysical factor of epidemic constitution held back epidemiological progress for two hundred years.

CHAPTER X

THE LAST OF THE PLAGUE TRACTATES

"Dr. Mead lived more in the broad sunshine of life than almost any man."—
SAMUEL JOHNSON

THE period of European history between 1650 and 1800 had a
quality all its own. To pass into this comfortable, assured,
sharply sunlit area seems like the entry to a different world.
Milton is succeeded by Pope, Spinoza by Kant, Rembrandt and Velasquez by Reynolds and Gainsborough. It is a world of crystallization
and formalism and satisfaction rather than of struggle and efflorescence
—a phase of fruition rather than flowering. In science, the period of tow-
ering giants like Newton and Harvey was passing, but their place was
taken by mathematical physicists and chemists of the order of Laplace,
Priestley, Cavendish, Lavoisier and Galvani and by the inventors, Fulton, Stephenson and Watt. In medicine, the systematist, Linnaeus, and
the inspiring teacher, Boerhaave, were perhaps the outstanding figures.

This world of two hundred years ago was a very pleasant place for
the more fortunate classes of society. It was what Wells has called the
period of the Grand and Parliamentary Monarchies, with George II of
England, Louis XIV of France and Frederick I of Prussia among its
prominent figures. The last quarter of the seventeenth and the first
quarter of the eighteenth century had been periods of many wars, yet
these wars did little to disrupt the course of economic and social life.
Leeuwenhoek continued to dispatch his communications to the Royal
Society of London in complete indifference to the fact that England and
Holland were at war. Economic conditions were on the whole favorable,
even for the lower classes. The world of thought was permeated by a
placid optimism which had its parallel in the later Victorian age of our
own youth. Gibbon, a little later, wrote, "Since the first discovery of
the arts, war, commerce, and religious zeal have diffused, among the
savages of the Old and New World, those inestimable gifts, they have
been successively propagated; they can never be lost. We may therefore
acquiesce in the pleasing conclusion that every age of the world has increased, and still increases, the real wealth, the happiness, the knowledge, and perhaps the virtue of the human race."

In England the world seemed particularly bright. Creative intellectual effort had not been encouraged under the Commonwealth; but with the restoration of Charles II in 1660 a new era set in. In contrast to the romantic spirit of earlier English letters it was dominated by the academic influence of France where the English courtiers had lived in their exile.

Central figure of our present chapter, Richard Mead, was born at Stepney in 1673, the son of a distinguished divine and a member of a wealthy Buckinghamshire family. He worked under Graevius at Utrecht and studied botany under Hermann and physick under Pitcairn at Leyden. He took his degree of doctor of philosophy and physick at Padua in 1695, returning in the next year, 1696, to begin practice at Stepney.

In 1703 Mead was appointed physician in St. Thomas' Hospital and later was asked to read the anatomical lectures in the hall of the Company of Surgeons. In 1707 he was made a doctor of physick of Oxford and in 1716 a fellow of the College of Physicians. He was also elected to the Royal Society of which he was a counselor and in 1717 served as vice president.

In 1714, when John Radcliffe, who had been physician to William III, and perhaps the leading physician in London, retired, shortly before his death, he turned over his practice to his young friend Mead. It was through Radcliffe's influence that Mead was summoned to the deathbed of Queen Anne in that year, and the foundation of his career was largely laid upon the prestige thus established.

Mead also received from Radcliffe the famous gold-headed cane, immortalized by William MacMichael, which was later to be the property of Askew, Pitcairn and Baillie, and which now retains an honored place in the library of the Royal College of Physicians.

In the year 1719 an outbreak of the plague at Marseilles was causing grave alarm (the great epidemic of 1665 being still fresh in London memory). Was this dread disease a contagion imported from abroad and to be excluded by quarantine, or was it a disease periodically generated in a given locality and beyond human control? The Lords of the Regency directed the Secretary of State to ask Mead for a report on this matter, and the document presented by him in response to this request was a vitally important contribution to epidemiology.

Mead was by now established as the leading medical practitioner in London. In 1726 he and Cheselden, the surgeon, were called in consultation by Sir Isaac Newton, recalling the line of Pope: "I'll try what

Mead and Cheselden advise." In 1727 on the accession of George II, Mead, who had attended him as Prince of Wales, was appointed Physician to the King. He died on February 16, 1754, at the age of 81, full of years and honors.

From a material standpoint Mead certainly had every reason to develop the psychology of success. At the height of his career he enjoyed an average income of £5,000 to £6,000, which had a purchasing power equivalent to approximately $100,000 today. He commonly charged a guinea as an office fee and 2 guineas or more for a home visit, and, like Radcliffe, he made it a practice while sitting in his coffee house (and without seeing the patients himself) to write prescriptions for half a guinea each for apothecaries who brought in verbal reports of cases.

Mead was as generous, however, as he was successful. The *Authentic Memoirs of the Life of Richard Mead, M.D.*, (Whiston and White) say of him:

"During almost half a century, he was at the head of his business, which brought him in one year seven thousand pounds and upwards, and for several years between five and six thousand pounds. His generous and benevolent Temper was constantly exercised in acts of charity. Clergymen, and in general all men of learning, were welcome to his advice, and his doors were always open every morning to the most indigent, whom he frequently assisted with his purse; so that notwithstanding his great gains he did not dye very rich, being persuaded, that what he got from the public could never be bestowed more honourably, than in the advancement of Science, and the encouragement of the Learned."

Mead enjoyed a remarkable reputation as a scholar and a patron of the arts. His library where his principal collections were housed was sixty feet long, and his house in Great Ormond Street is described as "a temple of nature and a repository of time."

In the *Authentic Memoirs* we read: "Nothing did more honor to this Patron of Learning than the free and constant access of men of different qualifications to his table, who were each employed the rest of the day, at his particular work or study. There no man's talents were misplaced, none was honoured with an undue preference: the Scholar took his place near the Naturalist, and the Mathematician near the Antiquarian or the Painter. Every one found himself surrounded with objects capable of instructing him, or exciting his emulation. Our Maecenas was frequently the only man in company, who was acquainted with all their different languages, and was able to perform the office of an interpreter to them all: he constantly questioned them in a most obliging manner, about their different occupations, taking great pleasure in commending their several performances and discoveries, and by this means, inspired them all with emulation and a reciprocal esteem for each other.

"No foreigner of any learning, taste, or even curiosity, ever came to London without being introduced to Dr. Mead; it would have been a shame to return home without having seen him. On these occasions, his table was always open, and united the Magnificence of Princes with the Pleasures of Philosophers."

Mead was a friend of Pope, Halley and Newton as well as of Garth, Arbuthnot, and the leading physicians of his time. He carried on a constant correspondence with Boerhaave, who had been a fellow student at Leyden. He represented to perfection the highest aims of the medicine of his day which visualized the physician as, above all, a cultivated gentleman.

Mead produced six literary works of major importance in addition to several minor ones. His earliest contribution entitled *A Mechanical Account of Poisons* was first published in 1702 six years after he began practice. It includes reports of elementary but highly courageous experiments made by the author upon snake venom, and it is notable that the author maintains throughout a mechanistic approach with an indomitable conviction that biological phenomena were governed by physical and chemical laws. He relies upon experiment to unveil those laws. And he is eager and open-minded in the attempt to utilize the newest results of the physical science of the day in explaining the reactions which occur in living tissue. If Mead had not become involved in the responsibilities of active practice, this work suggests that he might have made a real name for himself as an experimental physiologist.

His second work *On the Influence of the Sun and Moon upon Human Bodies and the Diseases Thereby Produced* is an attempt to explain celestial influences on health (which were of course accepted as real by all philosophers of the time) on the basis of Newtonian mechanics. There is a very interesting appeal for theoretical analysis as well as experimental observation in medicine.

Mead's third major work, *A Discourse on the Plague*, was published in 1720 and went through seven editions in one year. The eighth enlarged edition was published in 1723 with a new chapter on treatment, and the final revision in 1744.

After the first appearance of the *Discourse on the Plague*, when Mead was forty-seven years of age, there was a long period of twenty-seven years during which no new contributions to literature came from his pen. This, of course, corresponds to the height of his activity as a fashionable practitioner. At the age of 74 he began to find leisure for writing once more, and in 1747 published his fourth major work, *A Discourse on the Smallpox and Measles*, to which we shall refer again, in so far as it contributes to epidemiological theory.

Mead's fifth major contribution, *Medica Sacra*, appeared in 1749; and is an ingenious and suggestive attempt to interpret passages in the Bible dealing with medical matters. In this work, Mead's handling of Biblical events is reverent and dignified, but with a consistent effort to emphasize natural law and to minimize the idea of irrational divine punishments and the emphasis of many commentators on the influence of demons.

His sixth and last work was *Medical Precepts and Cautions*, published in 1751 when the writer was seventy-eight years of age. This distillate of a long life of medical practice and philosophical thinking is a general discussion of the symptoms and treatment of various diseases designed apparently for the general public; and it has been considered by many medical commentators to be Mead's most important contribution.

The *Discourse on the Plague* is, however, a more masterly example of logical and philosophical analysis than any of Mead's other works.

It is an interesting fact that this outstanding contribution of the eighteenth century to the theory of epidemiology was again concerned with the plague; and as the "Last of the Great Plague Tractates" is a lineal descendant of the long and distinguished series of documents dating back to Jehan Jacme of Lerida in 1348.

On the whole, epidemics of communicable disease were much less serious and much less widespread in the eighteenth century than in the seventeenth. Malaria, influenza and scarlet fever were common, as were diphtheria, pertussis and smallpox in somewhat lesser degree. The last disease was being fought by inoculation; and Mead played a considerable part in popularizing this practice in England, being appointed by George I to conduct experiments on condemned criminals to demonstrate its value. Typhus was prevalent as "Camp

Fever" and "Jail Fever." Epidemics of yellow fever occurred in various parts of the New World and attracted wide attention. Plague and syphilis were much less malignant than in the seventeenth century; but serious epidemics of the former pestilence occurred in Turkey, Russia, Scandinavia and Germany in 1709 and 1710. There was an outbreak in Southern France in 1719 and 1720; and the serious epidemic at Marseilles was the threat which led to the preparation of the *Discourse on the Plague.* As first published this was a small pamphlet of about 7,000 words, the first third devoted to "Nature of Contagion," the last two-thirds to "Methods to Prevent Contagion." In later editions it grew to much larger proportions with a preface of 6,000 words; Part I "On the Plague in General" (11,000 words), including chapters on the origin and nature of the plague and on causes which spread the plague; and Part II "On the Methods to be taken Against the Plague" (11,000 words), including chapters on preventing infection from other countries, on "stopping the progress of the plague, if it should enter our country," and on "the cure of the plague." In the analysis which follows, citations are chiefly from the second Dublin edition of 1721, which represents essentially the original form and from the final revision of 1744 as reprinted in the 1767 Dublin edition of Mead's collected works.

In the explanation of the mysterious phenomena of epidemic disease five different sorts of causes had been invoked ever since the days of the Hippocratic writings. These five causes may be briefly designated as (1) the wrath of the gods, (2) the general epidemic constitution of the atmosphere, (3) local miasmatic conditions due to climate, season and organic decomposition, (4) contagion and (5) variations in individual vital resistance. The first of these factors was dominant with Procopius but had been discarded by serious students since the Middle Ages and the fifth was a vague assumption to explain exceptional cases. A study of theories of epidemiology from Hippocrates to Pasteur centers, therefore, about the relative emphasis laid upon epidemic constitution of the atmosphere, local miasms and contagion.

To the modern scientist it is often difficult to realize why the development of the concept of contagion was so slow and, particularly, why it was generally emphasized by laymen while physicians laid stress upon epidemic constitution and miasmatic influence. Thucydides described the plague as contagious but Hippocrates considered it to be caused by a corruption of the atmosphere which he corrected by burning spices in the streets. The Princes of the Church instituted quarantine measures for the practical control of leprosy in the sixth century, and the maritime cities throughout Europe did the same for plague in the fourteenth. Yet even at this latter period, when the great pandemic of plague was devastating the whole world, the medical faculty of Paris represented a considerable body of orthodox opinion when it reported in 1348 that "the immediate cause of the present epidemic" was a malign conjunction of planets over the Indian Ocean which produced "corrupt vapors," "raised up and disseminated through the air by the blasts of the heavy and turbid southerly winds." When Marseilles suffered from the plague in 1720 (the outbreak which caused the Lords of the Regency to call upon Mead for his report) the anonymous author of the "Relation historique de tout ce qui s'est passé à Marseille pendant la dernière Peste" was a contagionist; but Chicoyneau and other leaders of the medical profession at Marseilles strongly upheld the miasmatic theory.

We cannot dismiss the resistance of the medical profession to the doctrine of contagion as merely an evidence of hidebound conservatism. There were sound reasons for this attitude. The layman perceived the broad truth of contagion as he watched the plague spread from country to country and from seaport to seaport; but the physician, knowing the facts more intimately, realized that no *existing* theory of contagion taken by itself could possibly explain those facts. Contagion, before the germ theory, was visualized as the direct passage of some chemical or physical influence from a sick person to a susceptible victim by contact or fomites or, for a relatively short distance, through the atmosphere. The physician knew that such a theory was clearly inadequate. Cases occurred without any possibility of such a direct influence. Cases failed to occur when such a direct influence was present. Epidemics broke out without the introduction into the locality of any recognizable case from without; and within the city or country they raged in a particular section and failed completely to spread beyond the borders of that area. Outbreaks began and outbreaks ceased without any causes that could be directly related to the presence or the absence of the sick. Until the theory of inanimate contagion was replaced by a theory of living germs and until to that theory were added the concepts of long-distance transmission by water and food supplies and, above all, of human and animal carriers—the hypothesis of contagion simply would not work. The task of the epidemiologist of this period was to supplement the conception of contagion by the simplest and most rational "x-factor" which would serve to explain the observed phenomena. It was this task which Mead accomplished more adequately than any other student of his time.

The theory of divine wrath as a cause of epidemic disease does not occupy much space in Mead's writings. He begins his later editions with reference to the conception that epidemics were judgments of God and counters with arguments based on Hippocrates' great dictum that no sickness is more divine than any other, all coming from the Gods but all owning natural causes. He recognizes, as almost all writers have done, the possible significance of individual resistance as influenced by personal hygiene, though without laying great stress upon this factor.

Most remarkable is the fact that the theory of a general, more or less world-wide epidemic constitution of the atmosphere (as distinct from purely local miasmatic conditions) finds almost no place in Mead's philosophy. This had been a current and accepted doctrine since the days of Hippocrates and it was to continue to play a major role in epidemiology through the whole of the eighteenth century. It was the dominant theory emphasized by the great Sydenham. Mead does not combat this theory. He scarcely alludes to it. It was characteristic of his naturalistic and experimental tone of thought that he seized upon the two immediate practical factors of contagion and local miasms and quietly ignored the more philosophical conception which he found unnecessary to explain the observed phenomena with which he was familiar.

He states his theory quite clearly in the first edition of the *Discourse* as follows: "Contagion is propagated by three causes, the air, Diseased Persons and Goods transported from infected Places." We may consider diseased persons and goods as merely two forms of contagion in the modern sense—so that Mead's three factors reduce to two, air and contagion, with major emphasis on the latter. In the later edition he begins with a discussion of the history of the plague in various countries and continues as follows:

"I have been thus particular in tracing the Plague up to its first origin, in order to remove, as much as possible, all objection against what I shall say of the causes, which excite and propagate it among us. This is done by contagion. Those who are strangers to the full power of this, that is, those who do not understand how subtle it is, and how widely the distemper may be spread by infection, ascribe the rise of it wholly to the malignant quality of the air in all places, wherever it happens; and, on the other hand, some have thought that the consideration of the infectious nature of the disease must exclude all regard to the influence of the air: whereas the contagion accompanying the disease, and the disposition of the air to promote that contagion, ought equally to be considered; both being necessary to give the distemper full force. The design therefore of this chapter, is to make a proper ballance between these two, and to set just limits to the effects of each."

We must first understand what Mead had in mind in his conception of the aerial or miasmatic factor in the causation of the plague.

Like the Hippocratic writers, he considers that the air may be corrupted by heat, rain and southerly winds. Above all, however, he lays stress on the influence of organic decomposition. He says,

"It has besides been remarked in all Times, that the Stinks of *stagnating Waters* in hot Weather, *putrid Exhalations* from the Earth; and above all, the Corruption of dead *Carcasses* lying unburied, have occasioned *infectious Diseases*.

"From hence it appears to be Concurrence of Causes, that produces Diseases of this Kind" (1721).

Plagues arise usually in southern countries: "Indeed *Plagues* seem to be of the Growth of the *Eastern* and *Southern* Parts of the World, and to be transmitted from them into colder Climates by the Way of *Commerce*. Nor do I think, that in this *Island* particularly there is any one Instance of a *Pestilential* Disease among us of great Consequence; which we did not receive from other *Infected* Places."

Hot, moist air is highly favorable. Air, however, does not carry infection from place to place without the aid of infection by people or fomites. This is proved by irregularities of spread. Mead says:

"I own it cannot be demonstrated, that when the Plague makes great ravage in any town, the number of sick shall never be great enough to load the air with infectious effluvia, emitted from them in such plenty, that they may be conveyed by the winds into a neighbouring town or village without being dispersed so much as to hinder their producing any ill effects; especially since it is not unusual for the air to be so far charged with these noxious atoms, as to leave no place within the infected town secure: insomuch that when the distemper is at its heighth, all shall be indifferently infected, as well those who keep from the sick, as those who are near them; though at the beginning of a Plague to avoid all communication with the diseased, is an effectual defence. However, I do not think this is often the case: just as the smoke, with which the air of the city of London is constantly impregnated, especially

in winter, is not carried many miles distant; though the quantity of it
is vastly greater than the quantity of infectious effluvia, that the most
mortal Plague could generate" (1744).

Miasmatic influences cannot cause plague—in England at least—
without the factor of contagion. Therefore Mead opposes Sydenham's
view that plague occurs from natural causes every thirty or forty years—
a fatalistic concept which would have rendered the practice of quarantine of little avail.

Mead's concept of the relation between endemic and epidemic diseases was again discussed in his monograph on smallpox and measles
(1747) where he says:

"Now upon mature consideration of the whole affair, I am inclined
to think that there are certain diseases, which are originally engendered
and propagated in certain countries, as in their native soil. These by
Hippocrates are called diseases of the country; and some of them, sprung
up in various parts of Europe and Asia, from peculiar defects in the air,
soil and waters, he has most accurately described; but the more modern
Greeks called them endemick diseases. These, in my opinion, always
existed in their respective native places, as proceeding from the same
natural causes perpetually exerting themselves.

"It is found by experience, that some of these are contagious, and that
the contagion is frequently propagated to very remote countries by
means suitable to the nature of this or that disease. For some not only
communicate the infection by immediate contact of the sound with the
morbid body, but have such force, that they spread their pernicious
seeds by emitting very subtile particles; which lighting on soft spongy
substances, such as cotton, wool, raw-silk, and cloathing, penetrate into
them, and there remain pent up for a considerable time: in the same
manner as I have elsewhere accounted for the wide progress of the
plague from Africa its original country. Others, on the contrary, are
infectious by contact alone. Wherefore the first sort may be spread by
commerce, but the latter by cohabitation only."

The causes which lead to generation of miasms and the relation of
various terrestrial phenomena to epidemic disease are discussed with
admirable restraint and good sense in *Medical Precepts and Cautions*
(1751) as follows:

"Now, this matter, in my opinion at least, stands thus: that the manifest qualities of the air have a considerable share in producing epidemick
diseases, is a point that admits of no doubt; but there are other conjunct

causes, which alter the force of those qualities, either by encreasing or diminishing them. These chiefly spring from the earth, as Lucretius wisely said,

> When she's grown putrid by the rains, and sweats
> Such noxious vapours, press'd by scorching heats.

"Now as this terrestrial putridity is chiefly occasioned by rotted vegetables, and sometimes also by the dead bodies of animals, and by minerals; so the waters, especially of lakes and morasses, which have their plants and animals, in the same manner frequently exhale pestilential vapours, which infect the circumambient air. In this class may be ranged, though rarely happening in our climes, inundations, earthquakes, eruptions from mountains, and all other remarkable and uncommon phaenomena of nature, which are capable of filling the air we breathe, with particles offensive to animal life. For these affect our bodies, and prepare them for the easy reception of diseases."

We may proceed next to a consideration of the interrelationship between atmospheric and contagionistic factors, which Mead states very clearly in the following paragraphs from the original discourse.

"But to return to the Consideration of the Air, which we left in a putrid State: It is to be observed, that Putrefaction is a kind of Fermentation, and that all Bodies in a Ferment emit a volatile active Spirit, of Power to agitate, and put into intestine Motions, that is, to change the Nature of other Fluids into which it insinuates itself.

"This is one Step towards *Contagion*. The next, as it seems to me, proceeds after this Manner. The Blood in all *Malignant Fevers*, especially *Pestilential* ones, at the latter End of the Disease, does like Fermenting Liquors throw off a great Quantity of active Particles upon the several *Glands* of the Body, particularly on those of the Mouth and Skin, from which the Secretions are naturally the most constant and large. These, in *Pestilential* Cases, although the Air be in a right State, will generally infect those, who are very near to the sick Person; otherwise are soon dispersed and lost: But when in an evil Disposition of This they meet with the subtle Parts, its Corruption has generated, by uniting with them they become much more active and powerful, and likewise more durable and lasting, so as to form an Infectious Matter capable of conveying the Mischief to a great Distance from the diseased Body, out of which it was produced.

"A corrupted State of Air is without doubt necessary to give these

Contagious Atoms their full Force; for ⟨
conceive how the Plague, when once it had
cease, but with the destruction of all the ⟩
accounted for by supposing an Emendatio
and the restoring of it to a healthy State ca
pressing the Malignity.

"On the other hand it is evident, that *I*
the Air itself, however predisposed, witho
thing emitted from Infected Persons" (17⟨

We may consider next Mead's argument⟨
contagion. In passing, however, it should be emphasized once more that
he was wholly right in recognizing that something more than contagion
alone was essential for an explanation of the epidemiology of plague (or
of cholera or typhoid or most of the other great epidemic diseases). To
account for the fact that outbreaks occur at one time or at one place and
not at another, it was necessary to assume another "x-factor." Such a
factor, or factors, we can now assume to be the presence of rats and fleas;
but in Mead's time, and with Mead's theory of contagion, a chemical
corruption of the atmosphere was by far the most logical influence to
invoke.

In arguing for the reality and importance of contagion, Mead in his
later editions is clear and vigorous as to one vital point—the individual
specificity of plague and other epidemic diseases. Sydenham had assumed that one disease could be transformed into another and for a
century after Mead the same doctrine was maintained by Webster and
Rush and LaRoche with regard to yellow fever. Mead's incisive practical
mind would tolerate no such assumption.

He says, in this connection, "I cannot but very much admire to see
Dr. Chicoyneau, and the other physicians, who first gave us observations
on the Plague, when at Marseilles, relate in the reflections, they afterwards published upon those observations, the case of a man, who was
seized with the Plague, upon his burying a young woman dead of it,
when no one else dared to approach the body; and yet to see them ascribe
his disease, not to his being infected by the woman, but solely to his grief
for the loss of her, to whom he had made love, and to a Diarrhoea,
which had been some time upon him. No question but these concurred
to make his disease the more violent; and perhaps even exposed him to
contract the infection: but why should it be supposed, that he was not
infected, I cannot imagine, when there was so plain an appearance of it.

oss to find any colour of reason for their denying
er case, they relate, of a young lady seized with the
the sudden sight of a pestilential tumor, just broke out
aid; not allowing any thing but the lady's surprize to be the
her illness."

ad argues that spread of the disease in families proves the impor-
nce of contagion as it does in smallpox and measles; and that it cannot
be fear that causes the sickening, since young children often suffer. He
also cites the protection of certain colleges and monasteries by strict
quarantine. The failure of some individuals to contract the disease when
exposed (always stressed by opponents of contagion) he explains by
variation in vital resistance.

The major argument for contagion is, however, based on the obvious
fact of its gradual progress from one country to another country. Mead
claims that the sweating sickness of 1485, and the plague of 1665 were
imported (the latter by cotton from Turkey); and he traces out in detail
the spread of contagion in the great plague pandemic of 1349. Like
most of his contemporaries, however, he cannot accept the theory of
living germs.

"The third Way, by which we mentioned Contagion to be spread, is
by Goods transported from infected Places. It has been thought so difficult to explain the Manner of this, that some Authors have imagined
Infection to be performed by the Means of Insects, the Eggs of which
may be conveyed from Place to Place, and make the Disease when they
come to be hatched. As this is a Supposition grounded upon no manner
of Observation, I think there is no need to have Recourse to it. If, as we
have conjectured, the Matter of Contagion be an active Substance, perhaps in the Nature of a Salt, it is not hard to conceive how this may be
lodged and preserved in soft, porous Bodies, which are kept pressed
close together."

In summary, Mead's theory of the epidemiology of plague is excellently summarized in the following paragraph:

"To return from this digression: from all that has been said, it appears,
I think, very plainly, that the Plague is a real poison, which being bred
in the southern parts of the world, is carried by commerce into other
countries, particularly into Turkey, where it maintains itself by a kind
of circulation from persons to goods: which is chiefly owing to the negli-
gence of the people there, who are stupidly careless in this affair. That
when the constitution of the air happens to favor infection, it rages there

with great violence: that at that time more especially diseased persons give it to one another, and from them contagious matter is lodged in goods of a loose and soft texture, which being packed up and carried into other countries, let out when opened, the imprisoned seeds of contagion, and produce the disease whenever the air is disposed to give them force; otherwise they may be dissipated without any considerable ill effects. And lastly, that the air does not usually diffuse and spread these to any great distance, if intercourse and commerce with the place infected be strictly prevented" (1744).

This is the gist of Part I of the *Discourse* which deals with the origin, nature and causes of the plague. It is this section which was expanded so greatly in the later editions of the work. Part II, on practical methods of control, was but little modified from the original presentation of 1720 (except for the addition of a chapter on treatment). It is as notable for its common sense and its humanity as is Part I for its good judgment and philosophic balance.

Mead first considers defense against the importation of the plague from abroad, since he was rightly convinced that it was not an indigenous disease in England. To avoid importation, he recommends that lazarettos should be built at every port for the reception both of men and goods. Passengers and crew on an infected ship should be quarantined for thirty to forty days, after the men have been washed and shaved and their clothing changed. Clothes "harbour the very Quintessence of Contagion."

If there has been no sickness on a ship from an infected port, the men should be washed and cloths and goods aired at the lazaretto for one week.

"But the greatest Danger is from such Goods, as are apt to retain Infection, such as Cotton, Hemp and Flax, Paper or Books, Silk of all sorts, Linen, Wool, Feathers, Hair, and all kinds of Skins. The Lazaretto for these should be at a Distance from that for the Men, and they must in convenient Ware-houses be unpackt, and exposed, as much as may be, to the fresh Air for 40 days" (1721).

In connection with the control of spread from place to place within the country, Mead recommends a quarantine of twenty days between towns but not absolute prohibition of travel. No goods or materials retentive of infection should, however, be transported.

All this was more or less standard practice on the continent; but, with regard to control methods within an area where plague had already been introduced, Mead outlined relatively new procedures. He reviews current practice as follows:

"The main Import of the Orders issued out at these Times was, As soon as it was found, that any House was infected, to keep it shut up, with *a large red Cross, and Lord have mercy upon us* on the Door; and Watchmen attending Day and Night to prevent any one's going in or out, except Physicians, Surgeons, Apothecaries, Nurses, Searchers, Etc. allowed by Authority: And this to continue at least a Month after all the Family was *dead* or *recovered*.

"It is not easy to conceive a more dismal Scene of Misery, than this; Families seized with a Distemper, which the most of any in the World requires Help and Comfort, lockt up from all their Acquaintance; left it may be to the Treatment of an inhumane Nurse (for such are often found at these Times about the Sick;) and Strangers to every thing but the melancholy Sight of the Progress, Death makes among themselves; with small Hopes of Life, and those mixed with Anxiety and Doubt, whether it be not better to Dye, than to survive the Loss of their best Friends, and nearest Relations.

"If Fear, Despair, and all Dejection of Spirits dispose the Body to receive *Contagion*, and give it a great Power, where it is received, as all Physicians agree they do, I don't see how a Disease can be more enforced, than by such a Treatment.

"Nothing can justify such Cruelty, but that Plea, that it is for the Good of the whole Community, and prevents the spreading of *Infection*. But this upon due Consideration will be found quite otherwise: For while *Contagion* is kept nursed up in a House, and continually encreased by the daily Conquests it makes, it is Impossible, but the Air should by Degrees become tainted, which by opening Windows, &c. will carry the Malignity first from House to House; and then from one Street to another. The shutting up Houses in this Manner is only keeping so many Seminaries of Contagion, sooner or later to be dispersed abroad: For the waiting a Month, or longer, from the Death of the last Patient will avail no more, than keeping a Bale of Infected Goods unpack'd; the Poyson will fly out, whenever the *Pandora's* Box is opened" (1721).

We cannot accept this theory of concentrated miasmatic poison; but we can readily agree that such harsh measures as those commonly in use were not only inhumane but must necessarily defeat their own ends by leading to the concealment of early cases of the disease. In place of the old methods, Mead suggests the following procedure:

"There ought, in the first place, a council of health to be established, consisting of some of the principal officers of state, both ecclesiastical and civil, some of the chief magistrates of the city, two or three physicians, &c. And this council should be intrusted with such powers, as might enable them to see all their orders executed with impartial justice, and that no unnecessary hardships, under any pretence whatever, be put upon any by the officers they employ" (1744).

"Instead of ignorant old Women, who are generally appointed Searchers in Parishes to enquire what Diseases People dye of, That Office should be committed to understanding and diligent Men, whose Business it should be, as soon as they find any have dyed after an uncommon Manner, particularly with livid Spots, Buboes, or Carbuncles, to give Notice thereof to the Magistrates; who should immediately send skilful Physicians to visit the Houses in the Neighbourhood, especially of the Poorer sort, among whom this Evil generally begins; and if upon their Report it appears, that a Pestilential Distemper is broke out among the Inhabitants, They should without Delay order all the Families, in which the Sickness is to be Removed; The Sick to different Places from the Sound; but the Houses for both should be three or four Miles out of Town; and the Sound People should be stript of all their Cloaths, and washed and shaved, before they go into their new Lodgings" (1721).

Mead in 1744 recommends the removal of the sick from their houses only in the early stages of an epidemic. When the disease has become more widespread he suggests that they be left in their homes and that even other persons resident in such houses may go freely abroad although it is suggested that "they should be obliged to carry about them a long stick of some remarkable colour, or other visible token, by which people may be warned from holding too free converse with them."

Compassion and care for the sick should animate the procedure at all stages and all expenses should be paid from the public purse.

With characteristic emphasis on fomites, Mead recommends in 1721 that after the occupants have been removed all goods in infected houses should be burned and the houses themselves also "if convenient." In 1744 he suggests that goods from infected houses should be buried instead of burned, to avoid danger of distributing infectious particles in smoke. He argues against the Hippocratic procedure of lighting fires in the streets, ingeniously suggesting that heat favors the spread of contagion. He recommends the deep burying of the bodies of the dead and, of course, urges general sanitary cleansing of the streets and abatement of nuisances. For the protection of individuals he advises keeping vital resistance at a high level by observing the rules of personal hygiene. Crowds should be avoided and those in actual attendance on the sick should not draw breath when in close proximity to the patient and should avoid swallowing their spittle.

In all this, of course, Mead's thinking was tremendously handicapped by the prevailing theories of contagion. No complete solution was possible until the concept of living germs replaced that of chemical *seminaria* of contagion. With the conceptions at his disposal, however, he constructed a rational and balanced theory which combined all that was known as to the respective effects of contagion and local influences. Between Galen and Pasteur, there were in my judgment two really outstanding and significant contributions to the theory of the causation of communicable disease—that of the Italian Fracastorius in the sixteenth century and that of the English Mead in the eighteenth. In his theories of epidemiology, as in all his life and work, Richard Mead showed a keen and ingenious mind, a sound practical judgment, and a warm and urbane humanity. He lived, as Johnson said, "in the broad sunshine of life"; and he worked in the clear light of reason. His personality was a fine flower of his nation, his generation and his profession. His *Discourse on Plague* has won for him a permanent place in the little group who through the ages have been classed as the fathers of epidemiology.

CHAPTER XI

THE ENIGMA OF YELLOW FEVER

"The subject of yellow fever has long attracted the attention of the medical profession on this and the other side of the Atlantic. Upon the origin, the mode of propagation, the pathology, and the appropriate treatment of that fatal disease, as much, perhaps, has been written, particularly within the last sixty years, as upon any other malady flesh is heir to."—LA ROCHE

THE early history of yellow fever is shrouded in obscurity. An epidemic, supposed to be this disease, occurred in Vera Cruz and San Domingo between 1493 and 1496; and, on the basis of rather dubious evidence of certain wall paintings, it has been suggested that the fall of the Mayan civilization was the result of yellow fever. More recent knowledge indicates the probability that infection was brought from West Africa by Negro slaves. After 1750, the disease was certainly widely prevalent in the West Indies, in South America and at various points in North America. As plague was the central problem for epidemiological speculation in earlier days, yellow fever was the outstanding enigma of the eighteenth century. It can serve us better than any other disease as a touchstone for the etiological thinking of the day.

On our own continent this problem was particularly pressing. Between 1702 and 1800, this terrible disease appeared in the United States thirty-five times (and even between 1800 and 1879 it visited this country every year, with but two exceptions). In particular, the city of Philadelphia suffered from epidemics of yellow fever in 1699, 1741, 1747 and 1762; while in 1793, it was the seat of one of the most devastating outbreaks of pestilence ever recorded on this side of the Atlantic. A tenth of the population of the city perished, and Matthew Carey in his vivid account of the epidemic says, "it is not probable that London, at the last stage of the plague, exhibited stronger marks of terror than were to be seen in Philadelphia from the 24th or 25th of August till pretty late in September."

In the 1790's, Philadelphia was the cultural, social and financial, as well as the political center of the young nation. Here the first medical school in America had been established in 1765; and here lived the leaders of American medicine, John Morgan, William Shippen, Jr., and Benjamin Rush—the greatest medical figure of his time on this side of the water. It is through his eyes that we may best visualize the problem of yellow fever.

Rush was born in 1745 on a farm near Philadelphia, of English Quaker stock. After graduating in 1760 from the College of New Jersey, he apprenticed himself to a prominent Philadelphia physician, John Redman (with whom Morgan also had worked); and in 1766 he went to Edinburgh to study under Cullen and Monro (as both Morgan and Shippen had done before him). In 1768 he received his medical degree at Edinburgh and next year opened his office in Philadelphia. He was at once elected professor of chemistry in the College of Philadelphia and succeeded Morgan as professor of practice in 1789, attaining the chair of the institutes of medicine when the college was merged into the University of Pennsylvania in 1791. He was named physician to the Pennsylvania Hospital in 1783, where he introduced clinical instruction. He was the chief agent in establishing the Philadelphia Free Dispensary in 1786, and one of the founders of the College of Physicians in 1787. He played a major role in the establishment of Dickinson College.

One of Rush's greatest distinctions was his attitude toward mental disease, in which he showed the same vision which characterized Galen and Sydenham but went far beyond them. Goodman rightly calls him the "First American Psychiatrist." In his work at the Pennsylvania Hospital he was a pioneer in developing humane and scientific treatment of the insane. Although he still stressed such violent methods as the "tranquilizer" and the "gyrator," he conceived of mental disease in pathological terms as a disease of the brain, he insisted on decent quarters and sanitary facilities for its unfortunate victims, and he employed hydrotherapy, occupational therapy, and emotional catharsis in treatment.

Unfortunately, Rush did not apply his knowledge of mental hygiene to the conduct of his own life. He was constantly engaged in vigorous and frequently acrimonious controversy, with his professional colleagues and with the political powers of the day. He returned from Edinburgh an ardent disciple of Cullen and, with characteristic aggressiveness, he was soon engaged in a virulent dispute with the majority of the local medical profession who supported the theories of Boerhaave. What this controversy (as to location of the seat of disease in the solids or fluids of the body) was about it is difficult for the modern to discern. Yet it was a burning issue in the eighteenth century. More comprehensible to us is the conflict between Rush and many of his colleagues in regard to treatment. He was a heroic purger and bloodletter and aroused so much resentment on this account that he lost his consultation practice and many of his own patients as well. Finally, Rush's championship of the theory of a local origin for the yellow fever epidemic of 1793 caused an even more violent clash of opinion.

Nor were Rush's battles limited to the field of medical theory. He was an ardent patriot (which did not endear him to many influential Philadelphians), rode to the First Continental Congress of 1774 in the same coach with John Adams and Robert Treat Paine, and in 1776 signed the Declaration of Independence, his name standing between those of Benjamin Franklin and Robert Morris in that immortal document. On the expiration of a term in the first Congress, Rush accepted a commission in the medical department of the Army, but in nine months resigned as a result of a bitter quarrel with the head of that department, Dr. William Shippen, Jr. He charged (with much supporting evidence) gross mismanagement of the army hospitals on Shippen's part; and when he failed to secure Washington's support, he attacked even the Commander-in-Chief. In 1779, Rush joined Dr. John Morgan (Shippen's predecessor in the Army post) in demanding a court-martial of Shippen; but Shippen was acquitted on the ground that the charges were not fully proved, discharged by Congress, and two months later reappointed! On which, Rush's comment was "If Shippen triumphs one day longer, then is virtue a shadow, and liberty only a name in the United States."

As if all this were not enough, Rush was a pioneer in at least three of the major social controversies of the century. In 1772 he began a campaign against alcohol with a tract entitled "Sermons to Gentlemen upon Temperance and Exercise"; and in 1790 he took on nicotine as well with "Observations upon the Influence of the Habitual Use of Tobacco upon Health, Morals and Property." In 1773, he appeared as one of the first advocates of Abolition in America, with an "Address to the Inhabitants of the British Settlements upon Slave-Keeping." In 1787 he entered the field of penal reform with a highly effective "Enquiry into the Effects of Public Punishments upon Criminals, and upon Society."

Benjamin Rush was a blood-brother to the passionate and unrelenting reformers of his day on the other side of the water, fellow to Bentham, Howard, Cobden, Chadwick and the rest. Often stubborn and always contentious, he was completely honest and unselfish, consumed with a flaming hate of injustice and wrongdoing. The marvel is that with all the enemies he made and all the vested interests he challenged he retained his position as one of the outstanding figures in American life and certainly the greatest physician of his country at this time. When he died in 1813 John Adams could well say of him, "As a man of science, letters, taste, sense, philosophy, patriotism, religion, morality, merit, usefulness, taken all together Rush has not left his equal in America; nor that I know in the world."

Benjamin Rush may therefore be taken as an excellent representative of late eighteenth century medicine; and the controversy between him and his colleagues in regard to the causation of yellow fever gives us a vivid picture of the epidemiological thinking of the time.

Rush's first contribution in this general field was a short but extremely interesting essay entitled "An Enquiry into the Causes of the Increase of Bilious and Remitting Fevers in Pennsylvania with Hints for Preventing Them" published in *The American Museum* for January 1787. He ascribes the increase of these maladies to three principal causes: (1) the establishment and increase of mill-ponds; (2) the clearing of forest land, without draining and cultivating it; and (3) inequalities of rainfall. Assuming, as must certainly have been the case, that he was speaking mainly of malaria, this represents reasonably keen observation. His two chief remedies are the planting of trees around all mill-ponds and cultivating land as soon as it is cleared. "Let every spot covered with moisture, from which the wood has been cut, be carefully drained, and afterwards, ploughed and sowed with grass-seed; let weeds of all kinds be destroyed, and let the waters be so directed as to prevent their stagnating in any part of their course." Among temporary measures of prevention, he mentions the building of large fires every evening ("Whether the matter which produces fevers be of an organic, or inorganic nature, I do not pretend to determine; but it is certain that fire, or the smoke or heat, which issue from it, destroy the effects of marsh miasmata"); the wearing of woolen clothing; a generous diet, avoidance of evening air and general cleanliness.

Rush's first major contribution to epidemiology was, however, his volume of nearly 400 pages entitled "An Account of the Bilious remitting Yellow Fever as it appeared in the City of Philadelphia in the Year 1793" published in 1794 and later constituting Vol. III of his *Medical Inquiries and Observations*. His first theories about the disease were apparently crystallized very quickly. It was on August 19, 1793, that he first came to the definite conclusion that a serious epidemic existed, and on August 24 he wrote to Dr. J. Hutchinson, who was acting as Port Physician ("the inspector of sickly vessels") as follows: "A malignant fever has lately appeared in our city, originating I believe from some damaged coffee which putrified on a wharf near Arch Street. This fever was confined for a while to Water Street, between Race and Arch Streets; but I have lately met with it in Second Street and in Kensington; but whether propagated by contagion, or by the original exhalation, I cannot tell."

Hutchinson, on August 27, reported to the Governor that the prevailing malignant fever "does not appear to be an imported disease"; but expressed some uncertainty as to the Arch Street putrid coffee being its original cause. On August 29 Rush wrote to the *American Daily Advertiser* to support Hutchinson on the contention that the disease had not been imported and to argue for Arch Street as the point of local origin. He says that "morbid exhalations, it is well known, produce fevers at the distance of two and three miles, where they are not opposed by houses, woods, or a hilly country. This is obvious to all the farmers who live in the neighborhood of mill-ponds. It is no new thing for the effluvia of putrid vegetables to produce malignant fevers. Cabbage, onions, black pepper, and even the mild potatoe, when in a state of putrefaction, have all been the remote causes of malignant fevers. The noxious quality of the effluvia from millponds, is derived wholly from a mixture of the putrified leaves and bark of trees, with water." "The publication," Rush says, "had no other effect than to produce fresh clamours against the author; for the citizens as well as most of the physicians of Philadelphia had adopted a traditional opinion, that the yellow fever could exist among us, only by importation from the West Indies." The mayor did, however, have the decayed coffee removed.

During the terrible days of this epidemic, when "almost every day, carts, waggons, coaches, and chairs, were to be seen transporting families and furniture to the country in every direction"; when President Washington had removed to Mount Vernon and most of the other officers of the federal government, the governor and "nearly the whole of the officers of the state," the magistrates of the city "except the mayor and John Barclay, esq." "had likewise retired," Rush labored in the care of the sick with complete courage and untiring devotion. He sometimes saw over a hundred patients a day and is said to have visited half the houses in the city. Three of the pupils who assisted him died of the disease, and Rush himself was stricken in October.

Rush, throughout his monograph, speaks of the "contagion" or "poison" of the fever as its "remote" cause, generally supplemented by "predisposing" causes (such as fatigue, heat, intemperance) and "exciting" causes (fear, grief, cold, sleep, immoderate evacuation). At this stage of his thinking, he recognizes contagion as a basic (or "remote") cause, distinct from putrid exhalations. He says, "There were for several weeks two sources of infection, viz. exhalation, and contagion. The exhalation infected at the distance of three and four hundred yards; while the contagion infected only across the streets. The more narrow the street, the more certainly the contagion infected. Few escaped it in alleys. After the 15th of September, the atmosphere of every street in the city was loaded with contagion." In another place, he says that "the contagion adhered to all kinds of cloathing and seemed to be propagated by them."

The heat, dryness and stillness of the air "favoured the accumulation of the contagion." It is mentioned that "moschetoes (the usual attendants of a sickly autumn) were uncommonly numerous"; but this fact (with the presence of dead cats and the appearance of a meteor) is clearly cited as supporting evidence for an unhealthy condition of the season and with no implication of any direct relationship to the epidemic.

Rush describes various methods in use for the purifying of houses, bedding and clothing (fumigating, burying, burning, whitewashing); but he himself thought that only airing and washing were necessary. He follows Sydenham in emphasizing the belief that such a disease as yellow fever "cannot spread without a corresponding constitution of the atmosphere."

The cessation of the epidemic is attributed, probably quite correctly, to rain and cooler weather in late October.

The really vital issue in the ensuing controversy was the question whether the disease had originally been imported or had arisen from local miasms. The College of Physicians (with Redman and two other members dissenting) took the former view. Under date of November 26, the College reported to the Governor that "No instance has ever occurred of the disease called the yellow fever, having been generated in this city, or in any other parts of the United States, so far as we know; but there have been frequent instances of its having been imported, not only into this, but into other parts of North America, and prevailing there for a certain period of time; and from the rise, progress, and nature of the malignant fever, which began to prevail here about the beginning of last August, and extended itself gradually over a great part of the city, we are of opinion that this disease was imported into Philadelphia, by some of the vessels which arrived in the port after the middle of July."

We now know the College was correct in its deductions, but Rush's reasons for disagreement were by no means without force—in the then existing state of knowledge. They may be summarized briefly as follows:

1. In the West Indies, yellow fever does not exist everywhere; it is endemic only in those regions where marsh exhalations from vegetable putrefaction are present and when the force of these exhalations is intensified by hot and dry weather.

2. The same causes (under like circumstances) must always produce the same effects. Therefore, since vegetable exhalations in hot, dry weather produce yellow fever in the West Indies, the same causes must produce it in the United States. Various epidemics of "Bilious Colic" are cited where no importation could have taken place.

3. The putrefaction of the damaged coffee was competent to produce disease as evidenced by citations from various authors who describe epidemics due to putrefied potatoes, cabbages, hemp, etc.

4. The rapid spread of the disease from the area affected by coffee effluvia supports the conception that this was the primary agent. "It is remarkable that it passed first through those alleys, and streets which were in the course of the winds that blew across the dock and wharf where the coffee lay."

5. Many persons who had worked or even visited in the neighborhood of the exhalation from the coffee, early in the month of August were indisposed "long before the air of Water Street was so much impregnated with the contagion as to produce such effects."

6. "The first cases of the yellow fever have been clearly traced to the sailors of the vessel who were first exposed to the effluvia of the coffee" and "their sickness commenced with the day on which the coffee began to emit its putrid smell."

7. "It has been remarked that this fever did not spread in the country, when carried there by persons who were infected, and who afterwards died with it. This I conceive was occasioned, in part by the contagion being deprived of the aid of miasmata from the putrid matter which first produced it in our city, and, in part, by its being diluted, and thereby weakened by the pure air of the country."

8. The fact that yellow fever in the United States has generally prevailed from August to October points to "a combination of more active miasmata with the predisposition of a tropical season."

9. Difference in symptoms from West India yellow fever and presence of cases among children (reported not to occur in the West Indies).

10. Assumed intimate relationship of the disease to cases normally occurring in Philadelphia; "it is only a higher grade of a fever, which prevails every year in our city, from vegetable putrefaction."

Points 1 and 2 undoubtedly have a certain logical force; and point 7 is, of course, highly pertinent, as proving that some factor of a local nature was effective. Point 10 illustrates the serious handicap from which Rush (like Sydenham) suffered in his refusal to admit the specificity of diseases. He says, "Science has much to deplore from the multiplication of diseases. It is as repugnant to truth in medicine, as polytheism is to truth in religion. The physician who considers every different affection of the different systems in the body, or every affection of different parts of the same system, as distinct diseases, when they arise from one cause, resembles the Indian or African savage, who considers water, dew, ice, frost, and snow, as distinct essences; while the physician who considers the morbid affections of every part of the body (however diversified they may be in their form or degrees) as derived from one cause, resembles the philosopher, who considers dew, ice, frost, and snow, as different modifications of water." In another place he says; "I shall not attempt to distinguish the yellow, from the common bilious fever. They are only different grades of the same disease. The following appears to be the natural order of a scale of such fevers as are derived from marsh miasmata: (1) The yellow fever; (2) The common bilious remitting fever; (3) The intermitting fever."

It might have been thought that Rush's vehement conviction as to the local origin of the fever would have led him to the view that it was not contagious; but, at this stage of his career, he was an ardent contagionist. He cites numerous cases to show that fevers generated by decaying cabbage, flax, and the like, spread afterwards by contagion. He even maintains that intermittent fevers are contagious. He says, of the theory that fevers produced by putrid exhalations are not contagious, "I hope I shall be excused by the physicians of other states for having employed a single page in combating an error which is so obvious to common observation. My only design in exposing it is to prevent a repetition of its fatal influence in the only city in the world in which it has ever been believed or propagated." In this passage, Rush was no doubt referring chiefly to the distinguished French physician, Jean Devèze, who was vigorously combating the concept that yellow fever could be contagious, chiefly on the ground that none of the doctors, nurses or attendants at the Bush Hill

Hospital contracted the disease—a very sound reason for doubting contagion in the current conception of the term.

Rush does admit that yellow fever may sometimes have been imported into the United States but thinks such occasions have been very rare; and he maintains that such has probably been the case in other lands with respect to the plague.

It will be noted that, at this period, Rush, like Mead, recognized both miasm and contagion, but his synthesis of the two factors was radically different. Mead visualized local circumstances as favoring a primary contagion; Rush conceived a primary miasmatic influence culminating in contagion.

In comments on the "Bilious Yellow Fever" of 1794, 1795 and 1796, printed in Volume III of later editions of Rush's *Medical Inquiries and Observations*, the same views are advanced. In commenting on the epidemic of 1794, he says, "the citizens of Philadelphia, having an interest in rejecting the proofs of the generation of the epidemic of 1793, in their city, had neglected to introduce the regulations which were necessary to prevent the production of a similar fever from domestic putrefaction." The disease appeared as a tertian fever, a remittent fever, a dysentery, an apoplexy and "disguised itself in the form of madness." It "blended itself with the scarlatina"; and "such was the predominance of the intermitting, remitting, and bilious fever, that the measles, the small-pox, and even the gout itself, partook more or less of its character."

In this essay, as it appeared in the first edition of *Medical Inquiries*, Rush was still a believer in contagion and advocated quarantine procedures. He says, "Let all the families which are within fifty yards of the infected person or persons be ordered instantly to remove into houses or tents, to be provided for them at the public expense. . . . Let chains be placed across the streets which lead to the sick, and let guards be appointed to prevent all access to the infected parts of the city, except by physicians and nurses and . . . other persons."

In the later editions of *Medical Inquiries* (of which I have used the fifth, 1818, edition), Volume IV is made up almost entirely of accounts of the bilious fever in Philadelphia in successive years from 1797 to 1809. From this volume, and from three other special monographs published by Rush, we may trace the development of his theories of epidemiology.

With regard to 1797, Rush says that after a disease prevailing among cats which indicated an unwholesome condition of the atmosphere, "there were no diseases to be seen but yellow fever" after the first week in September. Current ideas with respect to the working of the poison are suggested in the following passage: "During my intercourse with the sick, I felt the miasmata of the fever operate upon my system in the most sensible manner. It produced languor, a pain in my head, and sickness at my stomach. A sighing attended me occasionally, for upwards of two weeks. This symptom left me suddenly, and was succeeded by a hoarseness, and, at times, with such a feebleness in my voice as to make speaking painful to me. Having observed this affection of the trachea to be a precursor of the fever in several cases, it kept me under daily apprehensions of being confined by it. It gradually went off after the first of October. I ascribed my recovery from it, and a sudden diminution of the effects of the miasmata upon my system, to a change produced in the atmosphere by the rain which fell on that day."

Rush at this time was active in the establishment of a short-lived Academy of Medicine to combat the importation theory of the College of Physicians, but with small success. He wrote to Noah Webster on February 7, 1798: "Not more than 20 persons of any note believe the late epidemic was generated among us, and not more than 50 believe in its being generated at any time in the United States. The absurd idea of its being a specific disease is nearly universal in our city."

Among predisposing causes of the fever, Rush cites, in various passages, a broken leg, a toothache and disappointment in love.

In 1799, Rush published two vigorously-worded pamphlets in support of his miasmatist views. In the first, "Observations upon the Origin of the Malignant Bilious or Yellow Fever in Philadelphia," he again states that "This disease is the offspring of putrid vegetable and animal exhalations in all countries" and that "It prevails only in hot climates and seasons." The specific points of origin in Philadelphia are the docks, the foul air of ships, the common sewers, the gutters, dirty cellars and yards, privies, putrefying masses of matter and impure pump water. In explaining why yellow fever did not occur more frequently prior to 1793, he emphasizes the necessity for three concurrent causes: "(1) Putrid exhalations, (2) An inflammatory constitution of the atmosphere, and (3) An exciting cause, such as great heat, cold, fatigue from riding, walking, swimming, gunning or unusual labour, intemperance in eating or drinking, ice creams, indigestible aliment, or a violent emotion of the mind." (This is the first time that the epidemic constitution of the atmosphere is prominent in Rush's thinking.) In a later passage, he advances the view that simultaneous heat and moisture are essential to the generation of deadly miasmata.

In this essay, Rush has already begun to modify his views with regard to contagion. He states that there are two kinds of contagion. The first is "secreted as in the small-pox and measles, in which state it acts uniformly, and without the aid of exciting causes, upon persons of all ages and constitutions who have not been previously exposed to it, and is not contracted by the obvious changes in the weather." In other cases, in bilious fever, the contagion "is derived from certain matters discharged from the body which afterwards by stagnation, or confinement, undergo such a change, as to partake of the same nature as the putrid exhalations which produce the fever." (In this distinction, we can today clearly read the difference between diseases transmitted by direct contact and those which require an intermediate host—in which the agent "undergoes a change.") By this time, Rush believed that contagion was of little practical importance in yellow fever. "Out of upwards of one thousand persons who have carried this disease into the country from our cities, there are not more than three or four instances to be met with of its having been propagated by contagion." "The interests of humanity are deeply concerned in the admission of the rare and feeble contagion of the yellow fever." Furthermore, he is more dogmatic than ever on the question of importation. He says, "Can the Yellow Fever be Imported? I once thought it might but the foregoing facts authorize me to assert, that it cannot, so as to become epidemic in any city or country."

"A Second Address to the Citizens of Philadelphia" issued in the same year, contains "Additional Proofs of the Domestic Origin" of yellow fever. The seeds of this disease "cannot be retained in our beds or houses from year to year, much less can they be imported. As well might a coal of fire be brought from one of the West India islands to this country, or a lump of ice be conveyed from this country to one of the West India islands, in the open air, as the yellow fever be imported from thence so as to become general in our city." The epidemic constitution of the atmosphere and the influence of putrefying organic matter are heavily stressed, with many citations from other authorities; and the importance of contagion is denied more and more strongly. Rush's two strongest arguments (and they were valid arguments in the absence of any conception of an intermediate host) were the failure to spread in other areas to which patients were taken and the cessation on the onset of cold weather. Of the first of these phenomena he says that "the same disease when carried into the healthy parts of the city, and even terminating in death with symptoms of what is called general putrefaction, has perished without propagating itself in a single instance. To suppose it to be contagious under such circumstances, is to make a feather outweigh a mountain or to believe one to be more than a thousand." Of the cessation of the disease on the onset of cold weather, he says that this fact "is alone sufficient to decide the question in favour of the disease being derived exclusively from domestic exhalation, and existing in the atmosphere during the warm weather."

Rush is therefore now vehemently opposed to all measures of maritime quarantine which he compares to the attempt to check the plague in Moscow by placing an ikon upon the city gate.

In 1805, Rush published (in the second edition of his *Medical Inquiries*, and also as a separate pamphlet) two additional essays which complete his contributions to epidemiology. The first of these is "An Inquiry into the Various Sources of the Usual Forms of Summer and Autumnal Disease in the United States." The sources of such diseases are, first and foremost, decaying vegetable matter, of which the author lists 27 examples; marsh exhalations, cabbage, potatoes, pepper, Indian meal, onions, mint, anise and caraway seeds, coffee, chocolate shells, cotton, hemp flax and straw, old canvas, old books and paper money which has been wetted, timber of an old house, green wood confined in a close cellar, green timber of a new ship, stagnating air of the hold of a ship, bilge water, water in confined hogsheads at sea, stagnating rain water, stagnating cellar air, stagnating gutter sewer and sink water, foul and stagnating water, a duck pond, a hog-stye and moist heaps of cut weeds. Animal matters are less dangerous: but eight types of putrid animal substances are listed as causes of epidemics as follows; unburied human bodies on a battle field, salted beef and pork, locusts, raw hides, a whale on the shore of Holland, a large bed of oysters, the entrails of fish, and privies! The coming of an epidemic may be foretold by violence of diseases during the previous season, by the blackening of white lead paint, by sickness among birds and beasts, by changes in the prevailing types of insect life (disappearance of house flies and increase of "moschetoes"), and abnormal phenomena affecting vegetable life.

A long section deals with the protection of individuals against the disease which (aside from a primary recommendation to fly from the affected area) boils down to the avoidance of exciting causes. Rush next deals with the "means of preserving whole cities or communities from the influence of those morbid exhalations." This may be accomplished by covering putrid matters with water or earth; by impregnating the air with effluvia which destroy or neutralize the dangerous miasmata (killing dogs and cats and letting them putrefy in the streets, exposure to smoke or the exhalations of tan yards); absorption of miasmata by water ("What would be the effect of placing tubs of fresh water in the rooms of patients infected with malignant fevers?"); and closing of windows opening toward miasmatic winds (Varro). Rush thinks less well of strewing lime over putrid matters, of Guyton-Morveau's use of muriatic gas (to which we shall refer in a later chapter); of exploding gunpowder, washing floors with alkaline salts, and building fires in the streets (Hippocrates).

Next, Rush describes various methods of "exterminating malignant and other forms of summer and autumnal disease, by removing their causes. The removal or destruction of putrid matters is listed first, and the books of Deuteronomy and Exodus quoted as examples of sound practice. Next follow the construction of cities with ample open spaces and without narrow streets and alleys, elimination of marshy areas, surrounding mill ponds by trees, prompt cultivation of cleared forest areas, and discharging the air from the confined hold of a vessel carrying putrescent articles before access to a wharf.

This essay closes with a denunciation of quarantine procedures which have led to the waste of millions of dollars and to the sacrifice of thousands of lives from "that faith in their efficacy, which has led to the neglect of domestic cleanliness." Furthermore, "a belief in the contagious nature of the yellow fever, which is so solemnly enforced by the execution of quarantine laws, has demoralized our citizens. It has, in many instances, extinguished friendship, annihilated religion, and violated the sacraments of nature, by resisting even the loud and vehement cries of filial and parental blood." This argument is continued in a final essay "Facts intended to prove the Yellow Fever not to be Contagious."

This begins with a distinction between fevers communicated from one person to another (smallpox and measles by secreted matters and typhus fever by excreted matters) and fevers produced by putrefaction and becoming epidemic only by means of an impure atmosphere (the "bilious fevers" including in modern terminology, yellow fever, malaria and typhoid). There is thus a clear and sound distinction between diseases spread by rather direct personal contact (under which head louse-borne typhus may properly be included) and those in which external factors, such as insect vectors, polluted water and the like, play a major role. That yellow fever belongs to the second group, he demonstrates by a series of propositions which involve the main lines of evidence presented in earlier discussions. Yellow fever "does not spread in the country, when carried thither from the cities of the United States" and "does not spread in yellow fever hospitals, when they are situated beyond the influence of the impure air in which it is generated." This is, of course, a sound argument; and it is supported by interesting experimental evidence. "Dr. Ffirth inoculated himself above twenty times, in different parts of his body, with the black matter discharged from the stomachs of patients in the yellow fever, and several times with the serum of the blood, and the saliva of patients ill with that disease, without being infected by them; nor was he indisposed after swallowing half an ounce of the black matter recently ejected from the stomach." Occasional propagation simulating contagion may occur in small, filthy and close rooms or on exposure to foul linen but this is attributed to "an additional putrefactive process" rather than to contagion in the true sense; and the phenomenon is rare. Rush adds, "I am disposed to believe the linen, or any other clothing of a person in good health that had been strongly impregnated with sweats, and afterwards suffered to putrefy in a confined place, would be more apt to produce a yellow fever in a summer or autumnal month, than the linen of a person who had died of that disease, with the usual absence of a moisture on the skin."

In support of the claim that "the yellow fever is propagated by means of an impure atmosphere, at all times, and in all places," Rush cites its appearance only in hot and moist climates and seasons; and only in the presence of "marshes, millponds, docks, gutters, sinks, unventilated ships, and other sources of noxious air"; the destruction of the disease by long-continued and heavy rains (which as we now know, would, of course, wash out mosquito-breeding pools); and by frost, intense heat and high winds. If we recall that Rush was thinking chiefly of yellow fever and malaria, which he considered as forms of the same disease, all these observations are significant.

Rush here proceeds to consider the question why yellow fever is absent in certain countries, and in certain years, in spite of the presumable presence of putrid vegetable matter. This he explains chiefly on the grounds of the absence of the proper epidemic constitution of the atmosphere, leaning, of course, heavily on Sydenham. It is notable, however, that while the epidemic constitution was Sydenham's major factor, it is local miasms which Rush always places first. This leads him to the practical and helpful conclusion that by abandoment of the false concept of contagion and by removal of the local conditions which generate miasmata the menace of yellow fever may be effectively controlled. "Large cities shall no longer be the hot-beds of disease and death. Marshy grounds, teeming with pestilential exhalations, shall become the healthy abodes of men. A powerful source of repulsion between nations shall be removed, and commerce shall shake off the fetters which have been imposed upon it by expensive and vexatious quarantines. A red or a yellow eye shall no longer be the signal to desert a friend or a brother to perish alone in a garret or a barn, nor to expel the stranger from our houses, to seek an asylum in a public hospital, to avoid dying in the street. The number of diseases shall be lessened, and the most mortal of them shall be struck out of the list of human evils. To accelerate these events, it is incumbent upon the physicians of the United States to second the discoveries of their European brethren. It becomes them constantly to recollect, that we are the centinels of the health and lives of our fellow-citizens, and that there is a grade of benevolence in our profession much higher than that which arises from the cure of diseases. It consists in exterminating their causes."

All in all Rush presents us with pregnant and valid evidence against the practical contagiousness of such diseases as yellow fever and malaria and with a program of control which—in some respects at least—contained substantial elements of truth. He may be considered as a competent advocate of the miasmatic theories which were to dominate epidemiological thinking for half a century to come. The viewpoint of 1800 cannot, however, be understood without reviewing the work of a contemporary, a friend and correspondent of Rush, Noah Webster. Like the fiery leader of Philadelphia medicine, this Yankee schoolmaster and lexicographer was an ardent anti-contagionist; and Rush's own change of heart on this point was largely due to Webster's influence. The views of the Connecticut scholar were, perhaps, less practically fruitful than those of the Pennsylvania physician on account of the greater predominance of the epidemic constitution in the writings of the former; but Webster's scope was wider and his approach more philosophical.

Noah Webster was thirteen years younger than Rush, born at West

Hartford, Conn., in 1758, of pioneer New England farming stock, sixth in line from John Webster who accompanied the Rev. Thomas Hooker in his pilgrimage through the wilderness in 1656. Noah was a student at Yale College during the Revolutionary War and shouldered a musket for a brief period which was cut short by the surrender of Burgoyne. He graduated in 1778, studied law and was admitted to the bar in 1781. Legal prospects were not favorable, however, and he took up his natural career as a schoolmaster. While operating a school at Goshen, N.Y., he initiated his real life work by beginning the preparation of three school books on spelling, grammar and reading. The first of these, *The American Spelling Book*, had a phenomenal career, over fifteen million copies being sold in the author's lifetime. The success of the "speller" not only made it possible for Webster to pursue a life of productive scholarship but also crystallized his major objective, the purification and standardization of our tongue. In a campaign to secure a federal copyright law, (enacted in 1790) he spent nearly a year of time in journeying about the country, lecturing on the English language and becoming intimate with Washington, Franklin and other national leaders. He practiced law for a time in Hartford and later edited a Federalist journal in New York. In 1798 he abandoned his journalistic and political ventures and settled down in New Haven to more fundamental scholarly labors. Here he was one of the incorporators of the Connecticut Academy of Arts and Sciences in 1799. In 1812 he moved to Amherst, Mass., for reasons of economy. He served as a member of the Massachusetts General Court for three terms (as he had served for nine sessions as a member of the General Assembly of Connecticut); and was an active participant in plans for the Hartford Convention. He took a prominent part in the establishment of Amherst Academy and as chairman of the board of trustees called the meeting which led to the foundation of Amherst College. His main interest was the compilation of the dictionary which was to be his chief title to fame, and he had a huge table built in the form of a hollow circle within which he stood with dictionaries in twenty or more languages arranged in order about him, from one to another of which he would turn in pursuit of the laws of comparative philology.

In 1822, the Websters returned to New Haven and, in 1823 Noah and his son visited France and England. In Paris, S. G. Goodrich met him and describes his appearance as follows: "A slender form, with a black coat, black small-clothes, black silk stockings, moving back and forth, with its hands behind it, and evidently in a state of meditation. It was a curious, quaint, Connecticut-looking apparition, strangely in contrast to the prevailing forms and aspects in this gay metropolis."

It was during this trip, at Cambridge, England, that the monumental lexicographic undertaking was at last completed. The author says, "I finished writing my Dictionary in January, 1825, at my lodgings in Cambridge, England. When I had come to the last word, I was seized with a trembling which made it somewhat difficult to hold my pen steady for writing. The cause seems to have been the thought that I might not then live to finish the work, or the thought that I was so near the end of my labors. But I summoned strength to finish the last word, and then walking about the room a few minutes I recovered."

Three years later, in November 1828, the great dictionary was published in two quarto volumes by S. Converse of New York. It was indeed a monumental work, with 12,000 words and 30,000 or 40,000 definitions, which had not been found in any previous dictionary; and this entire task was completed by Webster's own hand as well as his own brain, for he had no regular assistant or amanuensis.

The rest of Webster's life was devoted to revisions of the *Dictionary* (the final one published in 1841); to an ambitious and not too well-judged revised edition of the Bible (published in 1833); and to minor literary activities. He died at the age of eighty-four on May 28, 1843.

By his school books which penetrated to every hamlet in the land, by his dictionary which was in itself so significant a demonstration of the possibilities of American scholarship, as well as by his political and social writings, Noah Webster contributed in no small degree to the upbuilding of the essential spirit of the American nation at this critical formative period. Warthin says, "Webster might well, nay, should, be ranged with the Fathers of this nation, since perhaps no other single individual of Revolutionary times contributed more to the welding of the diverse colonial states into a national solidarity than did this New England schoolmaster."

Aside from his primary work in linguistics, Webster, like other scholars of his time, enjoyed an astonishingly wide range of interests, moralistic, political and scientific. A volume of essays (somewhat in the vein of Poor Richard) published in his Hartford period over the signature of "The Prompter" had notable success. A series of essays in support of the Jay treaty, signed "Curtius" are said to have "contributed more than any papers of the same kind to allay the discontent and opposition to the treaty." He wrote treatises on dew and on the changes in the weather and on vital statistics.

Webster's major contribution to the natural sciences was, however, his study of epidemiology. His interest in the general subject was first aroused by epidemics which he himself observed in New England, of influenza in 1789 and 1790 and of scarlet fever in 1793. In both instances observations made by him during his travels led to the conclusion that the epidemics progressed from place to place and increased in malignancy as they did so. In the autumn of 1793 the "pestilential state of the air" associated with these earlier outbreaks "arrived to its crisis in Philadelphia" and aroused universal alarm. The appearance of the same disease in New Haven in 1794 and in New York, Baltimore and Norfolk in 1795, he says, "revived my curiosity with double zeal." Webster suspected the prevalent idea of infection to be unfounded and was already in ardent correspondence with Rush in regard to the question. In order to throw light on the problem of importation Webster sent out a circular letter to the physicians of Philadelphia, New York, Baltimore, Norfolk and New Haven under date of October 31, 1795. In this letter he says, "The first measure to be taken in this business seems to be to ascertain the following points—Whether the bilious remitting fever, commonly called the Yellow Fever, is of foreign or domestic origin; whether it is always imported or may be generated in our own country; whether it is an epidemic, or depends for propagation on specific contagion; or whether it partakes of the nature both of an epidemic and a contagious disease."

The information received in response to this questionnaire in the form of monographs and letters was published by Webster in 1796 with his own comments and conclusions under the title "A Collection of Papers on the Subject of Bilious Fever, prevalent in the United States for a Few Years Past."

The first essay in this collection is by Dr. Valentine Seaman on the 1795 outbreak in New York which caused 732 deaths, almost wholly in one restricted area of low land, between July and October. Seaman is a convinced anti-contagionist although he says that his thoughts are "decidedly opposed to the common sense of the faculty in general." He accepts Howard's definition of contagion as a force operating within a distance of ten paces and against the possibility of such contagion he sets forth three chief arguments.

1. Cases occurred which had never been in contact with preexisting

cases (some, for example, not having been out of their houses for several weeks).

2. Cases did not arise when contagion should have been expected. No further spread occurred from cases which had moved out of the city and (as in Devèze's experience at Bush Hill) attendants on the sick at Bellevue did not contract the disease unless they had visited the infected area.

3. The seasonal prevalence of the disease, even according to the more recent opinions of Rush, required the assumption of "the concurrence of a predisposing condition of the air."

Hence, Seaman concludes that the disease was caused by putrefying substances in the low water-logged lands and stagnant water of the affected area and he compares the doctrine of contagion with the delusion of the Salem witchcraft. "Nineteen persons were executed in and about Salem in 1692 from this demoniacal delusion, and no doubt, but ten times that number have been shamefully permitted to die of the yellow fever in Philadelphia and New York, in consequence of neglect from the fear of contagion, when perhaps the unhappy sufferers were as free from the power of afflicting their friends, as the New England witches were."

Dr. Elihu H. Smith of New York, like Seaman, is a vigorous anti-contagionist. He advances detailed arguments against the current belief that the infection had been introduced from Port-au-Prince on the ship *Zephyr*. He concludes that "no direct, no clear evidence ever has been, or can be produced, in favor of the opinion that the fever was imported.". Like most of the anti-contagionists, Smith denies the specificity of the disease, considering it only a "heightened" form of the usual summer fever.

He emphasizes strongly the localization of the epidemic in one particular area, "the lowest, flattest and most sunken part of the whole city." Much of this area was "swampy, and abounds with little pools and puddles of stagnant water." Heavy rains had occurred. The season had been so damp that "every article of household furniture, or in use about a house, susceptible of mould, was speedily and deeply covered with it." "Clouds of musketoes, incredibly large and distressing" characterized the summer.

Smith was, however, much more philosophical than most writers on the subject at this period. He notes that the question whether the disease be "epidemic" or "contagious" is largely a question of terminology. If by the query whether the disease is contagious "it is meant to inquire, whether the well became affected with the Fever, in consequence of the contact of a sick person or the clothing of a sick person, or from the performance of the offices of friendship, charity and meniality, to those who were sick—I answer that no such cases have come to my knowledge." Smith's own theory is that the primary cause of the malady is predisposition due to corruption of the atmosphere aggravated by breach of principles of personal hygiene, and perhaps further aggravated by exhalations from the bodies of the sick. With regard to importation he concludes, "The whole, therefore, that can be granted, or ought to be assumed by those who maintain the disease which prevailed in New York in 1795, to have been imported is—That infection may be brought into any place (and therefore into this city) from abroad; that, under certain circumstances of the place, where it is introduced, it becomes very active and destructive; but that when these circumstances do not exist, however the person immediately affected—if it be introduced by a sick person—may suffer, it is harmless, so far as the general health of that place is concerned. If the subject were viewed in this light, as most assuredly it ought to be, the question of importation, or non-importation, would sink into its merited insignificance; the efficient cause, the causa *sine qua non*, of such Fevers, would be clearly discerned as depending on local circumstances, capable of being wholly changed."

Here is an admirable statement, clear and logical and in essential accord with all the facts we know today.

Only letters from two local medical luminaries of New Haven, the Munsons, in regard to the 1794 epidemic in New Haven, set forth, in this volume, an opposing view. There had been no yellow fever in New Haven since 1743, but in 1794 there were 160 cases and 64 deaths between June and November. The elder Dr. Munson (Eneas) says:

"In a climate where the disease is not epidemical, and where it is not generated, we are under advantages to decide, with much more certainty, in respect to its infectious nature, than we should be in a hot climate; where the long-continued heat, in conjunction with a number of other causes, is productive of the disorder, and where it would, therefore, be very difficult to determine when the Fever was constitutional, and when propagated by contagion." He quotes authorities to show that fevers often do not occur when thousands of bodies putrefy on a battlefield or in the neighborhood of churchyards as weighing against a miasmatic origin.

The younger Munson (Elijah) describes the arrival of a sloop from Martinique infected with yellow fever at the beginning of June. The first local cases occurred in the Gorham family living on Long Wharf within a few rods of the mooring of this vessel. "No person had the Yellow Fever, unless in consequence of attending the sick, or of being exposed by nurses, infected houses, clothing or furniture." He concludes that the scarlet fever which previously prevailed was "an Epidemical disease, which originated in the constitution of the air—while the Yellow Fever was propagated only by contagion."

Webster, himself, sides unqualifiedly with the non-contagionists and expounds his views in a closing essay (written in December 1795). He says (taking as we may note the admirably balanced analysis of Elihu Smith as his basis):

"One thing may safely be averred, that, whether imported, or generated by local causes in our own country, the epidemic influence and destructive effects of this malignant bilious fever, are greatly increased by local causes, which are wholly within the command of human power. ... This circumstance lessens very much the importance of deciding the question whether imported or not; for if imported, it does not spread, unless its progress is favored by unwholesome air in this country." Webster classified diseases as (1) neither contagious nor epidemic (pneumonia); (2) propagated solely by contagion (smallpox); (3) epidemic but not ordinarily communicated by infection (colds and the intermittent fevers); (4) those which may be both epidemic and contagious, in varying degree (dysentery, scarlet fever, yellow fever). He says that influenza cannot be contagious because so many people are stricken "in a day without any intercourse with each other."

Pestilential epidemic diseases may be due to food and drink or to the air we breathe. In the latter case, morbid exhalations[1] are due to fermenting animal and vegetable substances. Heat and moisture favor putrefaction and air carries it. Exhalations proceed from a center in

[1] Webster in this volume presents an interesting summary of Professor S. L. Mitchill's opinion concerning the causes of epidemic distempers which shows how definitely chemical was the current concept of the miasms producing fevers. Oxygen, according to Mitchill, is the basis of vital air, azote of foul air. When azote, called also by Mitchill "septon," unites with "caloric," poisonous miasms result. Chills and fever are explained in great detail as specific reactions to this toxic air.

straight lines if not diverted by wind and become diluted as they pass outward from the center.

Danger can be avoided by removing putrescible substances and by ventilation to dilute the poison, "to remove the sources of the poison or to dissipate it as much as possible." Cities should be constructed so as to avoid low grounds or hollow places, to facilitate drainage and permit free ventilation.

His Concluding Observations are "(1) That the Yellow Fever, so called, is only the most malignant degree of ordinary bilious fever. (2) That this fever may be, and often is, generated in the United States, especially in the more filthy parts of populous towns. (3) That it is not ordinarily infectious, that is, attended with specific contagion; but may be rendered so, by peculiar circumstances that conspire to increase its malignancy."

He admits the operation of infection in New Haven and to a degree in Philadelphia but not in New York or Norfolk. He emphasizes that there is no danger of spread in rural areas. "The panic that seized the whole continent, when the disease appeared in Philadelphia, is now found to have been needless and without just cause; and it is presumed that such inhuman caution and barbarous measures as were adopted on that occasion, will never again disgrace our country."

The preparation of this volume of collected papers only whetted Webster's appetite for the topic which he at once began to study on a wider scale. Between October and December 1797 he wrote and published in the public press a series of twenty-five letters to Dr. Currie of Philadelphia in which he controverted the theory that the disease was of foreign origin. Rush wrote on November 27, 1797 to congratulate Webster on these letters and said, "They have made a greater impression upon our Citizens than anything that has ever been published in Philadelphia upon that subject."

By January 1798 Webster had already begun to collect literature, first on epidemics in America, then, throughout the world. He visited the libraries of New York and Philadelphia and of Yale and Harvard Colleges with this end in view. On April 10, just after his removal to New Haven, he writes in his diary, "Begin to write my History of Epidemic diseases, from materials which I have been three months collecting." Rush was always in close touch with him and their correspondence at this period was extensive. In March 1799, Rush wrote, "I long to see your book in circulation. It will prove I hope a weapon powerful as the Club of Hercules in overcoming error upon the subject of Epidemics. I have prepared my class (consisting of near 100 pupils) to receive and read it with avidity and attention. It ought to be published before the next season for the prevalence of bilious fevers." In a postscript he adds: "Since the former date of this letter, I have read the section you have sent me of your book. I now return it by Mr. Allen. Accept of my thanks for the instruction I have derived from it. It has *arranged* my floating and half-connected ideas upon the subject of Epidemics."

Webster's own position was steadily moving from his reasonably moderate position of 1796 to a more and more vehement denial of contagion and his thoughts were increasingly centering on the influence of the epidemic constitution of the atmosphere and its relation to meteorological and geological phenomena.

In December 1799 the *History of Epidemic and Pestilential Diseases* was published; and excited, as might have been expected, highly diverse reactions. Currie dismisses Webster's analysis with the comment that it is "as much the creature of the imagination as the tales of the fairies." Rush was, of course, greatly pleased with it on the whole, referring to Webster in a letter to Oliver Wolcott some years later, as "a Giant upon this subject."

The *Epidemic and Pestilential Fevers* had no great popular success— either medically or financially. Its two volumes represent, however, so far as I am aware, the best general summary of epidemiological opinion at the beginning of the nineteenth century which is extant; and few works surpass it as a compendium of earlier speculations in this field. The first volume begins with an analysis of the diverse opinions advanced by earlier writers in regard to the cause and origin of pestilence. Webster summarizes the three chief opinions as follows: "The philosophers of antiquity, attentive to changes in the seasons and to the revolutions of the heavenly bodies, attempted to trace pestilential diseases to extraordinary vicissitudes in the weather, and to the aspects of the planets. Modern philosophers and physicians, on the other hand, unable to account for pestilence on the principle of extraordinary seasons, and disdaining to admit the influence of the planets to be the cause, have resorted to invisible animalculae, and to infection concealed in bales of goods or old clothes, transported from Egypt or Constantinople, and let loose, at certain periods, to scourge mankind and desolate the earth. In both periods of the world, the common mass of people, usually ignorant and always inclined to believe in the marvellous, have cut the

Gordian knot of difficulty, by ascribing pestilence to the immediate exercise of divine power; under the impression that the plague is one of the judgments which God, in his wrath, inflicts on mankind to punish them for their iniquities."

The theory of divine wrath occupies little of Webster's attention; but he is vehement in his condemnation of that of infection. He is particularly bitter against Richard Mead. He says, "Dr. Mead's treatise on the plague has been much admired and celebrated; yet I will assert, that next to the 'Traité de la peste,' a treatise in quarto on the plague of Marseilles, published by royal permission, it is the weakest and least valuable performance on the subject now extant." Yet, as a matter of fact, the *Traité de la peste* is an excellent bit of descriptive epidemiology; and Mead's *Short Discourse concerning Pestilential Contagion* was probably the most significant contribution made since classic days with the exception of the writings of Fracastorius. Webster's mind was, however, by this time absolutely closed to any suggestion of the importation of infection. He says, "In opposition to all these great authorities, it will probably be proved, that the plague generally if not always originates, in the country where it exists as an epidemic." He repeatedly heaps scorn on such "vulgar notions" as "that the plague is conveyed from country to country in bales of goods."

Neither can Webster accept what he presents as the doctrine of the ancients with regard to the effect of season and weather. He quite rightly points out that there are contradictions in any theory which assumes that a particular kind of weather is inevitably and always associated with epidemics. He might have learned something from a statement he quotes from Ammianus Marcellinus in regard to various types of diseases associated with various seasons; but Webster was too firmly convinced of the fundamental identity of all epidemic diseases to pursue this fruitful line of thought.

Webster mentions the theory of Aëtius (and others) that the air may be vitiated by "the evaporation from putrid substances. These substances are multitudes of dead bodies after battles, marshes or stagnant water in the vicinity which emit poisonous and fetid vapors." He does not here stress the point, however.

The main cause which, even in this first chapter, Webster does emphasize is the general "epidemic constitution of the atmosphere" which Aristotle invoked as a necessary factor, in conjunction with the pestilential state of the air due to season and weather, to explain the most serious epidemics. He quotes Diemerbroeck's description of this epidemic constitution as˙ "a most malignant, poisonous, and to human nature, deadly pestilent germ (seminarium), like a subtle fermentum or leaven, in a very small quantity, diffusing itself through the air like a subtle gas, and rendering it impure. This gas, he supposes to spread over many regions its numerous particles, and to impress on the air an infection like poison, which often affects not only many persons but almost the whole world." It should be noted that the word "seminaria" is used in a much more general sense than that of Fracastorius. Webster thinks this explanation in part somewhat whimsical but he seems to accept it in general. He says, "that some such general cause exists in the atmosphere, at certain periods, will be rendered very probable, if not certain, by the facts hereafter to be related"; and he adds, "there must be an alteration in the chymical properties of the atmosphere to solve the difficulties that attend our inquiries into the cause of pestilence." He naturally cites Sydenham's analysis of the epidemic constitution of the air with approval.

The other seven chapters of Volume 1 of *Epidemic and Pestilential Diseases* comprise a chronological summary of the history of the subject from the earliest times (beginning with the books of Moses) to the year 1799. Throughout, Webster's essential argument is that epidemics occur in certain periods, generally in widely distributed places; that a pestilential state of air extends, at the same time, over many parts of the world; that if a violent plague is raging in one place, malignant diseases, if not plague, prevail in other places; and that such epidemic periods among human beings are associated with diseases among animals, plagues of locusts, earthquakes, volcanic eruptions and the appearance of comets. Of the plague at Athens, Webster says, after describing earthquakes, droughts, volcanic eruptions, etc., "When we attend to the violent concussions of nature, that accompanied and followed the pestilence, and in general prevalence in the world for a series of ten or twelve years, all attempts to trace its origin to infection, dwindle into puerilities; and the occasional causes of sickness, crowded population, heat and bad diet, tho powerful as auxiliaries, could not be adequate to the violent and continued effects in Athens, and the neighboring cities." In a later paragraph he says, "It will be found invariably true, in every period of the world, that the violence and extent of the plague has been nearly proportioned to the number and violence of the following phenomena—earthquakes, eruptions of volcanoes, meteors, tempests, inundations." Webster, however, has the good sense to warn against "the illusions of credulity and terrified imaginations." "I take no notice," he says, "of the monsters born and an ox's speaking on these occasions."

Webster is very careful to disclaim direct causal connection between any of the physical phenomena discussed. The comets did not cause the earthquakes and inundations. The earthquakes did not cause the epidemics. All were associated with some subtle atmospheric condition which was the effective agent in producing the various catastrophic results. We must remember that Webster assumed all epidemic disease to be alike and progressively increasing in seriousness over long periods. He specifically says, "When therefore we speak of pestilence, as prevailing in a particular year, we are to consider the epidemic as extending to a period of three, four or five years, perhaps to a much longer period, either in the form of plague, a deadly petechial fever, or other fatal disease." Also, that comets, earthquakes and epidemics might precede or follow each other in any order and in any place without interfering with conclusions as to their interrelationship. He says, "It is true that an extraordinary season does not always precede or attend pestilence, in a particular place; but by extending our view of the subject, to general causes, operating over whole quarters of the globe, and perhaps over the whole globe; and considering the causes as invisible, and acting for a series of years, the whole mystery is unfolded." With such leeway in space and time, it is not surprising that Webster was able to prove his point. Earthquakes and comets were pretty sure to occur before or after epidemics at some place on the earth's surface.

Even in the case of the Black Death, Webster denies any form of contagion and explains each plague epidemic as arising from locally preceding diseases of other sorts. Commenting on the epidemic at Avignon, he says, "It is remarkable, that the disease which is technically called *plague*, pestis, is always preceded by a similar fever. It is in fact *the plague in its first stages*, tho it does not exhibit the glandular swellings, which modern physicians contend are characteristic of true plague, and mark a generic or at least a specific difference between that and any other kind of typhus fever. This fact of a *progressiveness* in the disease, annihilates the favorite notion of deducing all plagues from infection; a notion which is bandied about between physicians and legislators like a tennis ball, tho unhappily for mankind, infinitely less harmless."

The Great Plague of London is discussed in considerable detail. Webster combats very successfully the specific theory, which seems based on very flimsy evidence, that the plague of 1665 was introduced by bales of cotton from Holland in the fall of 1664; and he makes the point—quite incontrovertible in the light of the current knowledge of the time—that the half-dozen cases of plague which occurred in 1664 could not possibly have caused the epidemic of 1665 on any known concept of infection. "The suspension of the disease, during six weeks, is evidence that infection had no agency in spreading the disease. It is a fact known and acknowledged, that infection cannot be preserved, for a tenth part of that time in the open air. Air dissolves the poison of any disease, in a very short time. Infection can only be preserved in confinement, as in close vessels or packages of goods. The walls of an infected house will be cleansed by the action of air, in a very few days, so as to be perfectly harmless. During the six weeks suspension of the plague in London, where was the infection concealed to preserve it from air and frost?"

Webster's own view, of course, is that the plagues of 1664 and 1665 arose from a general prevalence of malignant disease in general, beginning in 1661. He assumes that the 1664 cases occurred in highly susceptible persons and that "the severe frost doubtless suspended the operation of the pestilential principle." This is close and good reasoning. Surely a "pestilential principle" might much more plausibly be assumed to lie latent during the winter and become active again in the spring than an infectious agent, as such an agent was visualized in 1800. It needed the rat and the flea to make contagionistic theory fit the facts. The current conception of contagious influence is well illustrated in Chapter VII by an episode recounted in connection with an outbreak of typhus in the town of Bethlehem, Pa. "During this epidemic, a flock of quails flew over the chimney of a house, in which were several diseased persons, and five of them fell dead on the spot. This was thought ominous; but was a natural event, which may rationally be ascribed to deleterious gas emitted from the chambers of the sick."

Some space is devoted to the epidemic of plague at Marseilles in 1720 in contravention of the view that infection was introduced on a ship from Port Said. Deaths did occur on the ship but the plague was not recognized at Port Said until shortly after the ship sailed; so Webster says, "How in the name of reason, could men or goods be infected, when the disease did not exist in the place?" Furthermore, there was a period of six weeks between the last death on the ship and the recognition of the disease in Marseilles, "a circumstance that renders it clearly impossible that there could have been any propagation of the distemper by infection." Until the factor of rat plague was understood the argument against infection was quite sound.

Chapter VIII, the closing chapter of Volume I, completing the historical summary, deals intensively with the period 1788-1798. Here Webster writes from close and intimate study, but the argument is the usual one. This decade was one of peculiarly severe "epidemic constitution" ushered in by earthquakes and an eruption of Vesuvius. It was characterized by a progressive development of epidemic diseases of diverse sorts culminating in America in the yellow fever. He takes up each of the major outbreaks of this disease in turn and demonstrates to his satisfaction that each one was the climax of progressive local disease and was not due to importation.

The New Haven epidemic of 1794 is discussed in detail. The current view was that the outbreak was caused by a chest of clothes brought on a sloop from the West Indies. Webster deals with this theory in masterful fashion, showing that there had been no cases of diseases on the sloop since leaving Martinique, that the chest probably contained no clothing worn by the sailor who died at Martinique, and that the first person to be taken ill in New Haven, Mrs. Gorham, had never been near the famous chest. Here he is on solid ground, for without the knowledge of the role of the mosquito, how could he have recognized the significance of the fact that Mrs. Gorham lived on the adjacent wharf and that nearly all subsequent cases occurred in the immediate neighborhood? He quotes Lind and other authorities to the effect that infection operates only within a range of ten feet. He acknowledges that, once it had started, the New Haven outbreak was propagated by infection; but its original source was to be found in previous diseases of a different sort associated with sickly oysters, multitudes of caterpillars, etc., locally aggravated by garbage, decomposing clams and spoiled fish in the vicinity of the fatal wharf. "The condition of the elements accelerates putrefaction, and that putrefaction in turn increases the deleterious quality of the air."

At Providence in 1797 there was the same story. Always a ship from the West Indies and a local outbreak nearby. Always crude and unsatisfactory attempts by local authorities to visualize a chain of direct infection which Webster can break down with logical ease. Always the prior existence of other diseases which were assumed to develop a gradually increasing malignity. Webster is particularly effective, in this instance, in showing that the blankets from the schooner said to have produced infection had belonged to a sailor who had not been sick and had been kept by him in a chest and not used; while the blanket and clothing of the sailor who died were carried to his home where they produced no disease.

While this first volume is almost wholly historical and chronological, the second begins with a dash of statistics. Chapter ix is purely statistical, consisting of a long table of Bills of Mortality for the seventeenth and eighteenth centuries, complete for London, and with data for Augsburg and Dresden from 1623 to 1726, for Boston from 1701 to 1777, and for Paris, Dublin and one parish in Philadelphia for shorter periods. For each year the table gives data as to the severity of the seasons, comets, volcanic eruptions and prevalence of disease, aside from the figures of mortality. Chapter x is a comment on the foregoing tables, and on the historical data of Volume I. The phenomena most closely connected with pestilences appear to the author to be earthquakes. He says, "I question whether an instance of a considerable plague in any country can be mentioned which has not been immediately preceded or accompanied with convulsions of the earth." Of course the earthquakes need not occur where the pestilence does, but in "some parts of the earth, and especially those which abound most with subterranean fire." Volcanic eruptions are next in order of relationship, then severe winters, then the appearance of comets. Though the material at hand is largely statistical, there is no trace of statistical method. Webster says that out of every 13 comets recorded in his historical summary, 8 coincided with eruptions of Mt. Etna and 11 with pestilence. It never occurs to him, however, to make a control calculation of what happened when comets were not observed. Since out of the 200 years covered in the table in Chapter ix, 67 show records of comets, 85 of volcanic eruptions and 179 of special prevalence of disease the opportunity for coincidence is not inconsiderable! Yet neither physician nor layman could, perhaps, have been expected to use controls or apply real statistical methods of analysis in 1799.

Chapter xi reviews certain particular pestilential periods with a view to showing that diseases gradually progress and develop from measles and influenza to diseases of the throat or anginas and finally to pestilential fever; and that such pestilential periods are generally worldwide in their incidence. Chapter xii reviews in greater detail the history of influenza as "the disease most closely connected with pestilence and the least dependent on local causes." "This epidemic," he concludes, "is evidently the effect of some insensible qualities of the atmosphere; as it spreads with astonishing rapidity over land and sea, uncontrolled by heat or cold, drouth or moisture. From these circumstances, and its near coincidence in time with the violent action of fire in earthquakes and volcanoes, there is reason to conclude the disease to be the effect of some access of stimulant powers to the atmosphere by means of the electrical principle. No other principle in creation, which has yet come under the cognizance of the human mind, seems adequate to the same effects."

Chapter xiii deals with the "order, connection and progression of pestilential epidemics," which is really the basic assumption in Webster's whole philosophy. He bases his theories on Hippocrates and Sydenham and is chiefly preoccupied with the seasonal cycle of respiratory diseases in the winter, dysentery and similar mild intestinal disorders in summer, and yellow fever in autumn, which strongly suggests a "progression." Chapter xiv deals with the wide, and often world-wide prevalence of a "pestilential state of the air." Webster's thesis is that epidemics of various sorts are nearly contemporary in Europe and America which fact he concludes "demonstrates that such diseases are occasioned solely by a constitution of air, without the influence of contagion, although when the diseases (in this special case measles and the anginas) are formed they are contagious."

Chapter xv deals in greater detail with the sequence of events which determine epidemic periods. Webster again deplores the excesses of "judicial astrology" but argues on reasonably rational grounds for the physical influences of heavenly bodies. "We are naturally led to suppose that all parts of our system are connected by principles of attraction and that a certain order and equilibrium are necessary to keep all parts in due harmony." If the moon affects the weather, why not the planets and the comets? He reviews all the phenomena related to the epidemic constitution of the atmosphere, dark days, fogs, diseases among plants and animals. "In all the great plagues which have afflicted the human race, other animals, as horses, cattle, sheep, sometimes cats, dogs and fowls, together with the fish in rivers and the oceans, and even vegetables, have borne their share in the calamity. The pestilential principle has extended to every species of life. The beasts of the field perish with deadly epidemics, the fish die on the bottom of rivers and the sea, or become lean and sickly; while corn is blasted on the most fertile plains, and the fruits in gardens and orchards, wither or fail to arrive at their usual state of perfection." Plagues of noxious insects occur and fowls, perceiving the altered state of the atmosphere which precedes calamity, leave their accustomed haunts.

Webster does not attempt to define precisely the change in the atmosphere which causes all these catastrophes. He favors, on the whole, the theory of "a superabundant stimulus, occasioned by the shock of an earthquake, and an atmosphere surcharged with electricity." The internal fires of the earth are held to be the probable ultimate cause of the electrical disturbances.

Webster then proceeds to combat certain alternative theories with the usual arguments. He shows that hot, damp air and putrid exhalations do not *always* cause epidemics and that famines do not *always* cause epidemics. Therefore some other factor must come in—the general epidemic constitution. As to contagion he makes a point which is quite sound, if we have no knowledge of a biological cause susceptible of evolutionary transformation. He says, speaking of a disease of cattle, "Like the writers on the cause of the plague in Egypt, who trace it to Barbary or Syria, and there leave the subject; so Lancisius and Ramazzini tell us that the distemper which destroyed most of the cattle in Italy, came from one cow, in a drove from Dalmatia; and there they stop short, without a syllable to explain why the cow from Dalmatia was seized. All these contagion-sticklers resemble the Indian, who, when asked what the world stands on, replied, on an elephant—the elephant on a great turtle, and the turtle on the ocean. Here he stopped, and as to what supports the ocean, he leaves us in the dark."

In Chapter xvi "On Contagion and Infection," Webster proceeds to definitions of what he means by "contagion" and "infection" based on suggestions by Maclean and by Bailey of New York—which definitions are highly significant.

"Specific contagion," he says, "I define to be, a quality of a disease, which, within a suitable distance, communicates it from a body affected with it, to a sound body, with great certainty, and under all circumstances of season, weather or situation."

On the other hand, "That quality of a disease which may or may not excite it in a sound body within a suitable distance, or by contact; and which depends on heat, foul air, an apt disposition in the receiving body, or other contingent circumstances, and which may excite the disease in the same person more than once" is given the denomination of infection.

Now the particularly interesting thing about this distinction is that Maclean and Webster cited measles and smallpox as examples of the first type, plague, dysentery and epidemic fevers as of the second. In other words, they recognized as contagious the two most common diseases due to filterable viruses—the two in which neither well carriers nor infection by fomites are known. They even recognized the specially high degree of acquired immunity which characterizes these virus diseases.

Webster raises certain highly pertinent questions with regard to the assumed importance of the factor of infection. How is it that a few early cases can occur as in London in 1664 to be followed after temporary cessation by a great epidemic? This fact, according to Webster, totally overthrows the ideas of infection—"It being impossible that the operation of infection should be thus suspended, and afterwards revived." Surely this was a sound argument on any then-available theory of infection.

The development of virulence during the course of an epidemic was another strong argument against infection. How could infection as then understood vary in its force? Epidemic constitution could, however, as usual meet any exigencies of the situation.

The cessation of epidemics is even more strongly emphasized. Webster says, "But the most incontrovertible evidence, that infection is not the primary controlling cause of the plague, arises from the manner in which the epidemic ceases. If infection were the principal and specific cause of its propagation, it must rage forever, or as long as any of the human race should survive to receive it; for the longer the disease exists, the more extensive must it be. This conclusion is inevitable; for if infection spreads the disease so rapidly, that one or two persons diffuse it in a few weeks over a city, the same principle must, in a given time, extend it over the whole earth, unless its operation should be arrested by a superior cause. And as one diseased person is supposed to infect more than one healthy person, its progress must be accelerated, in a duplicate, triplicate and quadruplicate ratio to its distance from its source. Its velocity also must be increased, not only by numbers in a crowded city, but by an augmented virulence, until all the inhabitants should be destroyed."

Today we explain the cessation of epidemics in part by acquired immunity; but Webster, as we have seen, denied such immunity in the plague. We explain it in part by seasonal effects. Webster discusses this and shows that epidemics (of various kinds) sometimes cease at one season and sometimes at another and are sometimes unaffected by season. Even today, of course, we have no explanation—except on the assumption of a loss of virulence—of such a phenomenon as the waning of the 1918 epidemic of influenza.

For all these reasons Webster heaps scorn on the theory of importation and on the current concepts of the spread of disease by fomites. "The Egyptians," he says, "were like all modern nations—unwilling to believe the plague generated at home—they ascribed it to infection brought by flying serpents, as the moderns ascribe it to old clothes, bales of goods, and infected ships." In another place he says, "Chandler, in his travels, gives us wonderful discoveries on this subject. He says, the disease proceeds from certain invisible animalcules, burrowing and forming their nest in the human body. These are imported annually into Smyrna—they are least at the beginning, and later end of the season. If they arrive early in spring, they are weak, but gather strength, multiply and then perish." This seems to us a highly suggestive statement. To Webster it was so absurd as scarcely to need refutation.

He devotes considerable attention to the evidence for contagion based on maritime origin, quoting the College of Physicians of Philadelphia to the effect that pestilential fever "commences invariably in our seaports, while inland towns, equally exposed to the ordinary causes of fever, escape." Webster meets this argument not too effectively—first by claiming exceptions to the rule (exceptions based on his inclusion of all types of pestilential diseases as identical) and, second, by suggesting that the humidity of maritime and lake cities renders them particularly susceptible to infection.

Webster next proceeds to discuss the practice of quarantine, and here is on firmer ground. He demonstrates quite clearly the almost complete failure of quarantine procedures as actually practiced. This, indeed, was a rather strong ground for disbelieving in the current theories of infection, for unless one suspected the role of human and animal carriers it was hard to see why quarantine regulations so often failed of their purpose. "The application of quarantine laws to our epidemic pestilential fever, is just as useless as the order of the Sultan, Achmet I in the wasting plague of 1613, for transporting all the cats in Constantinople to the island of Scutari."

On the other hand, Webster does acknowledge the value of quarantine in certain instances, particularly with regard to jail and ship fever (typhus). He says that such diseases are propagated by infection among crowded populations, spreading by contact or near approach and never assuming the complexion of an epidemic.

Here, Webster makes a new distinction, the effect of which is to transfer certain maladies from the pestilential to the communicable class. He says, "hence the necessity of distinguishing carefully between *epidemic* pestilence, proceeding principally from general causes in the elements, and marked by other epidemic diseases, by the failure of vegetable productions and by the sickness, or death of cattle, fish and other animals— and *diseases merely infectious*, generated by artificial means, which *may* be communicated, which may happen in jails, ships and camps, in the healthiest state of the elements, and which cease as soon as the infection can be dissipated by purifications and fresh air."

Thus, we may assume, Webster for practical purposes places ship and jail fever with smallpox and measles as at times a communicable disease.

For all the rest (including the petechial fevers which he seems not to identify with ship and jail fevers) he assumes three factors: infection (a minor one, operating only in certain circumstances), local harmful conditions due to climate, season or putrid exhalations and, above all, the general epidemic constitution of the atmosphere.

Infection, as a rule, he conceives as secondary. He says of its part in originating an outbreak, "I will admit the *bare possibility*, that imported infection may kindle the flame of pestilence, in a place fitted for it by local causes, where no pestilence would appear without a spark from infection. This is as much as I can admit to be possible and more than I believe. . . . Of the nature of the infecting principle in disease we know very little. . . . It is supposed that the diseased body discharges certain fine poisonous particles which are suspended and diffused in the air, and being imbibed by the pores of the skin and with the breath, excite the same species of distemper in a healthy body." The infecting principle in smallpox and plague must be very different, since the first always operates and the second only under certain circumstances. The infection in the case of plague and other autumnal diseases "appears to consist of a species of air, which is one of the elementary parts of all vegetable and animal substances. It may be what Dr. Mitchill denominates, the *septic acid*; that fluid which is discharged from flesh in the process of putrefaction. . . . It operates, in producing disease, no otherwise than all the morbid exhalations extricated from every species of vegetable and animal substances in the putrefactive process."

It is of interest to note that Webster recognizes clearly the seasonal characteristics of certain forms of disease and speculates as to why the effluvia of smallpox, measles and angina should be independent of temperature, while those of dysentery, plague and typhus fevers are excited by heat and destroyed by cold.

Next come the local pestilential factors which, like infection, increase the effect of the epidemic principle. "The infection of the plague, dysentery and the like seems therefore, to be nothing more than an *access of noxious matter, to the local causes, morbid exhalations.* The noxious airs of filthy streets, docks and tenements, are secondary and augmenting causes of the plague; when the disease appears, the effluvia from the disease still *augment* these other local causes." Infection, local morbid exhalations and epidemic constitution are all cooperating chemical changes in the air.

In ordinary healthy periods, marsh effluvia produce the common intermittent and remittent fevers (malaria and typhoid). When the epidemic pestilential constitution of the air supervenes, they produce "bilious plagues of the country" in combination with marsh effluvia; "bilious plagues of American cities" in combination with vegetable and animal effluvia jointly; and the "inguinal plague of the east" in combination with animal exhalations.

An epidemic disease—that is, a disease due to the general epidemic constitution of the atmosphere—can be distinguished from one due to infection or specific contagion by two characteristics. First, it is always "preceded by influenza, affections of the throat or acute and malignant fevers." Second, it "predominates over other diseases; totally absorbing them or compelling them to assume its characteristic symptoms." "In every possible case, a plague that banishes other diseases, as I believe it always does, is an epidemic generated in the place where it exists; for it is not possible that this expulsion of other diseases, could take place, unless the epidemic depended solely on the elements."

Quarantine may be effective and is justifiable when we are dealing with infectious diseases such as smallpox and jail fever but is useless when dealing with what Webster calls an epidemic—that is, one due to the general atmospheric principle. "In nine cases of ten, in which quarantine is enjoined, human efforts are opposed to the great laws of nature, and are therefore useless. In all cases, where the air of a country exhibits evidences of a pestilential constitution, in an increase of the number and violence of the symptoms of common diseases; in the production of certain epidemics, as catarrh, anginas, measles, petechial fevers and the like; in the death of fish or the unusual diseases of cattle and other animals; in the production of insects, uncommon in size, in kind or numbers, and other remarkable phenomena before mentioned; in all such cases, the pestilence which invades man will be found to arise solely from the uncontrollable laws of the elements; and quarantine will be utterly unavailing."

Nothing could well be more fatalistic than this conclusion; but Webster was essentially a practical and an optimistic person. So it is in accord with psychology, if not with logic, that he returns to the factor of local noxious exhalations for final major emphasis. Indeed his most vigorous criticism of Mead's deadly fallacies is based not on the needless interferences with commerce caused by unjustified quarantine. "These," he says, "are not the worst effects. The erroneous system of specific contagion has misled mankind into a fatal security, on the subject of the local causes of diseases. Supposing the laws competent to guard public health, men have not attended to the best modes of constructing houses and cities, and to the means of watering and cleansing them—means by which all the slighter pestilences might be avoided, and the more severe ones greatly mitigated. . . . Had Mead, and other eminent physicians taken the same pains to lead mankind into truth, as into error, we should long ago have introduced improvements into the arrangement and structure of our cities which would have secured our citizens from nine-tenths of the infectious diseases, by which they have been alarmed and distressed."

Chapter xvii draws more detailed practical conclusions as to "the means of preventing or mitigating pestilential diseases." This is to be accomplished by public sanitation and personal hygiene. It is essential in order to control the lesser plagues and mitigate the greater ones to eliminate putrescible substances by municipal scavenging and particularly by liberal use of water in streets and houses. Marshes should be drained; and Webster presents an idealistic program of city planning, including the use of a sloping terrain, proper design of wharves and docks, straight streets at right angles, lots at least 60 by 250 feet with not over 40 per cent of the frontage built upon, a garden behind each house, and an alley running behind the gardens through each block. The streets with their footwalks should be 100 feet wide and planted with three rows of trees. The city should be supplied with fresh running water.

As elements in personal hygiene, he stresses avoidance of excesses of diet, extreme exposure to the heat of the sun, and undue fatigue. Special emphasis is laid on the importance of bathing. The practice of "leaping into river or sea water" is condemned, as is long immersion in very warm water, both being considered as debilitating and the first highly dangerous in hot weather. "The most safe, easy, pleasant and beneficial mode of using water, is, to bathe or wash the body in a private apartment at home. This may be done in several ways—either in a large vessel immersing the whole body at once; or, what is less troublesome with a single pail or bowl of water in a bed chamber. The washing may be done with the hand, or a sponge, in a few minutes, as the person rises in the morning or retires at night." Webster in a concluding appeal reemphasizes his belief that "The only means of avoiding or mitigating epidemic pestilence are first to withdraw the aid of local causes; secondly to fit the body, by modes of living, to resist its causes; and thirdly, on failure of these, to remove from the place where it exists."

In reviewing Webster's theories of epidemiology, it is evident that he added no new principle and that the difference between his etiology and that of other writers whom we have quoted (except Sydenham) lies chiefly in his predominant emphasis on the factor of epidemic constitution.

Webster and his contemporaries were, of course, perfectly sound in arguing that in the case of such diseases as the remittent and intermittent fevers, typhus, plague and yellow fever, the factor of infection as then understood could not possibly account for observed phenomena. To them, the theory of infection involved the simple assumption that (a) a previous recognized case of disease causes (b) a second recognized case of disease. This was often manifestly untrue. Today, we should say that either (a) a clinical case or (a_1) a human carrier sometimes plus (a_2) an insect or animal carrier or an inanimate carrier such as water or milk causes (b) the second clinical case. It required knowledge of the germ and, particularly, of the human carrier to make the theory of infection plausible. This is why the medical profession, from Hippocrates to Pettenkofer and Murchison, fought against the layman's fundamentally correct concept of communicability. The layman perceived the broad relationships; but the physician, knowing more, realized that there were fatal exceptions to any doctrine of communicability which could be formulated, until the role of the human and animal and inanimate carriers was understood.

Unfortunately, as Webster's studies progressed, he tended to move farther and farther away from a sound balancing of two independent factors, infection and local causes, which were so well recognized by Dr. E. H. Smith and by Webster himself in his earlier volume. More and more he came to minimize the role of infection and the danger of communicability. His attitude and that of Rush, LaRoche and other strong anti-contagionists, is largely, I think, to be explained by their concept of the nature of infection. They conceived it, and often defined it, as something which operated with absolute inevitability and within a very narrow spatial range. Webster puts the maximum possible range of infection sometimes at ten feet, sometimes at ten paces. The infectious agent was visualized as a chemical gaseous agent (septic acid). It was natural that such an agent should be assumed to be either present or absent, operative when present on all within the fatal radius, incapable of influence beyond that radius, and insusceptible of modification by climate or season or local circumstances.

It is this sort of infection or contagion (for he uses the words quite indiscriminately throughout most of the text) which Webster denies in yellow fever and in most other epidemic diseases. His chief arguments, like those of other non-contagionists, may be summarized as follows.

1. Cases occur without exposure to a preexisting case of disease. Here, of course, was a perfectly sound argument. Webster is most effective in demolishing many detailed attempts of the contagionists to demonstrate actual routes of infection by fomites. He shows that at New Haven and Providence the blankets and clothing supposed to cause the primary cases could not have been infected and that the soiled blankets of an actual patient failed to produce results. He shows that the sufferers had generally not been in direct contact with previous cases and in certain instances had not been out of their houses for weeks. Until the role of the carrier was understood, such arguments were incontrovertible.

2. In many epidemics the spread has been so rapid as to preclude the possibility of infection as the primary cause. The violence and explosiveness of influenza certainly lent plausible color to this criticism.

3. Direct exposure to cases of disease frequently—and, in the case of yellow fever, generally—fails to produce infection. The absence of secondary cases at the Bush Hill Hospital was Devèze's chief argument, and the fact that patients from New York and Philadelphia who moved into the country never caused secondary cases was a powerful argument, definitely proving the necessity for some second factor, if it did not demonstrate the absence of any factor of communicability. A similar type of evidence was the failure of certain epidemics to spread from one community to another.

4. Many epidemic diseases, and particularly yellow fever, remain strictly localized in restricted areas of the city.

5. Most epidemic diseases are definitely associated with particular seasons, which again argues strongly for some factor other than infection.

6. Epidemics, particularly of plague, often show a few cases and then an intermission and then a recrudescence. Sometimes, as in London in 1664-1665, the latent period extends over a winter. How could such a phenomenon be consistent with infection until the animal carrier was known? A chemical poison in the air could scarcely remain latent and then break out again.

7. Epidemics run their course and then die out. Yet, if a chemical infection were the cause it should multiply in geometrical ratio until the human race were extinct. We explain this phenomenon partly by acquired immunity (which Webster denied in plague and yellow fever) and partly by seasonal influences. In the case of such a disease as influenza we assume a cyclical change in the virulence of the organism. But chemical infection as understood in Webster's day could hardly be supposed to show such a change.

8. Finally, Webster raises the ingenious and pertinent question as to the ultimate origin of infection. If it spreads from Egypt to France and from Syria to Egypt, how did it first come into being in Syria? Through some other cause? Then why not through the direct action of that same cause in Egypt and in England?

It was these arguments which led Webster to maintain that (except in smallpox and measles and sometimes in typhus fever) infection played a relatively minor and secondary role. Above all, he was always vehement in his criticism of any assumption that disease had been imported from one country to another and almost emotional in his repeated flings at Mead, whom he evidently regarded as the chief advocate of the importation theory. He allows that quarantine may operate with regard to a disease like typhus when in an infectious stage, but considers quarantine regulations as in general quite ineffective. He objects to them (except in special instances) as placing an unwarranted burden on commerce and, above all, as diverting attention from the really important factors of local sanitation and personal hygiene.

The second major factor recognized in the eighteenth century as contributing to the prevalence of epidemic disease was a mephitic condition of the air due to climate and season or to local pollution by decomposing organic matter. This was the factor commonly opposed to that of infection in the yellow fever controversies, and it was always recognized by Webster, although with varying emphasis. The fact that infection sometimes operated and sometimes failed to do so, the seasonal incidence of various diseases, and particularly the localization of epidemics in certain areas—usually low and waterlogged and uncleanly—pointed clearly to local influences. Webster considered such influences as determining with regard to the regular summer fevers (malaria, dysentery, typhoid, etc.) and as contributory in the greater pestilences (plague and yellow fever). He recognized the vicinity of marshes as of special importance, supporting this conclusion particularly with evidence from Italy and the United States where malaria was prevalent; and, in general, laid stress on dampness and accumulations of decomposing organic matter. Like Rush, he thought human and animal feces less important than decomposing vegetable and animal matter.

In the *Collection of Papers on Bilious Fevers* these local miasmatic influences received major emphasis, and here the reasoning of Webster and his contemporaries was essentially sound. They were quite right in believing that the infection of malaria and typhoid, of plague and yellow fever, would not spread unless local conditions permitted. In the greater part of the *Epidemic and Pestilential Diseases*, however, the factor of local miasms does not loom very large. Webster is chiefly concerned with proving the need for still a third factor, and emphasizes the fact that putrefaction and dampness and season often fail to produce the effects which would be expected.

This third factor—the one which Webster throughout the *Epidemic and Pestilential Diseases* chiefly emphasizes—is the general epidemic constitution of the atmosphere. From the time of Hippocrates belief had persisted in such an influence, quite aside from local miasms, as accounting for the pandemic prevalence of the major plagues.

The epidemic constitution, according to Webster was generally a world-wide condition and it was associated with other biological and meteorological phenomena of which the most important were epidemic diseases of cattle, fish and other animals, diseases of plants, disappearance of birds who perceived and fled before the approaching calamity, plagues of noxious insects, storms, cold winters, hot summers, "dark days," floods, earthquakes, volcanic eruptions, and the appearance of comets and meteors. Such associations, or some of them, were accepted by the majority of medical writers from the days of the Greeks to the middle of the nineteenth century; but the *Epidemic and Pestilential Diseases* is certainly one of the most exhaustive summaries of evidence in support of their existence.

It should be clearly emphasized, first, that Webster was not thinking of any mystical astrological influence but of a strictly physical one; and, secondly, that the various catastrophic phenomena listed were not supposed to cause each other but were all brought about by a deeper underlying condition of the atmosphere. "There must be an alteration in the chymical properties of the atmosphere to solve the difficulties that attend our inquiries into the cause of pestilence." Webster was inclined to believe that the basic factor was electrical and associated with changes in the inner fires of the earth. Mephitic vapors might play a secondary role, but only electricity could account for all the mysteries involved; and Webster suggests that its influence on the human body may be exerted chiefly by producing excessive stimulation followed by debility.

It was this basic condition of the atmosphere which was the true cause of great pestilences; but its most terrible effects were produced only when reinforced by local miasms and were sometimes supplemented by infection. The cooperation of the three forces was easy to visualize. The epidemic constitution was a physical and chemical state of the atmosphere. Local miasmatic conditions added other deleterious chemicals (septic acid). Finally, contagion might contribute other chemical effluvia of much the same nature, generated by the diseased body in its immediate vicinity, much as the local miasms were produced over a wider area in the neighborhood of marshes and accumulations of putrefying organic matter.

There were valid reasons for the persistence of the theory of epidemic constitution. Hippocrates and Sydenham were not fools—and neither was Noah Webster. Great epidemics, as distinguished from ordinary endemic prevalence of disease, could not and cannot be accounted for solely by infection (even as we understand it today) or by infection combined with local environmental factors. Why did bubonic plague become pandemic in 1894 and influenza in 1918? We do not know. The recognition of an unknown "x-factor" is logically essential. We assume, on theoretical grounds, a change in virulence or a symbiotic action of two germs. Hippocrates and Sydenham assumed an epidemic constitution of the atmosphere. In 1800 their view was still the more plausible.

What was unfortunate about Webster's thinking was the relative weight which he attached to the three major factors in the problem. He minimized the influence of direct communicability, denying it any important part except in measles and smallpox; and he enormously exaggerated the third or "x-factor" to which he attributed nineteen-twentieths of the plagues and pestilences which afflict mankind.

We owe to the Greeks the basis of all scientific thinking, for it was they who first established the principle of scientific causation and gave us faith in the orderly objectiveness of natural phenomena. The Greek thinkers freed us from anthropomorphism; but they left us an unhappy though less sinister heritage in their fondness for intellectual abstractions. The epidemic constitution is a case in point. Known factors were indeed inadequate; but epidemic constitution was an abstract theoretical concept, having no tangible properties and hence insusceptible of scientific analysis or experimental proof or disproof. With its protean and elusive possibilities, it infected medical thought for twenty centuries and furnished a plausible explanation which really explained nothing but which turned the mind away from the search for more valid causes. It was a tempting mirage of a high road which led nowhere but diverted attention from the narrower and more difficult paths by which truth could be approached. It was the chief source of Webster's errors. It is interesting to note that Webster quotes the statement of Mead, in regard to assumed atmospheric changes, "It may be justly censured in those writers that they should undertake to determine the specific nature of these secret changes and alterations which we have no means at all of discovering": and says that this sentence is "very exceptionable, as it is calculated to check a spirit of free inquiry—a spirit to which mankind are greatly indebted for improvements in science." Yet Mead was here expressing the sound scepticism of the experimental thinker with regard to an assumed abstract principle incapable of scientific proof or disproof.

It is, of course, obvious that Webster's belief in the epidemic constitution was largely conditioned by his denial of the specificity of the various epidemic diseases. The fallacious assumptions that one disease progresses into another and that one disease replaces another might be attributed to the fact that Webster was a layman. Yet these views were held by the ablest physicians from Hippocrates to Sydenham. Even LaRoche fifty years later assumes a transition between the ordinary remittents and intermittents and yellow fever. The specificity of tuberculosis was not accepted till Koch discovered the tubercle bacillus in 1882. The distinction between diphtheria and other "anginas" was not clearly drawn till bacteriological methods of diagnosis were applied ten years later. The discovery of the germ and the demonstration of the carrier were essential to a sound theory of etiology.

The writings of Rush were, on the whole, far sounder than those of Webster in their greater emphasis on local miasmatic factors as distinguished from the epidemic constitution of the atmosphere, but the two writers were at one in their denial of importation and contagion and in their practical stress on sanitary measures for the control of the environmental factors which favor the spread of epidemic disease. Webster was, perhaps, the last distinguished exponent of the epidemic constitution as Hippocrates and Sydenham had understood it; but the views which he and Rush shared as to the importance of miasms was to dominate epidemiological thought for nearly a century. LaRoche in his classic monograph on *Yellow Fever*, published in 1855 devotes but 30 pages to facts and arguments in favor of the contagious character of the disease and 330 pages to "facts and arguments against contagion" and "proofs of non-contagion." Even in 1898 an official bulletin of the United States Marine Hospital Service could say that, in yellow fever "one has not to contend with an organism or germ which may be taken into the body with food or drinks but with an almost inexplicable poison so insidious in its approach and entrance that no trace is left behind."

The enigma of yellow fever had to wait till the eve of the twentieth century for its solution.

CHAPTER XII

THE GREAT SANITARY AWAKENING

"It has been among the oldest and most universal of medical experiences that populations, living amid Filth, and within direct reach of its polluting influence, succumb to various diseases which under opposite conditions are comparatively or absolutely unknown."—SIMON

THE first half of the nineteenth century was marked by the inception of the modern public health movement. Under the stimulus of a group of enthusiastic humanitarians, a campaign for sanitary reform was launched in England and spread throughout the world to lay the foundation for our modern war against disease. The theoretical basis of this campaign is therefore of vital interest in tracing the evolution of epidemiological thought.

The problems of the nineteenth century were very different from those of the seventeenth and eighteenth. Plague, which for four hundred years had constituted a major menace, had almost disappeared from Western Europe; and even typhus fever had become far less prevalent than in earlier centuries. Yellow fever continued as the great threat to the New World; but in Europe cholera and typhoid were the outstanding problems. It was the intestinal diseases with which the sanitarians of the early nineteenth century were chiefly concerned; and these, of course, were precisely the diseases in which environmental sanitation was of fundamental importance. Therefore the concept of local miasms fitted the case remarkably well. As we shall see, however, the nineteenth century Filth Theory of Disease was a relatively precise and scientific form of the old doctrine of miasms. It was backed up by statistical and epidemiological evidence; and it actually accomplished results in the practical control of epidemic disease.

As a connecting link between the old phase and the new we may consider the contributions to epidemiology of the very first of the pioneer English sanitarians, John Howard (1726-1790). Appointed Sheriff of Bedfordshire in 1773, he discovered the most appalling conditions of mismanagement and exploitation in the jails for which he was theoretically responsible. He took this responsibility with admirable seriousness and set out, at his own expense, to inspect jails in other counties of England and, finally, on the continent. "Howard presented his exhaustive findings in prosaic but overwhelmingly convincing form, to the House of Commons in 1774. He received the official thanks of Parliament and had the greater satisfaction of seeing passed forthwith a bill for the abolition of the fee system of paying gaolers and another for the betterment of the sanitary condition of prisons. Prisons were to be whitewashed yearly, regularly washed and ventilated; rooms were to be set apart for the sick, hot and cold water baths provided, and in cases of necessity clothes were to be lent to prisoners; surgeons and apothecaries were to be appointed. Very moderate steps forward; yet they not only set in motion the whole modern movement for prison reform but formed the thin edge of the wedge in introducing into the mind of the British public the fundamental conceptions of sanitation."

In the jails of the time, typhus fever was the outstanding problem. The interest aroused in Howard's mind by this disease led him in 1785 to undertake a tour abroad for a study of the quarantine stations of France and Italy. An illuminating report on "The Principal Lazarettos in Europe with various papers relative to the Plague," published in 1789, gives an excellent picture of the theory and practice of the day.

So far as maritime quarantine stations were concerned, plague—which still prevailed in the Near East—was the chief danger in view. Howard therefore prepared himself with a questionnaire on the epidemiology of this disease, and submitted it to the physicians whom he visited at the various ports. One chapter of his book is devoted to the opinions of these authorities. In answer to the question, "Is the Infection of Plague frequently communicated by the Touch?" all answer in the affirmative, most believing that very near approach or direct contact is essential, while one held that "those who approach the atmosphere of a pestiential body may receive the infection by respiration." As to the question whether the plague ever arises spontaneously, nearly all answer in the negative and believe wholeheartedly in importation and spread by contact. Two, out of eight authorities, however, accept the idea of possible spontaneous origin. The distance at which the air may be infected around the patient is estimated at "a few paces," "some paces," "five geometrical paces," and "two ells"; but several believe that the range of contagion varies with the virulence of the disease. Control is to be sought by avoidance of contact, purification of goods (by exposure to the air for forty days), and fumigation of the air with aromatics and sulphur, also sprinkling with vinegar. Howard's own observations give a vivid picture of the way in which the quarantine regulations were actually carried out at various seaports. At Venice, it is provided that "The prior and his substitute must carefully avoid touching either goods or passengers in quarantine, and for that end, in their walks and visits always carry a cane to keep passengers at a proper distance; but if by an unfortunate accident they should be contaminated by touch, they must perform the quarantine from whence the suspicion of infection was derived, and others would be appointed in their room, *pro tempore*." At Malta, it is noted that "a letter brought by a ship just arrived from Turkey was, I saw, received with a pair of iron tongs, dipped in vinegar, and then put into a case, and laid for about a quarter of an hour on wire grates, under which straw and perfumes had been burnt." The "expurgation" of goods at Venice is described in detail. Wool, flax, feathers and similar materials were aired for forty days, by removing them from their containers and mixing and turning over the heaps twice a day by porters working with hands and arms bared. Woollen and linen cloths were periodically unfolded and refolded and sometimes hung on cords for better exposure to the air. Furs were considered specially dangerous and were "very often waved and shaken." Such articles as beeswax, sponges and candles were purged by immersion in salt water for forty-eight hours. Salted hides, grains, salt, minerals, and the like were considered non-infectible.

Thus we see that at the end of the eighteenth century plague, at least, was recognized as communicable, and that an elaborate quarantine system had been built up for dealing with that disease—involving many cumbrous and unnecessary procedures (and ignoring the vital factor of the rat) but undoubtedly of some substantial efficacy in controlling the unrecognized factor of flea-borne infection. Howard himself was thoroughly convinced of the contagiousness of this disease; but it must be remembered that his contact was with the officials of quarantine stations who were naturally believers in the value of their own work. Howard cites at least one authority, Dr. Maximilian Stoll of Vienna, as advocating the same non-importationist views advanced by Rush and Webster in America.

Howard has given us a picture of the officially-accepted practices employed for the control of plague; but we naturally ask, "What were the fundamental theoretical conceptions underlying such practices?" "How did the sanitarian of 1800 visualize the actual nature of 'contagion'?" For answer to these questions, we may profitably turn to a distinguished

French savant, whose influence on this point was perhaps as great as that of any other authority of his time.[1]

L.-B. Guyton-Morveau (1737-1816) was trained as a lawyer at Dijon but early developed a keen interest in chemistry and was instrumental in introducing instruction in natural sciences at his native university. He collaborated with Lavoisier and Berthollet in developing a new nomenclature in chemistry and took an active part in combating the theory of phlogiston. When the storm of the Revolution broke, he became an active member of the Party of the Mountain, president of the Committee of Public Safety, and commissioner general of the Army of the North. He was appointed professor of chemistry at the newly-organized Ecole Polytechnique in 1794, under the rule of the Convention. In 1797, he retired from political life. He became a member of the reconstituted Institute, and in 1798 was appointed director of the Polytechnic School. In 1800, under Napoleon, he was made administrator of the Mint. In 1803, he received the cross of the Legion of Honor (officer in 1805) and in 1811 was made a Baron of the Empire.

The work of Guyton-Morveau in which we are here interested is summarized in a volume on methods of disinfecting air and preventing contagion and arresting its progress, published in 1802. The aim of this treatise is to elaborate on the value of hydrochloric acid as an agent for disinfection. Chaptal in a preliminary note says that in 1801 "The British House of Commons has just voted a grant of 5000 pounds sterling to Doctor Smyth, the originator of an important discovery, which makes it possible to disinfect the vitiated air of prisons, hospitals, etc."; and claims priority for France in this field on the strength of Guyton-Morveau's discoveries, dating back to 1773. James Carmichael Smyth had advocated nitric rather than hydrochloric acid and his studies began at Winchester in 1780.

Guyton's process was based on the logical theory that, since putrefaction is accompanied by the production of great quantities of ammonia, hydrochloric acid is the natural agent to neutralize the dangerous products of putrefaction. He demonstrated the reaction experimentally by

---

[1] To illustrate how concretely our forefathers conceived infection we may cite a passage from one William Grant quoted by Murchison: "If any person will take the trouble to stand in the sun and look at his own shadow on a white-plastered wall, he will easily perceive that his whole body is a smoking dunghill, with a vapour exhaling from every part of it. This vapour is subtle, acrid, and offensive to the smell; if retained by the body it becomes morbid; but if re-absorbed, highly deleterious. If a number of persons, therefore, are long confined in any close place, not properly ventilated, so as to inspire and swallow with their spittle, the vapours of each other, they must soon feel its bad effects."

the cloud of ammonium chloride produced in this reaction; and applied it first to the air of the burial vaults of the church at Dijon (in 1773) by liberating the fumes from a mixture of salt and sulphuric acid. This was apparently the initiation of the use of chlorine as an atmospheric deodorant. Later, a similar procedure of acid fumigation was utilized by Guyton in hospitals and prisons; by Smyth and his colleague Menzies on British and Russian ships, by Cruickshank in England and by Manthey in Denmark. Guyton reviews a large number of possible chemicals which might be used for disinfecting air. He considers aromatic fumigants and vinegar, the lighting of fires and firing of cannon, as of little value. Pure acetic acid and sulphurous fumes may be useful; but the mineral acids are most efficacious. These views are not based on fine-spun theory but on specific, well-conducted experiments, of which forty-two are fully reported in the text. In each of these experiments he tested in the laboratory the power of a specific fumigant to destroy or neutralize the odors produced in an enclosed vessel by putrefying material. The mineral acids proved by far the most efficacious of the materials studied; and it is of special interest to note that Guyton really comprehends the fact that the fumes of these acids act essentially as oxidizing agents. He considers their power of destroying organic effluvia themselves as primarily dependent on a process of oxidation; and he also believes that, in a less clearly understood fashion, oxygen tends to increase the vital powers of the human body in resistance against disease. (It is of interest to note that when chlorine was first used for water purification in this country thirty years ago, its concentration was expressed in terms of "potential oxygen.") In summary of this section, Guyton says, "Thus, oxygen, and above all, the gaseous liberators of oxygen, manifestly produce two effects which contribute toward the same end: they exercise upon the contagious miasms an affinity which decomposes those miasms; and they aid nature to resist that power of assimilation which constitutes their danger."

Guyton then proceeds to consider the question how far the conclusions drawn from his laboratory experiments may be applicable in actual sanitary practice. He says,

"145. Since the experiments which I have reported have been only concerned with the products of animal putrefaction and with the air infected by such putrefaction, one has the right to ask whether the agencies whose efficacy I have demonstrated would exert the same power upon contagious germs [*germes contagieux*] of a different nature. It would, I am convinced, be going beyond the evidence to assume that all the maladies which may be communicated from the sick to the well have the same material as a common cause; in view of the fact that the symptoms which these diseases manifest indicate particular individual characteristics, and that there are many of them, such as scabies, small-pox, venereal disease, plague, rabies, etc., whose propagation manifestly depends on a specific virus [*virus spécifique*]; but such a first glance at the question can not give us its ultimate solution.

"146. We may admit the distinction, properly established, between those diseases which arise from certain emanations generally distributed throughout the atmosphere, which we call epidemic because they attack a multitude of people who are exposed to them and those other diseases which are contracted only by immediate contact with a material which is also often invisible but less volatile, sometimes by the introduction into the body of a morbific ferment [*levain morbifique*]. Yet it must be recognized that it is the first class of diseases which are the most widely prevalent, against which defense is most difficult, and for which the need of preservatives and anti-contagion procedures is most keenly felt. It is in this class that we must place the fevers of hospitals and prisons, those of seamen and those which occur in the neighborhood of marshes where putrefaction is fermenting,' to use the expression of Jancourt—in a word all the malignant fevers which owe their existence to putrid exhalations."

Guyton assumes without question that the epidemic diseases carried primarily by the atmosphere must be capable of control by fumigants which destroy odors of putrefaction; but he also maintains that the line between epidemic and contact-borne diseases cannot be too sharply delineated. He points out that in the case of yellow fever, considered by most authorities as not contagious, others hold to the conception of a specific ferment ("*levain*"). Guyton discusses the characteristics of such a ferment in an extremely suggestive passage, as follows.

"A principle, any ferment of contagion whatever, is not a simple sub-stance; simple substances cannot multiply or reproduce themselves: yet how can we doubt the fact of reproduction when the pus from a small-pox patient or the bubo of a plague patient gives birth to other germs [*germes*] of the same type, capable of infecting thousands of individ-uals? But, if it is a compound substance, the elements of which have been assembled by the organized forces of the animal body, it should obey the law common to all such products, it is impossible that it should resist combustion."

Becoming somewhat more speculative, our author goes on to suggest that it may be "no unknown material, no new element which impresses its character on the contagious virus. It is merely an increase of one of the simple principles which all animal substances contain within themselves in such abundance." The essence of this change may be the presence of "condensed but feebly-bound nitrogen." It is this which is destroyed by oxidizing agents; and therefore, the diseases spread by more or less contact, as well as those transmitted through the general atmosphere, may be expected to be controllable by the use of acid fumigants.

It is clear that Guyton-Morveau, while he used such suggestive words as "*levain*" and "*germes*" held—as truly as Fracastorius—a fundamentally chemical theory of contagion. His views probably represent as clearly as those of any other authority the best thinking of the early nineteenth century—thinking immensely superior in its scientific concreteness to the philosophical abstractions of Sydenham and Rush and Webster. How those conceptions were applied in the field of practical sanitation must be the next subject of our inquiry.

In this connection, the oustanding figure is, of course, Edwin Chadwick (1800-1890), the author of the great sanitary awakening in England. Chadwick came of a land-owning and manufacturing family of Lancashire, and his father was a journalist of some distinction who edited *The Statesman* in London for a time and later emigrated to follow his profession in New York. Edwin himself, like Guyton-Morveau, was educated for the law. Very shortly, however, he developed a keen interest in social problems and became an intimate disciple of Jeremy Bentham. The study of problems relating to life insurance led him to a consideration of the preventability of disease. In the words of B. W. Richardson, his biographer, "as the labour progressed, a new train of reasoning came into his mind, which, in the end, developed into what he called the 'sanitary idea,' that is to say, the idea that man could, by getting at first principles, and by arriving at causes which affect health, mould life altogether into its natural cast, and beat what had hitherto been accepted as fate, by getting behind fate itself and suppressing the forces which led up to it at their prime source." It is difficult for us today —when the power of man to control his material environment is universally accepted—to realize how revolutionary a view this was in the early nineteenth century. In Chadwick's early days a distinguished authority wrote an essay to show that, if the death rate from one disease decreased, the death rate from some other disease must automatically increase, on the principle that nature abhors a vacuum. Though less crudely expressed, such fatalism was characteristic of the thinking of the time; and perhaps Chadwick's greatest service was in replacing this fatalism by a new faith in the power of scientific control of the physical environment.

Chadwick's personal researches into the conditions of London slums led to an attack of typhus fever. Fortunately, however, he recovered; and in 1832, when a commission was appointed to inquire into the existing program of poor relief, he accepted appointment as one of its assistant commissioners (later becoming chief commissioner) and definitely abandoned a normal legal career for one of social reform. In 1834 a new Poor Law Board was appointed as a result of the 1832 inquiry, and Chadwick was made secretary of the new board, whose creation, according to Lord John Russell, had "saved the country from great social evils, if not absolutely from social revolution." In this post Chadwick carried on for twelve years a most extraordinary series of studies on poor relief, education, child labor, crime control and intemperance, most of which led to concrete administrative reforms. His contributions to the cause of public health began in 1838, when an epidemic in Whitechapel caused him to appoint Doctors Neil Arnott, Kay and Southwood Smith to report on general sanitary conditions in the metropolis. At this time, too, Chadwick effected a most salutary medical reform by securing a new law for the registration of causes of death, and selecting William Farr to administer its operation.

In 1839, as a result of the London study, Lord John Russell ordered the Poor Law Commissioners to conduct a wider inquiry into conditions affecting the health of the laboring classes of Great Britain as a whole— an inquiry which we must later consider in some detail.

As a result of internal friction and external pressure, the Board of Poor Law Commissioners was dissolved in 1846; but two years later—as a result of the 1839 inquiry—a national Board of Health was created; and as a member of this board Chadwick continued his work, with Lord Carlisle, Lord Shaftesbury, and Dr. Southwood Smith as his colleagues. When the Board of Health was merged in the Local Government Board in 1854, he retired from official life but continued, up to the time of his death at the age of ninety, to battle for various good causes, such as civil service and for sanitary reform in the Army and the colonial possessions.

The report on the *Sanitary Condition of the Labouring Population of Great Britain*, published in 1842, was Chadwick's most important single literary contribution. It was the basis for the wave of sanitary reform which swept over the civilized world in the middle of the nineteenth century; and it gives us the best example of the epidemiological thinking upon which that wave of reform was based.

The first thing to notice about this epoch-making document is that it is no arm-chair production but a report of a survey, with full details of existing conditions and a serious and continued attempt to correlate those conditions with local mortality experience. As with Guyton-Morveau, the nineteenth century demanded facts as well as theories. The first part of the report presents data with regard to several specific types of insanitary conditions, "Yet almost all will be found to point to one particular, namely, atmospheric impurity, occasioned by means within the control of legislation, as the main cause of the ravages of epidemic, endemic and contagious diseases among the community, and as aggravating most other diseases."

To understand why miasms generated by organic filth played so large a part in Chadwick's day, it is necessary to realize the extreme degree of insanitation with which he had to cope—conditions which had their counterpart in every country and were to be faithfully duplicated in Stephen Smith's survey of New York City in 1865. At Inverness, the local observer reports, "There are very few houses in town which can boast of either water-closet or privy, and only two or three public privies in the better part of the place exist for the great bulk of the inhabitants." At Gateshead, "The want of convenient offices in the neighborhood is attended with many very unpleasant circumstances, as it induces the lazy inmates to make use of chamber utensils, which are suffered to remain in the most offensive state for several days, and are then emptied out of the windows." A surveyor reported on two houses in London, "I found the whole area of the cellars of both houses were full of night-soil, to the depth of three feet, which had been permitted for years to accumulate from the overflow of the cesspools; upon being moved, the stench was intolerable, and no doubt the neighborhood must have been more or less infected by it." In Manchester, "many of the streets in which cases of fever are common are so deep in mire, or so full of hollows and heaps of refuse that the vehicle used for conveying the patients to the House of Recovery often cannot be driven along them, and the patients are obliged to be carried to it from considerable distances." In Glasgow, the observer says, "We entered a dirty low passage like a house door, which led from the street through the first house to a square court immediately

behind, which court, with the exception of a narrow path
leading to another long passage through a second house, was
entirely as a dung receptacle of the most disgusting kind. Be,
court the second passage led to a second square court, occupie
same way by its dunghill; and from this court there was yet a third passage leading to a third court and third dungheap. There were no privies
or drains there, and the dungheaps received all filth which the swarm of
wretched inhabitants could give; and we learned that a considerable
part of the rent of the houses was paid by the produce of the dungheaps."
At Greenock, a dunghill in one street is described as containing "a hundred cubic yards of impure filth, collected from all parts of the town. It
is never removed; it is the stock-in-trade of a person who deals in dung;
he retails it by cart-fuls. To please his customers, he always keeps a
nucleus, as the older the filth is the higher is the price. The proprietor
has an extensive privy attached to the concern. This collection is front-
ing the public street; it is enclosed in front by a wall; the height of the
wall is about 12 feet, and the dung overtops it; the malarious moisture
oozes through the wall, and runs over the pavement. The effluvia all
round about this place is horrible. There is a land of houses adjoining,
four stories in height, and in the summer each house swarms with
myriads of flies; every article of food and drink must be covered, otherwise, if left exposed for a minute, the flies immediately attack it, and it
is rendered unfit for use, from the strong taste of the dunghill left by the
flies."

We can well understand today how such conditions spread disease, by
direct contact with filth, and by fly transmission; but in 1842 it was
natural to postulate atmospheric effluvia as the vehicle of dispersal.
Thus Dr. Barham of Truro says, "I have repeatedly noticed in the country that the occurrence of fever has been connected with *near proximity
to even a small amount of decomposing organic matter*; and it is certain
that all measures for effecting improvement in the sewerage of streets,
the supply of water, and ventilation may be rendered nearly inoperative
for the obviating of the causes of disease, if a little nidus of morbific
effluvia be permitted to remain in almost every corner of the confined
court; where the poor man opens his narrow habitation in the hope of
refreshing it with the breeze of summer, but gets instead a mixture of
gases from reeking dunghills, or, what is worse, because more insidious,
from a soil which has become impregnated with organic matters imbibed long before; and now, though perhaps, to all appearance dry and

..ar, emitting the poisonous vapour in its most pernicious state." The medical officer of the Ampthill union in discussing an epidemic of "typhus"[2] says, "The cottages in which it first appeared (and to which it has been almost exclusively confined) are of the most wretched description; a stagnant pond is in the immediate vicinity, and none of the tenements have drains; rubbish is thrown within a few yards of the dwellings, and there is no doubt but in damp, foggy weather, and also during the heat of summer, the exhalations arising from these heaps of filth must generate disease, and the obnoxious effluvia tend to spread contagion where it already exists."

The remedy for such conditions was, of course, the elimination of excretal deposits, the cleansing and flushing of the streets, and the introduction of water-carriage and sewerage systems. Even where plumbing was available the sanitarian of 1840 was, however, obsessed by the fear of sewer-gas. Chadwick warns against the danger existing "in some of the best quarters of the metropolis, where the supplies of water are adequate, and where the drains act in the removal of refuse from the house, but where from want of moderate scientific knowledge or care in their construction, each drain acts like the neck of a large retort, and serves to introduce into the house the subtle gas which spreads disease from the accumulations in the sewers." Again, he says, "In the course of the present inquiry instances have been frequently presented of fevers and deaths occasioned by the escape of gas from the sewers into the streets and houses. In the evidence given before the Committee of the House of Commons, which received evidence on the subject in 1834, one medical witness stated that of all cases of severe "typhus" that he had seen, eighttenths were either in houses of which the drains from the sewers were untrapped, or which, being trapped, were situated opposite gully-holes; and he mentioned instances where servants sleeping in the lower rooms of houses were invariably attacked with fever." This was a natural but unfortunate corollary of the miasmatic theory of contagion.

The contributors to the report do not make any very clear distinction between the effects of stagnant water as such and the effects of stagnant water contaminated with excreta. Apparently the former, as well as the latter, was considered dangerous—and, of course, justly so. The assistant commissioner for Cornwall and Devon "reports, that he found the open drains and sewers the most prominent cause of malaria." Reports from

---

[2] Quotes are added by the author to remind the present-day reader that the physician of 1842 made no distinction between typhoid and typhus.

Scotland are full of evidence of the good results accomplished by drainage. Improved health as well as improvement of agriculture are noted as a result of drainage in parish after parish in such terms as the following: "So much draining that now no swamps; formerly agues common, now quite unknown"; "health improved from draining"; "since the land was drained, scrofula rare and ague unknown." Similar experiences are reported from England. At Newhaven, "of late very extensive improvements have taken place in the drainage of these levels, and in consequence of that change, the diseases constantly engendered by marsh miasmata, viz. 'typhus' and intermittent fevers, are not more common than in other districts which present to the eye a fairer prospect of health."

A third major evil revealed by the Survey was the lack of an adequate supply of pure water for drinking and washing. Chadwick quotes an interesting case of an epidemic of dysentery at the barracks in Cork, which was stopped when a polluted water supply from the River Lee was replaced by a pure spring water. It is interesting to note, however, that Chadwick's emphasis on drinking water as a vehicle of disease is relatively slight as compared with his stress on filth in general. Even water supply is considered more as a means of promoting general cleanliness than as a vector of disease. From Edinburgh comes the tale of a "question and answer more than once exchanged, 'When were you last washed?' 'When I was last in prison.'"

A fourth major evil stressed in the Survey is overcrowding. At Gateshead, in certain streets, "each small ill-ventilated apartment of the house contained a family with lodgers in number from seven to nine, and seldom more than two beds to the whole." At Durham, a laborer was asked by the Canon how he was going to dispose of his family of eleven in a new dwelling. "He told me they were to inhabit one of these hind's cottages, whose narrow dimensions were less than 24 feet by 15, and that the eleven would have only three beds to sleep on; that he himself, his wife, a daughter of six, and a boy of four years old would sleep in one bed; that a daughter of eighteen, a son of twelve, a son of ten, and a daughter of eight would have a second bed; and a third would receive his three sons of the age of twenty, sixteen, and fourteen."

The problem of ventilation is also discussed in some detail in a section on work places and it is concluded that "the effects of bad ventilation, it need not be pointed out, are chiefly manifested in consumption."

The report on sanitary—or insanitary—conditions, district by district, is followed by a highly suggestive analysis of variations in mortality rates in relation to economic status. At Truro, the mean age of death was 40 years for professional persons or gentry; and 28 years for laborers and artisans. At Derby, the corresponding figures were 49 years and 21 years, respectively. Studies of various districts in Manchester and its suburbs showed mortality rates for males varying from 23 to 38 per 1,000, while for Leeds and its suburbs the corresponding figures were 17 and 35 per 1,000. The variations corresponded closely to the degree of poverty and insanitation prevailing in each district.

These comparative studies are supported by a review of the results accomplished in the reduction of excessive morbidity rates in prisons, in the Navy and in certain model industrial villages by the application of the principles of sanitary reform.

The major conclusions of the Survey are finally summarized in the following three brief paragraphs, two dealing with extent and operation of the evils concerned, and the third, with the means of improvement.

"That the various forms of epidemic, endemic, and other disease caused, or aggravated, or propagated chiefly amongst the labouring classes by atmospheric impurities, produced by decomposing animal and vegetable substances, by damp and filth, and close and overcrowded dwellings prevail amongst the population in every part of the kingdom, whether dwelling in separate houses, in rural villages, in small towns, in the larger towns—as they have been found to prevail in the lowest districts of the metropolis.

"That such disease, wherever its attacks are frequent, is always found in connexion with the physical circumstances above specified, and that where those circumstances are removed by drainage, proper cleansing, better ventilation and other means of diminishing atmospheric impurity; the frequency and intensity of such disease is abated; and where the removal of the noxious agencies appears to be complete, such disease almost entirely disappears.

"The primary and most important measures, and at the same time the most practicable, and within the recognized province of administration, are drainage, the removal of all refuse of habitations, streets, and roads, and the improvement of the supplies of water."

There in a nutshell is the law and the gospel of the epidemiology of the Great Sanitary Awakening. It was based on a concept of disease which was notably incomplete. Yet the doctrine of miasms was no fanciful theory but a sound deduction from observed relationships. As Chadwick says, at one point in the Survey, "The medical controversy as to the causes of fever; as to whether it is caused by filth and vitiated atmosphere, or whether the state of the atmosphere is a predisposing cause to the reception of the fever, or the means of propagating that disease, which has really some other superior, independent, or specific cause, does not appear to be one that for practical purposes need be considered, except that its effect is prejudicial in diverting attention from the practical means of prevention."

Blessed was the rugged common sense of the nineteenth century! The theory was indeed incomplete. "Filth," as has been said, "is not the mother but the nurse of disease." Yet the theory of miasms had enough truth in it to work. When the sanitary reformers cleaned up the masses of putrefying filth through which our great-grandfathers moved, the epidemics of typhoid and cholera and typhus and dysentery actually ceased. The miasmatic theory was the first generalization of epidemiology to be actually—and on a world-wide scale—justified by its fruits.

It should not be inferred, however, that there was no theoretical speculation as to the *modus operandi* of the miasm. Southwood Smith, for example, gives us a clear picture of his conception of the way in which minute particles of morbific matter diffused in the atmosphere might enter the body. He says, "When diffused in the air, these noxious particles are conveyed into the system through the thin and delicate walls of the air vesicles of the lungs in the act of respiration. The mode in which the air vesicles are formed and disposed is such as to give to the human lungs an almost incredible extent of absorbing surface, while at every point of this surface there is a vascular tube ready to receive any substance imbibed by it, and to carry it at once into the current of the circulation. Hence the instantaneousness and the dreadful energy with which certain poisons act upon the system when brought into contact with the pulmonary surface. . . .

"Now that substances mixed with or suspended in atmospheric air may be conveyed with it to the lungs and immediately enter into the circulating mass, any one may satisfy himself merely by passing through a recently-painted chamber. The vapour of turpentine diffused through the chamber is transmitted to the lungs with the air which is breathed, and passing into the current of the circulation through the walls of the air vesicles exhibits its effects in some of the fluid excretions of the body, even more rapidly than if it had been taken into the stomach."

If the miasmatic theory of Chadwick had been understood for what it was—a realization of the empirical fact that insanitary conditions played a vitally important role in the causation of epidemic disease—all would have been well. Unfortunately, the human mind has an incurable tendency to what we may call "the fallacy of a single cause." If factor A, under a certain set of circumstances, is demonstrated to be causally related to a certain phenomenon, we rashly conclude that, under no circumstances, can factor B be causally related to that phenomenon. Yet we should have learned that multiple rather than unique causation is the general rule in the complex world in which we live. If Factor B be universally present, the presence or absence of Factor A may be determining; but if Factor A be universally present, the reverse is the case.

The sanitarians of the middle nineteenth century—like the students of yellow fever fifty years before—were the victims of this fallacy. Since, in actual experience, it had been proved that elimination of filth decreased certain forms of epidemic disease, they concluded that filth was the unique cause of such disease and that, therefore, contagion was a non-existent factor. So there ensued another long and fruitless controversy between miasmatist and contagionist, with the heavy artillery in the hands of the former.

An excellent example of this trend is to be found in the first and second reports of the Metropolitan Sanitary Commission published in 1848. This Commission consisted of Lord Robert Grosvenor, Chadwick, Southwood Smith, Richard Owen, surgeon and anatomist, and Richard Lambert Jones; and its appointment was chiefly motivated by rumors of a spread of cholera from the Near East. It followed the usual practice of taking the testimony of experts, and supplemented the opinion thus obtained by extensive citations from continental authorities. There can be no doubt that it represented the generally accepted conclusions of the time.

These conclusions, so far as they concerned the etiology of disease, were essentially two in number, one of them sound, the other unsound.

The Commission was essentially right in its first basic assumption—that decomposing filth and undrained marshy areas were major factors in the causation of epidemic disease. Thus, the First Report says that cholera "generally first appeared in the neighborhood of rivers or marshes, and principally raged in low and damp localities, particularly where there were also the outlets of filth." At Manchester, "Where the cholera broke out (as often happened) in places apart from the canals and streams, it was noticed that this, in most instances, was in yards, courts, and narrow streets, polluted by offensive cesspools, pigsties and other sources of malaria (some of which were too disgusting to be described), or by open or obstructed sewers." Evidence from India is quoted to show that "when a regiment has been encamped, one part on high and dry land and the other part on a morass, or on the bank of a river, the former has remained healthy, while the latter has suffered severely." In London "as in every town and city, the places in which 'typhus' is to be found, from which it is, rarely, if ever, absent, and which it occasionally decimates, are the neglected and filthy parts of it; the parts unvisited by the scavenger; the parts which are without sewers, or which, if provided with sewers, are without house drains into them; or which if they have both sewers and house drains are without a due and regulated supply of water for washing away their filth, and for the purposes of surface cleansing and domestic use." So, "while cholera manifested a decided preference to follow the track of rivers and water-courses, it made those portions of this track which were at the same time the outlets of filth the chief places of its attack; and that therefore in towns and cities it was remarkably prevalent and fatal in the neighbourhood of sewer mouths." There is much emphasis throughout the report on lack of drainage and resulting dampness; but "the whole of the evidence, however, appears to lead to the conclusion that it is the combination of impurity with humidity of the air which so powerfully predisposes to cholera; cleanliness being apparently capable of counteracting the influence of mere humidity; thus the remarkable exemption enjoyed by Holland from the visitation of cholera, is generally and probably correctly attributed to the scrupulous cleanliness of the houses and habits of the people." Poverty and under-nutrition are recognized as contributory factors; "but it is now universally admitted that a far more powerful predisponent is the habitual respiration of an impure atmosphere." Therefore, "there is but one safeguard against this malady [cholera] as against other diseases of the same class. That safeguard consists in sanitary arrangements." Similar opinions are expressed in the Second Report; and there is a supplementary aid to control suggested in the use of disinfectants, such as chlorine and other acid gases and nitrate of lead. The earlier enthusiasm for gaseous disinfectants seems, however, to have noticeably waned.

All this is fundamentally sound empirical epidemiology; but the second conclusion running through these reports is the corollary that contagion is a factor of no importance whatever. The type of evidence supporting this conclusion (strikingly similar to that reviewed in an earlier chapter with regard to yellow fever), as we find it scattered through both reports may be ranged in logical order as follows:

The fundamental thesis is "That there is no evidence that cholera spreads by the communication of the infected with the healthy."

This thesis is supported first by evidence that where the fullest opportunity for direct contact exists cholera often wholly fails to extend its influence. "In the hospitals at Newcastle and Gateshead, where, were there such an agent as contagion, it must have been present in its most concentrated form, no case has occurred of illness arising from attendance on the sick, either in the persons of the nurses, the resident apothecaries, or the attending or numerous succession of visiting members of the medical profession." The city of Birmingham remained entirely free from the disease in spite of constant intercourse with the suburban area of Bilston, where "cholera prevailed more virulently than in any town of the kingdom." Except for one witness, all who had studied the disease in London agreed "that the disease did not spread from the communication of the infected with the healthy." In the Second Report there is special note of "the non-extension of the disease through families, in which the seizure in the great majority of instances, and except under peculiar circumstances, is confined to individual members." Evidence from Russia is quoted to the effect that "among all the physicians of Moscow, there is certainly not one who believes that a cholera patient communicates the disease by the touch. Daily experience is too decided on this head." From India, Dr. Parkes testifies, "I have never observed any indication of contagion. In common with the great majority of Indian writers, my evidence is on the negative side."

Thus, experience indicates that direct exposure to infected persons fails to spread the disease. A second line of evidence shows that, in the absence of such exposure, the disease does spread freely. In one epidemic "it was proved that no one of those who were taken ill had seen or attended on or been near the man who was alleged to have brought the disease from Orenburg, but on the contrary, several persons who had visited this man, and attended on him during his illness escaped." At Sunderland, "numerous cases have occurred simultaneously at distant points, where no communication could by possibility have taken place." The first case in an epidemic at East Smithfield occurred on a ship in port which "had lain in the river three weeks prior to its being attacked. There was no cholera in the place from whence this ship had sailed." The rapidity of extension in certain epidemics[3] is also cited as obvious evidence against spread by contagion. Thus in St. Petersburg "when once cholera broke out in that city, a few days sufficed for its dissemination over the capital, and that so widely and so generally as to preclude all idea of mere communication with infected persons, as the cause of its propagation."

Additional evidence on this point is adduced from the failure of quarantine measures attempted in Turkey and Russia. Two Swedish physicians appointed to investigate the Russian cholera situation report that the Moscow authorities "had altogether abandoned the old theory of the spread of the disease by contagion, a theory which had led in 1830 to the most extravagant hopes from the benefits to be derived from cordons and quarantines."

On similar grounds, the Commission is more than sceptical as to the value of hospital isolation. They note that "The measure of alleviation chiefly relied on during its last visitation was the establishment of district cholera hospitals; but the experience of the results of these establishments is by no means favorable to their re-adoption, except under particular circumstances and modifications." Much stress is rightly laid on the danger to the patient of removal to a hospital in a disease so rapid and debilitating as cholera; and there is (as we have seen in the discussions of yellow fever) emphasis on the inhumanity engendered by fear of contagion.

The First Report concludes, "That when cholera first appeared in this country the general belief was that the disease spreads principally, if not entirely, by communication of the infected with the healthy, and that therefore the main security of nations, cities, and individuals, consists in the isolation of the infected from the uninfected—a doctrine which naturally led to the enforcement of rigorous quarantine regulations; the establishment of military and police cordons; the excitement of panic; and the neglect, and often the abandonment of the sick even by relations and friends.

"That since opportunities have been obtained of a closer observation of the character of this disease, and of the mode in which it spreads through continents, nations, cities, towns, and families, facts have been

---

[3] Today, we should, of course, interpret these as water-borne epidemics.

ascertained which are incompatible with the foregoing view of its mode of dissemination, and of its prevention.

"That the disease is not, as it was then generally supposed to be, contagious, and that the practical application of that doctrine did no good, but was fraught with much evil."

The Second Report takes note of the fact that the Swedish Commissioners in their survey of Russia, and the Metropolitan Board of Health of London in 1832, both accepted the idea that the first case of cholera in a given community is often definitely traceable to an individual who has come from a previously infected area. The Report, however, believes that such occurrences are few in number and susceptible of other explanation, if not accidental coincidences; and appeals to experience in regions where cholera is normally prevalent, in which (naturally enough) no such evidence is presented. It concludes that the "specific contagion emanating from the bodies of the sick" is harmful only when highly concentrated in confined spaces.

It must be recognized that the negative non-contagionist arguments—as well as the positive miasmatic arguments—had much empirical support. Cholera is not, of course, very readily communicated from person to person. Without a conception of the role of indirect transmission by water and food and without knowledge of the well carrier, the conclusions reached were almost inevitable—so far as cholera was concerned. The 1848 Reports, however, also discuss the problem of influenza; and here we have an example of the misleading influence of extreme miasmatic conceptions when carried to their logical extreme.

The Report does not deny in so many words that influenza may be spread by contagion; but it does imply this conclusion very clearly. Thus, the Second Report, after discussing the abandonment of the idea that cholera was contagious, continues, "Fifty years ago, it was the general belief among medical men that influenza was contagious, and the evidence adduced to support the opinion was precisely similar to that which is now relied on to establish the contagious character of cholera." On another page we read that "The result of our investigations is in accordance with that presented by the history of epidemic influenza, wherever an authentic account of its progress has been recorded, namely, that its spread is intimately connected with an unusual degree of humidity, combined with sudden and great alterations of temperature." Data in regard to seasonal and local incidence are cited to support this hypothesis. "From returns which enable us to ascertain the comparative degree in which the several districts have suffered from the visitation of disease, we find that the cholera districts, the 'typhus' districts, and the influenza districts are the same, and that the local conditions which favor the spread and increase the intensity of these, and all kindred maladies are everywhere similar."

Finally, through the whole discussion runs the undertone of Sydenham's insidious theory of the transmutability of various diseases. It is the "assimilating power of a predominant epidemic that renders the present prevalence of diarrhoea a subject of apprehension; because though in the absence of Asiatic cholera, diarrhoea like 'typhus' is a distinct species of disease, it is very readily converted into cholera on account of its close resemblance to that malady." In another place, we are told that "influenza has preceded and accompanied the great and mortal epidemics which have devastated this country at distant periods"; and the Black Death of the fourteenth century, the Great Plague of London, and various epidemics of "typhus" and cholera are cited as specific examples.

The development of sanitary theory during the third quarter of the nineteenth century can be clearly traced in the official writings of John Simon (1816-1904), who took over from Chadwick leadership in the practical development of the British sanitary program. As a young lecturer on pathology, he was appointed medical officer of the City of London in 1848; and in 1855 he was named for the newly created office of central medical officer to the General Board of Health of the nation, a post which—with various changes of administrative responsibility (involving attachment to the Privy Council and finally to the Local Government Board)—he held until 1876. Except for W. H. Duncan of Liverpool, he was the first professional public health administrator and one of the wisest, most persuasive, and most enthusiastic health teachers of all time.

In his first London report of 1849 he emphasizes the danger from the cesspool gases. "These gases," he says, "which so many thousands of people are daily inhaling, do not, it is true, in their diluted condition, suddenly extinguish life; but, though different in concentration, they are identically the same in nature with that confined sewer-gas which, on a recent occasion, at Pimlico, killed those who were exposed to it, with the rapidity of a lightning stroke." An earnest plea is made, in this report and in that of 1850, for an adequate supply of water; and although Simon's discussion of quality of water relates chiefly to the problem of hardness, he also refers to the danger of excremental impurities.

In another part of the first London report, Simon gives the following unequivocal statement of the Filth Theory of Disease, which reminds us how far that theory was removed from our modern distinction between conditions which are merely offensive and those which tend to the transmission of infection. He says, "The atmosphere in which epidemic and infectious diseases most readily diffuse their poison and multiply their victims is one, as I have already often stated, in which organic matters are undergoing decomposition. Whence these may be derived signifies little. Whether the matter passing into decay be an accumulation of soaking straw and cabbage leaves in some miserable cellar, or the garbage of a slaughter house, or an overflowing cesspool, or dead dogs floated at high water into the mouth of a sewer, or stinking fish thrown overboard in Billingsgate dock, or the remains of human corpses undergoing their last chemical changes in consecrated earth; the previous history of the decomposed material is of no moment whatever. The pathologist knows no difference of operation between one decaying substance and another; so soon as he recognizes organic matter undergoing decomposition, so soon he recognizes the most fertile soil for the increase of epidemic diseases

In Simon's fifth London report for 1853, the threat of cholera was again dominant. An epidemic was occurring on the continent. "Perhaps from the eastern centres of its habitual dominion—from the alluvial swamps and malarious jungles of Asia, where it was first engendered amid miles of vaporous poison, and still broods over wasted nations as the agent of innumerable deaths; or perhaps from the congenial flats of Eastern Europe, where it may have lingered latent and acclimatised; the subtle ferment was spreading its new infection to all kindred soils." The "soils" to which "infection" is likely to be spread are, of course, characterized by dampness and the presence of polluting material. "It would, therefore, appear that in certain lowlying levels—to constitute them favorable soils for the disease, there must be joined to their first condition of lowness (with the mere watery dampness which it implies) some other second condition; one, which is of extreme frequency in such districts, though not essentially present there. This second condition impends wherever there dwells at such levels a certain density of population; it *mainly varies with the degree in which that dense population lives in the atmosphere of its own excrements and refuse.*" The evils of the miasma of decay may be felt for great distances. "From the polluted bosom of the river steam up, incessantly though unseen, the vapours of a retributive poison; densest and most destructive, no doubt, along the sodden banks and stinking sewers of lowest level; but spreading over miles of land—sometimes rolled high by wind, sometimes blended low with mist, and baneful even to their margin that curls over distant fields."

A later paragraph attempts to explain the "specific causation" of cholera, in a fashion reminiscent of Mead (though much less clear and logical than Mead's analysis): "What may be the exact chemistry of this process, I do not pretend to say: urging only that in all human probability, the poison arises in specific changes impressed by some migratory agent upon certain refuse-elements of life. . . . that which comes to us from the East is not itself a poison, so much as it is a test and touchstone of poison. . . . Past millions of scattered population it moves innocuous. Through the unpolluted atmosphere of cleanly districts, it migrates silently, without a blow; that which it can kindle into poison, lies not there. To the foul, damp breath of low-lying cities, it comes like a spark to powder. Here is contained that which it can swiftly make destructive —soaked into soil, stagnant in water, griming the pavement, tainting the air—the slow rottenness of unremoved excrement, to which the first contact of this foreign ferment brings the occasion of changing into new and more deadly combinations."

Ten years later, we note at least one important modification of this straightforward and simple miasmatic conception. In a special report on London cholera epidemics, prepared by Simon as medical officer of the General Board of Health in 1856, we find (as a result of the epidemiological studies of John Snow to be discussed in a later chapter of the present volume) a distinct recognition of the fact that the vital causative factor might, in certain epidemics, be drinking water. In view of this evidence Simon draws the somewhat grudging but practically important conclusion that "under the specific influence which determines an epidemic period, fecalized drinking-water and fecalized air, equally may breed and convey the poison."

In a special report of 1858 on *The Sanitary State of the People of England*, Simon recognizes smallpox, whooping cough, measles and scarlet fever as nearly universal contagious diseases which are relatively insusceptible to control. Cholera, diarrhea and dysentery, on the other hand, show marked inequalities in local prevalence; they occur where "the population either breathes or drinks a large amount of putrefying animal refuse"; hence, these maladies can be controlled by sanitation. By this time, the distinction between typhus and typhoid fevers was recognized. Both were considered by Simon to be associated with filth, "Yet not both essentially associated with the same kind of filth. One of them (the *typhoid* fever of modern observers) has intimate affinity to the cause last mentioned—the faecal pollution of air and water. The other (which is now distinctively called *typhus*) more nearly associates itself with overcrowding, especially of destitute persons, and probably has its essential source in the putrefaction of their undispersed exhalations." Simon quotes Jenner as unqualifiedly convinced of the contagiousness of typhus fever proper. In this distinction, there is more than a glimmer of sound, empirical epidemiology; but even in the case of typhus, Simon emphasizes the connection with overcrowding and filth. Tuberculosis is attributed chiefly to conditions of occupation.

It was at this period, 1854-1858, that Florence Nightingale (1823-1910) effected her magnificent reforms in sanitation and hospital management on the Crimea and laid the foundation for her wider campaign against insanitary and unhygienic conditions affecting the health of the British Army in India and elsewhere. She drew a suggestive contrast between the diseases most prevalent at Scutari in winter—the "scorbutic type" (frost-bite, rheumatism and scurvy)—which she attributed to bad food, dampness, deficient clothing, exposure and fatigue; and those prevalent in spring and summer—the "malarial type" (cholera, continued, remittent and typhoid fevers)—which were caused by bad drainage, bad ventilation, dampness, malaria, nuisances, organic effluvia and overcrowding. Diarrhea and dysentery appeared in both of her seasonal lists. Miss Nightingale says of the latter group, "Zymotic Diseases, Fevers, Diarrhea, Cholera, Dysentery, etc., are known in Civil life to be most intense in their activity where certain local conditions are present." Bad air, contaminated by moisture and exhalations from the skin, caused by overcrowding and defective ventilation is the primary factor involved. Next in importance are "emanations proceeding from animal excretions or from decaying vegetable matter, together with moisture. The want of drainage and the foul state of the latrines and urinals in Barracks . . . are sufficient illustrations of this class of causes." The evils of overcrowding were, of course, associated in her mind with miasmatic pollution. She says, "If nothing is done in the walls of wards, the respiration and exhalations from patients contaminate them with a still greater impregnation of organic matter for the next series of inhabitants. If nothing is done for the ventilation, the hospital atmosphere becomes more and more fatal."

It was in 1858, too, that Charles Murchison (1830-1879) first coined the term "pythogenic" for the fever "produced by emanations from decaying organic matter" (typhoid fever).

In Simon's later reports to the Privy Council (1858-1870) we find continued emphasis on "the tainting of the atmosphere with the products of organic decomposition, *especially of human excrement*"[4] and "the habitual drinking of impure water" as causes of diarrheal diseases. Emphasis grows on the influence upon tuberculosis incidence of industrial dusts and bad ventilation of workshops. The 1863 report contains an analysis of the relation of marsh districts to "ague and other malarious diseases"—another example of the clearer definition emerging from growing recognition of the specificity of diseases. Twenty years before, all the "fevers" had been lumped together.

Another section of Simon's report for 1863, dealing with hospital hygiene, gives us a fascinating picture of the moment of transition from miasmatic to parasitic concepts of disease etiology. This is so important that both the text and Simon's footnotes must be quoted verbatim.

"First, as regards the *spread of communicable diseases*: each communicable disease has its own laws of communicability—laws which must be properly understood if the danger of contagion is to be guarded against. The communication of some diseases (of scabies, for instance, and favus) is not by any true product of the human body, but consists in the migration of parasites, or germs of parasites, animal or vegetable, from one person's body to another—a migration which of course the recipient may to any extent facilitate by dirty personal habits, and which, as regards some parasitic diseases, can scarcely be conceived to occur otherwise than in consequence of such habits. Other communicable diseases (and for hospital purposes they are the greatly important group for consideration) communicate themselves by that process which is distinctively called *zymotic*:* in the first affected body, and by or with a specific chemical transformation of some of its material, there is generated or multiplied a specific *zyme, contagium*, or ferment; which, if transferred while active to a second (not accidentally insusceptible) body, will there, according to the common law of ferments, excite the same morbid phe-

---

[4] Italics, mine—to illustrate gradual modification of the earlier dogma that all organic decomposition was alike in its effects.

nomena, the same chemical changes, as those amid which itself was begotten.† The several zymotic diseases are aetiologically quite distinct from one another.‡ Also they differ widely in their manifestations, and have widely different degrees of importance; some of them being comparatively trifling local ailments, while others are fevers and fluxes of more or less considerable danger to life. The different ferments by which they severally are communicated have respective peculiarities of their own—peculiarities which are primarily governed by the nature and anatomical relations of the morbid process in which each particular ferment originates: all of them are essentially unstable and transitory but, while some of them tend under ordinary circumstances to undergo a rapid extinction, others of them can with comparative ease retain their power for long periods of time, and some apparently have not their full force till some time after they have left the diseased body;—some of them associate themselves indistinguishably with one or more of the common excretions and exhalations of the body, others are separately tangible in vesicles and pustules or at ulcerating or suppurating surfaces, and may or may not also exist in other products of the body;—some of them are evolved in small quantity, others in very large quantity, or with very large natural admixture;—some of them are fixed, others but very scantily volatile, others as volatile as if they were vapours;—some of them operate easily on a second body by mere contact (more or less prolonged) with the outer or inner surface to which they are applied, others are not found to act unless they come into contact with accidentally abraded surfaces, or be thrust into the bodily substance by inoculation. Thus, in vaccine lymph and in the matter of chancres respectively, there is a contagium which we know only in a fixed form, and only as communicable by intentional or accidental inoculation:—also ophthalmia and gonorrhoea and glanders are communicable by the fixed contagium which their pus contains; but this contagium does not need inoculation to infect the mucous membrane to which it is applied; and as regards ophthalmia, there are reasons for suspecting that to some extent the contagious pus may retain its activity when dry enough to float as dust in the air:—in some forms of milzbrand (including, probably, the so-called 'malignant pustule' which is the best known human form of the disease) the highly virulent fluids can, it is alleged, infect by soakage through the cuticle:—in diphtheria, the characteristic exudation is capable of infecting by contact; and though often the disease is communicated from person to person without any manifest transplantation of matter, it may be that in such cases particles of the decomposed false membrane are conveyed as a volatile contagion:—cholera and typhoid fever send forth their respective contagia for the most part, if not exclusively, as matter dissolved or suspended in the evacuations which pass from the patient's bowels; and probably these evacuations (which, at least in cholera, gradually develop their full infective force after their discharge from the body) can under some circumstances bring into similar contagious fermentation the excrement with which they are mingled in privies, drains, and cesspools, and can thus convert the effluvia and leakage from such sources into means of extensive secondary infection of air and water:—the volatile contagion of hooping cough is probably disengaged in large quantities by the air-passages, and as it forms is sent forth with the breath:—in typhus, small-pox, measles and scarlatina, the diffusion of volatile contagium occurs to a vast amount, probably with all exhalations from the body; and in addition to this, contagium, more or less fixed, collects abundantly about the patient's person and bedding; and, in a far less degree, something of the same sort probably occurs in erysipelas."

* I take the present opportunity of suggesting, as in my opinion a most desirable amendment of present uses, that, in sanitary discussions, the word "zymotic" should never be employed but in its exact pathological sense.—J.S.

† Some of the above expressions are meant to hesitate between two particular assertions. In this respect they correspond to the uncertainty which at present prevails as to the exact nature of some or all morbid ferments. A few years ago it might have seemed permissible to describe without reserve the contagia of the zymotic diseases, as but some changing organic material of the first affected body. At present, however, reserve on that point is necessary. That the power of contagiousness is associated with such changing organic material is certain;—but whether the power be *proper to the material*, or be only *contingently* its attribute, seems to require further investigation. The recent very interesting experiments of Professor Schröder in Germany, and of M. Pasteur in France (published respectively in Wöhler and Liebig's Annalen der Chemie, and in the Comptes Rendus de l'Académie des Sciences) aim at proving, most extensively, an essential dependence of specific fermentatory and putrefactive changes on the presence, in each case respectively, of some characteristic molecular living thing; and they give it to be understood that, if certain fermenting or putrefying organic matters tend by their contact to bring a given quiescent organic compound into chemical excitement like their own, this contagious power of theirs depends on their carrying with them those distinctive microscopical animal or vegetable forms which in each case respectively are the true agents of change. The conclusiveness of those experiments in the field to which hitherto they have been confined is still matter of the warmest scientific controversy; and while therefore it would be at least premature for me to insist upon them as evidence even in that field, it would be yet more premature for me to speculate on the possible results of an extension of similar researches to the pathology of zymotic diseases. But it is impossible to ignore their very important bearing in that direction. . . .—J.S.

‡ How their respective first contagia arose, is, as regards nearly all of them quite unknown. This, in pathology, is just such a question as in physiology is "the origin of species." Indeed, regard being had to matters mentioned in the last footnote, it is hardly to be assumed as certain that these apparently two questions may not be only two phases of one. Hourly observation tells us that the contagium of small-pox will breed small-pox, that the contagium of typhus will breed

typhus, that the contagium of syphilis will breed syphilis, and so forth,—that the process is as regular as that by which dog breeds dog, and cat cat, as exclusive as that by which dog never breeds cat, nor cat dog; and, prospectively, we are able to predict the results of certain exposures to contagion, as definitely as the results of any other chemical experiment. But, retrospectively, we have not the same sort of certainty; for we cannot always trace the parentage of a given case of small-pox or measles. And here, notwithstanding the obvious difficulties of proof either way, some persons will dogmatize that there must have been an overlooked inlet for contagium, while others will dogmatize that there must have been in the patient's body an independent origination of the specific chemical change. Presuming (as may pretty confidently be presumed) that in the history of mankind there was once upon a time a first small-pox case, a first typhus case, a first syphilis case, etc., and admitting our entire ignorance as to the combination of circumstances under which those first cases respectively came into existence, we have no scientific reasons for denying that new "spontaneous generations" of such contagia may take place. But, as regards some of the diseases, there are conclusive reasons against supposing that this is of frequent occurrence. Where we can observe isolated populations, we find very long periods elapse without any new rise of certain "species" of disease. For instance, in 1846, the contagium of measles was imported by a sick sailor into one of the Faroe Islands, and led to an epidemic which attacked more than 6,000 out of the 7,782 inhabitants; sparing only the persons who previously had had the disease, and 1,500 who were kept out of reach of contagion; but before that time *there had not for 65 years been, in those islands, a single case of measles*. And the statistical return to which I have already often referred (Parliamentary Paper, 1864, No. 12) contains another very striking illustration of the same sort of thing:—England has 627 registration districts. During the 10 years 1851-60, scarlatina, small-pox, and measles were (as usual) prevailing more or less throughout the country, producing among children under five years of age an average annual mortality of 802 per 100,000; *i.e.* by scarlatina 419, by small-pox 103, and by measles 280. In 626 of the registration districts there were deaths (and, for the most part, in not inconsiderable quantity) from one or more of those causes;—not quite invariably from all of them; for 43 of the 626 (thanks no doubt, to vaccination) had not any death by small-pox, and among the 43 districts which thus escaped mortality by small-pox, there was one which also had not even a single death by measles;—but, with these exceptions, all the 626 districts had deaths from the three diseases—deaths by measles, deaths by small-pox, deaths by scarlatina. But the 627th district had an entire escape. In all the 10 years it had not a single death by measles, nor a single death by small-pox, nor a single death by scarlet fever. And why? Not because of its general sanitary merits, for it had an average amount of other evidence of unhealthiness. Doubtless, the reason of its escape was that it was insular. It was the *district of the Scilly Isles*; to which it was most improbable that any febrile contagion should come from without. And its escape is an approximative proof that, at least for those 10 years, no contagium of measles, nor any contagium of scarlet fever, nor any contagium of small-pox had arisen spontaneously within its limits. I may add that there were only 7 districts of England in which no death from diphtheria occurred, and that, of those 7 districts, the district of the Scilly Isles was one. Still to say that a disease is contagious is not to say that it may not arise without contagion. Indeed I shall presently adduce evidence to show the circumstances under which the "spontaneous generation" of the traumatic infections takes place. And the statements which were published in 1862 by Dr. Salisbury in the American Journal of the Medical Sciences, as to the producibility of measles by inoculation and other infection with *straw fungi*, deserve to be borne in mind.—J.S.

Simon then reviews the results obtained by Semmelweis in the control of puerperal fever in Vienna, by a process which clearly embodied the practice of asepsis. Yet he still maintains that any putrefying wound may generate the contagium of erysipelas *de novo* and assumes the spread of that contagium through the atmosphere. In a later sentence, he says, "If typhus spreads from bed to bed in a ward, or if traumatic infections prevail there, presumably the ventilation is not proportionate to the number and kind of case under treatment." Hence, ventilation is still the main procedure to be relied upon.

By 1865, Simon's thinking had progressed far enough to warrant the conclusion, "That many of our worst diseases acquire diffusion and local perpetuity by means of specific infective influences which the sick exercise on the healthy is an elementary truth of medicine; and among persons who are competent to distinguish the certainties from the uncertainties of science, there is no more doubt broadly as to that truth than there is doubt as to the diurnal and annual movements of the earth." Local conditions (both sanitary and "cosmical") influence the spread of such infective influences.

"The doctrine on this subject which in my opinion deserves, in the present state of knowledge, to be accepted as practically certain—sufficiently certain, I mean, to be made the basis for precautionary measures, may be stated in the following propositions:—that, when cholera is epidemic in any place, persons who are suffering from the epidemic influence, though perhaps with only the slightest degree of diarrhoea, may, if they migrate, be the means of conveying to other places an infection of indefinite severity; that the quality of infectiveness belongs particularly, if not exclusively, to the matters which the patient discharges by purging and omitting, from his intestinal canal; and that these matters are comparatively non-infective at the moment when they are discharged, but subsequently, while undergoing decomposition, acquire their maximum of infective power; that choleraic discharges, if cast away without previous disinfection, impart their own infective quality to the excremental matters with which they mingle, in drains or cesspools or wherever else they flow or soak, and to the effluvia which those matters evolve; that if the cholera-contagium, by leakage or soakage from drains, or cesspools, or otherwise, gets access, even in small quantity, to wells or other sources of drinking-water, it infects in the most dangerous manner very large volumes of the fluid; that in the above-described ways even a single patient with slight choleraic diarrhoea may exert a powerful infective influence on masses of population among whom perhaps his presence is unsuspected; that things, such as bedding and clothing, which have been imbued with choleraic discharges, and not afterwards fully disinfected, may long retain their infectious properties, and be the means of exciting choleraic outbreaks wherever they are sent for washing or other purposes."

In the report for the next year (1866) references begin to appear on the "so-called cholera fungus" as discussed at a medical conference held at Weimar in August 1867. In the report for 1867, Villemin's experiments are noted; and in the report for 1868, the disinfection of prostitutes is discussed as a practical public health problem. Laboratory research has, by this time, become a recognized part of the work of Simon's staff. In the report for 1869 he summarizes studies by Burdon Sanderson "shewing experimental reasons, which we think conclusive, for believing that each contagium, as regards its physical form, consists essentially of *extremely minute separate solid particles*; and arguing on grounds which we think scarcely less certain, that these effective particles of each specific contagium are *living self-multiplying organic forms*."

Thus, when Simon summarized the studies of a long professional life in a report on *Filth Diseases and Their Prevention* in 1874 and in an article on "Contagion" prepared for Quain's *Dictionary of Medicine* (prepared in 1878), he had arrived at a theory of disease etiology essentially sound and scientific.

In the first of these classic documents, he says, "that the chief morbific agencies in Filth are other than those chemically-identified stinking gaseous products of organic decomposition which force themselves on popular attention. Exposure to the sufficiently concentrated fumes of organic decomposition (as for instance in an unventilated old cesspool or long-blocked sewer) may, no doubt, prove immediately fatal by reason of some large quantity of sulphide of ammonium, or other like poisonous and foetid gas, which the sufferer suddenly inhales; and far smaller doses of these foetid gases, as breathed with extreme dilution in ordinary stinking atmospheres, both give immediate headache and general discomfort to sensitive persons temporarily exposed to them, and also appear to keep in a somewhat vaguely depressed state of health many who habitually breathe them; but here, so far as we yet know, is the end of the potency of those stinking gases. While, however, thus far there is only the familiar case of the so-called *common chemical poison*, which hurts by instant action and in direct proportion to its palpable and ponderable dose, the other and far wider possibilities of mischief which we recognise in Filth are such as apparently must be attributed to *morbific ferments* or *contagia*; matters which not only are not gaseous, but on the contrary, so far as we know them, seem to have their essence, or an inseparable part of it, in certain solid elements which the microscope discovers in them: in living organisms, namely, which in their largest sizes are but very minute microscopical objects, and at their least sizes are probably unseen even with the microscope; organisms which, in virtue of their vitality, are indefinitely self-multiplying within their respective spheres of operation, and which therefore, as in contrast with common poisons, can develop indefinitely large ulterior effects from first doses which are indefinitely small. Of ferments thus characterised, the apparently essential factors of specific chemical processes, at least one sort—the ordinary septic ferment*—seems always to be present where putrefactive changes are in progress, as of course in all decaying animal refuse; while others, though certainly not essential to all such putridity, are in different degrees apt, and some of them little less than certain, to be frequent incidents of our ordinary refuse. As, apparently, it is by these various agencies (essential and incidental) that Filth produces 'zymotic' disease, it is important not to confound them with the foetid gases of organic decomposition; and the question, what infecting powers are prevalent in given atmospheres, should never be regarded as a mere question of stink. It is of the utmost practical importance to recognise in regard of Filth, that agents which destroy its stink may yet leave all its main powers of disease-production undiminished."

In the article on Contagion, he discusses, first, recognized parasites (scabies, trichiniasis and other worm-infections) and then passes on to "the true or metabolic contagia," which, "in their respective and specific ways, operate *transformingly* on the live bodily material which they affect, are perhaps the most important of all the incidental physical influences which concern mankind. Whether they may all, at some time hereafter, admit of being named, like the parasitic contagia, in terms of biological classification, is a question which needs not in the first instance be raised; for meanwhile the identity of each separate true contagium is settled in experimental and clinical observation by the uniformity of the operation of each on any given animal body which it affects. Each of the diseases propagates itself in its own form in as exact identity, as if it were a species in zoology or botany; and in each such repetition of the disease there is a multiplication—always a large, and sometimes an inconceivably immense multiplication, of material which has the same infective property. Evidences innumerable to that effect are under daily clinical observation in this climate in instances of small-pox, measles, scarlatina, whooping cough, enteric fever, mumps, typhus, syphilis, cow-pox, diphtheria, erysipelas, hospital gangrene, purulent

* For convenience I use the singular number, but have no intention of implying that ordinary putrefactive changes have only one ferment which can be considered habitual to them.—J.S.

ophthalmia and gonorrhoea, venereal soft-chancre and phagedaena, etc.: for, barring fallacies, no man ever sees any one of those diseases produced by the contagium of any other of them; and any man who has before him a case of any of them can see that, however minute may have been the quantity of contagium by which the disease was started, the patient's diseased body (part or whole) yields for the time an indefinitely large supply of the specific agent."

These official papers of Sir John Simon give us, as in a mirror, a perfect picture of the evolution of epidemiological theory between 1849 and 1878; and it is fascinating to see the vision clarify itself during this period of thirty years, just as a landscape is gradually illumined by the rising of the sun.

The miasmatic theory of disease emerged into practical vitality during the fifth decade of the nineteenth century. It was based on a sound empirical recognition of the relation between filth and disease; and this relationship had sufficient validity to make possible the achievement of phenomenal results in the control of epidemic disease by the practical application of the theory.

At first, this theory was a crude one and involved the assumption that the cause of "zymotic" disease was organic decomposition *per se*, and that the relationship was non-specific, both as to the nature of the substance decomposed and the nature of the particular disease produced. Step by step, however, evidence accumulated as to the role played by drinking water in the transmission of such diseases and as to the importance of the preexisting case as a source of infection. Gradually, too, there crept into the discussion of this subject a realization of the specificity of the diseases themselves. Filth was recognized as the medium by which contagion was transmitted rather than as the primary source of that contagion. Finally, the conception of the contagious element as a particulate living organism clarified the entire picture.

The chief factors which brought about this transformation were two in number—the careful studies of a few pioneer field epidemiologists on the one hand, and the development of the germ theory by Pasteur on the other. These fundamental contributions will be discussed in succeeding chapters.

CHAPTER XIII

THREE PIONEER EPIDEMIOLOGISTS

"Epidemiology at any given time is something more than the total of its established facts. It includes their orderly arrangement into chains of inference which extend more or less beyond the bounds of direct observation. Such of these chains as are well and truly laid guide investigation to the facts of the future."—W. H. FROST

THE replacement of the miasmatic by the contagionistic theory of disease was to be dramatically completed through the triumphant advances of bacteriology. These triumphs, however, should not obscure the fact that the citadel of Miasma had really been effectively overthrown before the days of Pasteur. If the germ-theory of disease had not been established by bacteriologists for a hundred years thereafter, the brilliant contributions of three pioneer epidemiologists had—by 1860—provided a sound basis for comprehension and control of communicable disease.

The Delta Omega Society has shown excellent discrimination in selecting the three public health classics whose reprinting it has sponsored. Beginning with Budd's *Typhoid Fever* in 1931, going on to Snow's *Cholera* in 1936 and then to Panum's study of measles in 1940, the society has given us modern convenient reprints of the three outstanding contributions of the middle nineteenth century to epidemiology (one of which was very rare and another unavailable except in Danish). These monographs are among the most brilliant achievements in the history of this science. They deserve detailed review, both from their theoretical significance and as admirable examples of the uses of epidemiological techniques.

The first of these contributions in point of time was the work of a Danish physician and physiologist, Peter Ludwig Panum. Panum was born in 1820 and received his medical qualification in 1845. Before he had completed his hospital training (in 1846), he was sent by the government, in company with A. Manicus, to cope with a serious epidemic of measles raging in the Faroe Islands; and in 1847 he published his classic study of this epidemic in a Danish journal. He went to Germany for graduate study, and there Virchow persuaded him to prepare a second report of his Faroe Islands investigation for the first volume of

Virchow's new *Archiv*,[1] and to France where he worked under Claude Bernard.

In 1850, Panum was sent to Bandholm to deal with an epidemic of cholera. In 1852 he was appointed professor of physiology, medical chemistry and pathology at Kiel, and in 1863 was called to Copenhagen, where his field included physiology, physiological chemistry and comparative anatomy. He emphasized the new viewpoints of Bernard, Virchow and Koelliker in his teaching and made important contributions to physiology and pathology. In 1884, when the Eighth International Medical Congress was held at Copenhagen, he served as its chairman and was perhaps the leading figure in Scandinavian medicine at that time. He died in the next year.

The epidemic in the Faroe Islands which Panum studied offered unique material for the epidemiologist; and perhaps no young graduate in medicine was ever given such an opportunity. In the first place, these islands, lying between the Shetlands and Iceland, had been free from measles since 1781, so that, when the epidemic of 1846 struck their non-immune population, more than 6,000 of the 7,782 inhabitants came down with the disease. In the second place, the population of the area was so separated in the coastal valleys of seventeen islands that each tiny settlement was an isolated community whose disease history could be studied independently. The largest community, Thorshavn, had only 800 inhabitants. Furthermore, intercourse between villages was so rare that the arrival of a visitor was an event of note, recorded in the calendar. Panum truly says in his German paper that "the circumstances under which the disease was observed were so favorable that similar ones were rarely, if ever, presented to an observer."

The original report begins with an elaborate analysis of the climate of the islands, of the diet and housing and occupation of the islanders and of their morbidity and vital statistics. Rheumatism, bronchitis, skin diseases and mental diseases and defects were found to be unduly prevalent and it is interesting to note that the latter were attributed by Panum to influence of the forbidding landscape and the fog. Tuberculosis and syphilis, however, he believed to be rare; and smallpox, scarlet fever and measles had been wholly absent for many years. In spite of highly unfavorable hygienic conditions, the average length of life in the Faroe Islands was over 44 years as compared with 36 in Denmark; and Panum

[1] An English translation of this second report was published in 1935 by Gafafer. It is chiefly an abstract of the Danish report but contains valuable new interpretive comment.

concludes "that the entire or partial exemption of the Faroe Islands from a number of diseases, especially those which are infectious, which decimate the populations of other countries, is the most important of all reasons for the favorable rates on these islands, and the high limit of life of the inhabitants."

Into this non-immune Eden entered the infection of measles in 1846. The initial case on the islands was a carpenter who arrived from Copenhagen on March 28 after visiting several persons in that city who were ill with measles. Two of his intimate friends were the first local victims.

The most significant evidence presented by Panum was obtained by visits to fifty-two of the isolated villages where he obtained complete records of the spread of the epidemic. One example may be cited as typical, since the phenomena were everywhere the same.

On June 4, ten fishermen from Tjörnerig took part in a grind[2] catch at Westmannharn, where they were intimately associated with measles cases. On June 18 all these men came down with measles. Twelve to sixteen days later most of the population of Tjörnerig succumbed and a third crop of cases appeared at a similar interval after the second. Only 20 out of the 100 inhabitants escaped.

By such observations as this, repeated in village after village, Panum established the incubation period of measles at thirteen to fourteen days. He concluded that infection had generally occurred when the primary case was in the early eruptive stage. A few cases reported contact only in the prodromal catarrhal period, but Panum was doubtful as to the accuracy of this observation. He was inclined to doubt the common view that the period of desquamation was infectious, having failed to find a single case traceable to exposure after the disappearance of the rash.

Panum was inclined—though with some hesitation—to accept the spread of the contagion by clothing and other fomites; and he furnishes good evidence of the lasting immunity acquired in measles, having himself interviewed ninety-eight old persons who had had previous attacks and all of whom escaped in 1846.

Panum has no curiosity as to the nature of the infective agent—certainly no conception of a *contagium animatum*. He apparently holds to the conventional view of contagion as due to gaseous emanations— "exhalations from the patient which are strongest during eruption and on the first day of efflorescence, and the peculiar acidulous odor of which

---

[2] A dolphin-like animal appearing in schools which was hunted by large numbers of fishermen from different neighborhoods.

is most characteristic at this time." He refers to typhus fever as originating spontaneously at times; but does not find any evidence that such generation of measles occurs on the Islands.

On one point, however, he was quite clear, as expressed in the major conclusion of his German paper. He there says "If among 6,000 cases, of which I saw and treated 1,000 myself, there was not a single one in which it was justifiable to attribute the affection to a miasmatic origin, while at the same time it was everywhere clear that the disease had spread from man to man and from village to village by means of the contagium (be it by direct contact with an ill person or by infected clothing and the like) then one is certainly justified at least to doubt very much the miasmatic nature of the disease."[3]

Panum conducted a workmanlike investigation of an unusual epidemic. After all, however, measles had for centuries been recognized as a disease spread primarily by direct human contact. Therefore, this work, though a brilliant study, did not involve any radical change in epidemiological theory.

The intestinal fevers, cholera and typhoid, furnished the real battleground of nineteenth century epidemiology. Here, the chain of infection was often—indeed, generally—obscure. New cases arose without any demonstrable exposure to a previous case, and sometimes in sudden epidemics affecting whole communities within a period of days. Here, environmental conditions seemed to play a major role, so that emphasis on non-specific filth was natural and reasonable.

It is true, of course, that very early in the century a few pioneers—particularly in France—had emphasized the importance of contagion and had recognized transmission by drinking water as the cause of certain local epidemics of typhoid fever. Stallybrass cites (at second hand) Dupré as having been perhaps the first to suggest the possibility of the spread of this disease by water in 1823. In 1828, Leuret of Nancy "traced, first the importation of the disease into a town by sick persons arriving there, and secondly the subsequent spread from person to person."

Bretonneau of Tours, in 1829 described an epidemic in which every individual in a girl's boarding school suffered from fever with no other cases in the neighborhood. He asks, "On what, except the contagious

<hr>

[3] A. Manicus, the colleague of Panum in the Faroe Islands study, published a report of his own which comes to similar conclusions, although his emphasis is chiefly clinical rather than epidemiological. His paper is translated as Appendix C of the Delta Omega reprinting.

nature of the disease, could such a difference in incidence depend?" The great Louis says, "The contagious power of typhoid fever seems to me demonstrated by the facts and I accept it with no hesitation." Gendron de l'Eure in 1834 concluded that typhoid cases generally arose from direct or indirect contact with the sick, "either through living in the same atmosphere" or "indirectly by means of the clothing or utensils that have been handled by the patient."

The growth of the pythogenic theory, however, had obscured these earlier observations, so that, as we have noted in the preceding chapter, this conception was generally dominant in the middle of the nineteenth century. It was in England that the half-truths of the miasmatic concept brought forth their first important fruits; and it was at the hands of two English epidemiologists, John Snow and William Budd, that convincing evidence was brought forth which replaced that theory by the fuller light of our modern doctrine of contagion.

John Snow, the first of these two pioneers in point of time and the most remarkable as an epidemiologist, was born in 1813, the son of a farmer near York. He served as apprentice to a surgeon at Newcastle and then to several other medical men in rural practice. He removed to London in 1836 where he studied at the Hunterian School of Medicine and the Westminster Hospital. He was entered as a member of the Royal College of Surgeons in 1838 and by 1844 was an M.D. of the University of London. As early as 1841 he began to present scientific contributions on asphyxia and, when American experiments on ether anesthesia reached England in 1846, he devoted his major effort to work in this field. When Simpson introduced chloroform he welcomed and applied this new advance and became the leading anesthetist of London.

At the same time, Snow became interested in the problem of cholera, and promptly arrived at the conclusion that early intestinal symptoms indicated an alimentary rather than an atmospheric origin. In 1849, he published a 31-page pamphlet, "On the Mode of Communication of Cholera," which he followed up with two series of articles in the *Medical Times* (1851) and the *Medical Times and Gazette* (1852). In 1852 he developed his general theories in an address as orator at the eightieth anniversary of the Medical Society of London under the title, "On Continuous Molecular Changes," and in 1855 he attained the presidency of that distinguished organization. In 1854, he used the London cholera epidemics of that year to excellent purpose for the testing of his theories, and in 1855 published a much enlarged and definitive edition of his 1849 essay.

Snow died in 1858, at the early age of forty-five, leaving behind him a notable reputation in both his fields of interest, anesthesia and epidemiology. He was a typical Victorian, in the mold of Chadwick and so many of his distinguished contemporaries, combining fervent humanitarian idealism—he was a life-long vegetarian and total abstainer—with hard-headed scientific thinking.

Snow's major theories in regard to the epidemiology of cholera were the same in 1849 as in 1855; but the second edition of his treatise contains far more supporting evidence. It is this second edition (as reprinted under the auspices of the Delta Omega Society in 1936) that we shall use as the basis for the present discussion.

Snow begins his treatise with a description of the general progress of cholera from one community to another. This disease "travels along the great tracks of human intercourse, never going faster than people travel, and generally much more slowly. In extending to a fresh island or continent, it always appears first at a seaport. It never attacks the crews of ships going from a country free from cholera, to one where the disease is prevailing, till they have entered a port, or had intercourse with the shore. Its exact progress from town to town cannot always be traced; but it has never appeared except where there has been ample opportunity for it to be conveyed by human intercourse." Snow confirms this conclusion by the citation of a whole series of case-histories—observed by himself and by other British physicians during the epidemic of 1848. In each instance, an infected individual coming into a given locality initiated a new chain of infection.

"Diseases which are communicated from person to person are caused by some material which passes from the sick to the healthy, and which has the property of increasing and multiplying in the systems of the persons it attacks. In syphilis, small-pox, and vaccinia, we have physical proof of the increase of the morbid material." The particular mode of infection, however, differs in various cases. "The itch, and certain other diseases of the skin, are propagated in one way; syphilis, in another way; and intestinal worms, in a third way." In the case of cholera, the agent of infection must be present in the discharges from the alimentary tract.

The incubation period of a disease (24-48 hours in the case of cholera) is "in reality, a period of reproduction, as regards the morbid matter;

ınd the disease is due to the crop or progeny resulting from the small quantity of poison first introduced."

Snow then proceeds to an acute analysis of the various ways in which "minute quantities of the ejections and dejections of cholera patients must be swallowed." He shows how uncleanly habits and the scarcity of water lead to the soiling of the hands of attendants; "and unless these persons are scrupulously cleanly in their habits, and wash their hands before taking food, they must accidentally swallow some of the excretion, and leave some on the food they handle and prepare." The rapid spread among pauper lunatics and in coal mines where privies are lacking[4] is particularly emphasized in this connection.

Then Snow proceeds, with admirable perspicacity, to a second mode of communicability. "If," he says, "the cholera had no other means of communication than those which we have been considering, it would be constrained to confine itself chiefly to the crowded dwellings of the poor, and would be continually liable to die out accidentally in a place, for want of the opportunity to reach fresh victims; but there is often a way open for it to extend itself more widely, and to reach the well-to-do classes of the community; I allude to the mixture of the cholera evacuations with the water used for drinking and culinary purposes, either by permeating the ground, and getting into wells, or by running along channels and sewers into the rivers from which entire towns are sometimes supplied with water."

Snow then proceeds to describe small water-borne epidemics at Horsleydown, Wandsworth Road and Rotherhithe in London, at Salford, at Ilford and at Locksbrookall in 1849, at Newburn in 1832, at Cunnapore, India, in 1814 and in the Black Sea Fleet in 1854. These are cited for the most part at second hand, though in the Wandsworth Road case Snow examined some of the suspected water and found in it "various substances which had passed through the alimentary canal, having escaped digestion, as the stones and husks of currants and grapes, and portions of the thin epidermis of other fruits and vegetables"—an interesting example of elementary water analysis. These citations are, however, altogether overshadowed by Snow's own classic study of the epidemic centering about Broad Street, Golden Square, in 1854.

This epidemic is described by Snow as "the most terrible outbreak of cholera which ever occurred in this kingdom." Within a radius of 250

---

4 Snow says "The mining population of Great Britain have suffered more from cholera than persons in any other occupation."

yards, over 500 fatal cases of cholera occurred within a period of ten days. Grouping the fatal cases by date of onset, there were 9 cases in the area in question originating between August 19 and August 29; 8 cases on August 30; 56 cases on August 31; 143 cases on September 1; 116 on September 2. Then the daily toll decreased to 5 on September 11—with a total of 540 new cases originating between August 30 and September 11. From September 12 to September 30, there were only 22 new cases.

On the outbreak of this epidemic, Snow at once suspected a street-pump in Broad Street supplying the affected area, and obtained record of 83 deaths registered on the first three days of September, which from their location bore out his theory. Out of 77 of these cases for which information was obtainable, he found that 59 used the water of the well in question. On September 7, he persuaded the local Board of Guardians to remove the handle of the Broad Street pump, and the epidemic, already on the decline, shortly ceased.

The major evidence presented by Snow in his final report is an excellent spot-map showing the location of the various pumps supplying the Golden Square area and adjacent districts of London with each fatal case of cholera plotted at its place of residence. This is, so far as I am aware, the first use of the spot-map in epidemiology; and it offers by itself most suggestive evidence of the responsibility of the Broad Street pump for the epidemic as a whole. Snow, however, adds many details which make the strength of his conclusions overwhelming.

A workhouse in Poland Street was more than three-fourths surrounded by houses in which cholera deaths occurred, yet but 5 cases appeared among its 535 inmates; this workhouse had its own private well. A brewery in Broad Street near the pump, but never using its water, had no cases among its 70 workers. On the other hand, a gentleman came from Brighton to the home of his brother who had died of cholera in Poland Street, remained in the house only twenty minutes (drinking the local water) and was attacked at his home in Pentonville the next evening. Most striking of all was a lady who had not visited the district in months but who had once lived in it and had a special fondness for the Broad Street water. A carter brought daily to her home in Hampstead a bottle filled from the Broad Street pump, and on August 31 she came down with the disease. A niece who was visiting the old lady also drank the water at Hampstead and returned to her home in Islington to die of cholera. There were no other cases of the disease in either of these communities.

Snow's observations were later extended by studies of the Rev. H. Whitehead and Mr. J. York, a surveyor, which are summarized in Sedgwick's *Principles of Sanitary Science and Public Health*. Whitehead, after a careful canvass of the dwellings on Broad Street, found that 90 cholera deaths had occurred among 896 persons. York opened up the Broad Street well itself and found that the main drain from No. 40 Broad Street was only 2 ft. 6 in. from the well and 9 ft. 2 in. above the level of water in the well. The discoloration of the soil and the washed appearance of the gravel clearly indicated an avenue of pollution.

After describing the Golden Square outbreak, Snow then proceeds to a wider analysis of the relation of cholera in London to the public water supplies which served various parts of the metropolis. He shows that in 1832, the highest cholera mortality was found in the districts supplied by the Southwark Company with water drawn directly from the Thames at London Bridge. In 1849, the Southwark Company had moved its intake up river to Battersea Fields, which was, however, by that time a source as polluted as London Bridge had been in 1832. Again, the users of this water had a mortality rate much higher than the customers of other companies. The same general relationship was manifest once more in 1853.

These data were available in the general registration reports and were highly suggestive; but in 1854, Snow conducted a special study which really clinched the argument. At this time the water supplied by what was now the Southwark and Vauxhall Company was still highly polluted, while that furnished by the Lambeth Company was from Thames Ditton, far above the sewage of the city. These two companies supplied most of London south of the river. One section was provided with Southwark water, one with Lambeth water, and in a considerable area the pipes of the two companies ran side by side so that each individual dwelling used the water of its choice. When the 1853 epidemic was continued in 1854, Snow seized upon the unique epidemiological opportunity offered by this situation. With the assistance of Dr. J. J. Whiting, every house where a cholera death occurred was visited to ascertain the source of the water; and where information was uncertain the tap water was tested for chlorides which were present to the amount of about one grain of NaCl per gallon in the Lambeth water as compared with 38 grains in the Southwark supply.[5] The result of this study showed for the four-week period in question the following rates.

Southwark and Vauxhall Supply	71 deaths per 10,000 houses
Lambeth supply	5 deaths per 10,000 houses
Rest of London	9 deaths per 10,000 houses

As the epidemic progressed, the difference between districts became somewhat less marked since, as Snow points out, secondary spread by other means than water supply would naturally go on in all areas. Even in the second seven weeks of the epidemic, however, mortality continued to be five times as high among Southwark as among Lambeth customers.

Snow then proceeds to buttress his conclusions by a review of the relation of cholera incidence to water-supply in various other British cities (Exeter, Hull, York, Glasgow, Newcastle and others) as well as in Paris and Moscow.

Finally, Snow discusses effectively certain objections raised to his theories. He deals admirably with the common criticism that not all the persons who drink polluted water come down with the disease: "This objection arises from mistaking the department of science to which the communication of cholera belongs, and looking on it as a question of chemistry, instead of one of natural history, as it undoubtedly is. It cannot be supposed that a morbid poison, which has the property, under suitable circumstances, of reproducing its kind, should be capable of being diluted indefinitely in water, like a chemical salt; and therefore it is not to be presumed that the cholera-poison would be equally diffused through every particle of the water. The eggs of the tapeworm must undoubtedly pass down the sewers into the Thames, but it by no means follows that everybody who drinks a glass of the water should swallow one of the eggs." This is certainly one of the earliest clear statements of the particulate character of contagion, whose recognition cleared up so much that had been confusing in the past.

The summer prevalence of the disease in England is attributed to greater use of unboiled water at that season, and Snow adds, "It is not unlikely that insects, especially the common house-flies, aid in spreading the disease."

Snow is less fortunate in a later section, attributing plague and yellow fever and malaria also to polluted water—on the ground of their sup-

---

[5] Influenced by mixture of sea water.

posed association with river valleys and low alluvial soils. He is on much
stronger ground in evidence which he presents relating dysentery and
typhoid fever to polluted water. In the latter case, he cites the study by
Austin Flint of the epidemic at North Boston (to which later reference
will be made). In connection with malaria, he makes the following
extremely acute observation: "The communication of ague from person
to person has not been observed, and supposing this disease to be communicable, it may be so only indirectly, for the *materies morbi* eliminated from one patient may require to undergo a process of development
or procreation out of the body before it enters another patient, like certain flukes infesting some of the lower animals, and procreating by
alternate generations."

Snow's "Oration on Continuous Molecular Changes" (delivered in
1852) is an illuminating discussion of the basic philosophical principles
underlying his theories of disease causation in their broad biological
relationships. He conceives the fundamental quality of all vital processes
to be a self-propagating chain of molecular changes. "The most characteristic property, indeed, of vital actions probably is, that they are always
caused by similar processes which have preceded them, whilst all other
molecular changes may arise, occasionally at least, from other causes. A
species of plant or animal consists, in fact, of a number or collection of
continuous molecular actions." By a perception which cuts deeper than
mere analogy, he considers the interchange of human thought by speech
and writing as a sort of extension of the power of "molecular changes
taking place in the brain"; and points out that "By the aid of literature,
indeed, knowledge committed to writing may lie dormant for centuries,
like the ears of wheat in the hand of the Egyptian mummy, and then
again take up the process of growth, to increase and spread in another
part of the world."

To Snow, there was "no distinct line of demarcation between vital
processes and those which are not vital. Vinous fermentation, for instance, has been generally looked upon as a merely chemical change;
yet it has great claims to be entitled a vital process. It is always accompanied by the formation of the cells or sporules of the yeast fungus—
the decomposition of the sugar into alcohol and carbonic acid bearing
a direct relation to the quantity of yeast produced."

The "communicable diseases"—a term which Snow prefers, as we do
today to "contagious" diseases are listed by him as "syphilis, small-pox,
measles, scarlet fever, typhus, typhoid and relapsing fevers, erysipelas,

yellow-fever, plague, cholera, dysentery, influenza, hooping-cough, mumps, scabies and the entozoa." The "material cause" of each of these diseases "resembles a species of living being in this, that both one and the other depend on, and in fact consist of, a series of continuous molecular changes, occurring in suitable materials. The organized matter, as we must presume it to be, which induces the symptoms of a communicated disease, except in the case of the entozoa, can hardly ever be separately distinguished, like the individuals of a species of plant or animal; but we know that this organized matter possesses one great characteristic of plants and animals—that of increasing and multiplying its own kind." The incubation period of such a disease is a "period of reproduction" of the *materies morbi*.

Snow then reviews early theories of epidemiology. "For want of knowing any other cause, epidemics were attributed, by the ancients, to the atmosphere, without any evidence; just as political and social events were believed to be occasioned by the stars." Later on, "when the communication of diseases began to be recognized, it was thought to depend, in most cases, on effluvia given off from the patient into the surrounding atmosphere: even syphilis, for some time after its appearance in Europe, was believed to be propagated in this way, and persons suffering from it were driven out of the towns and villages to live or die in the fields, lest they should infect others with their breath." These earlier views must be abandoned in favor of "specific causes of disease." The specific causes of various diseases have their specific modes of transmission. "It is not improbable that the specific cause of influenza and measles is drawn in with the breath, as these diseases affect chiefly the respiratory organs, and spread almost equally amongst all classes of the community; but the great aid that want of personal cleanliness lends to the extension of many communicable diseases points to another mode of communication. . . . There is evidence tending to show that typhoid fever, yellow fever, and plague, as well as cholera, are communicated by accidentally swallowing the morbid excretions of the patients, and that these latter may sometimes be conveyed to a distance with the drinking water or other articles of diet, without losing their specific properties."

Finally, he adds: "It may very fairly be asked whether communicable diseases do not sometimes arise spontaneously—that is, from other causes than their communication, just as ordinary combustion, putrefaction, and some other continuous molecular changes, very often commence anew, from various causes, without any continuity with previous changes of the same kind, and it is not improbable that some communicable diseases may arise, so to say, spontaneously. The erysipelatous inflammation, for instance, which attacks the neighbourhood of wounds, probably arises now and then without being communicated; otherwise we must suppose the material which causes it to be almost as widely diffused as the spores of some of the fungi. There is, however, great reason to believe that the larger number of communicable diseases never arise from any other cause than the communication of the specific virus from a previous patient."

Benjamin Ward Richardson in his memoir on Snow in the *Asclepiad* (1887) says, "It was my privilege, during the life of Dr. Snow, to stand on his side. It is now my duty, as a biographer who feels that his work will not be lost, to claim for him not only the entire originality of the theory of the communication of cholera by the direct introduction of the excreted cholera poison into the alimentary system; but, independently of that theory, the entire originality of the discovery of a connection between impure water supply and choleraic disease."

A more modern commentator, Wade Hampton Frost, in his introduction to the Delta Omega reprint of Snow's most important contributions rightly says, "A nearly perfect model is John Snow's analysis of the epidemiology of cholera which led him to the confident conclusion that the specific cause of the disease was a parasitic micro-organism, conforming in all essentials of its natural history to what is now known of the *Vibrio cholerae*."

What Snow did for cholera was accomplished for typhoid fever by his eminent contemporary, William Budd. The doctrine of contagion was commonly known as Snow's Theory, and Frost states that "Among English writers of distinction Budd seems to have stood nearly if not quite alone in prompt and unqualified acceptance of Snow's theory as well as his facts." Yet Budd was more than an intellectual disciple. His first published paper did, it is true, appear seven years after Snow's, but his own observations dated back to 1839 and "for many years" before the date of the 1856 paper he "had taught these doctrines" in his "lectures at the Bristol Medical School and had acted upon them in practice, in the prevention of the fever." He was an independent investigator who, in the study of typhoid, reached the same conclusions at which Snow arrived in the study of cholera.[6]

William Budd was born at North Tawton in Devon in 1811. After four years of study in Paris (where he was, no doubt, influenced by the teachings of the French contagionists) he took his M.D. at Edinburgh and assisted his father in rural practice. He began the study of typhoid in his native village in 1839—having himself an attack of the disease from which he nearly died. In 1842 he removed to Bristol, where he taught at the local medical school and served on the staff of the Royal Infirmary. He published important monographs on variola ovina— sheep's smallpox—on scarlet fever and its prevention, on cholera and disinfection, and on typhoid fever. He retired from practice on account of ill-health in 1873 and died in 1880.

Budd's first published contribution to epidemiology was a brief communication to the *Lancet* in 1856—in the form of comment on a recently-reported institutional epidemic at St. John's Wood and on an earlier outbreak of a similar kind in France. He identifies the disease in both instances as that recently differentiated by Louis (typhoid fever). "This species of fever," he says, "has two fundamental characteristics. The first is, that it is an essentially contagious disorder; the second, that by far the most virulent part of the specific poison by which the contagion takes effect is contained in the diarrhoeal discharge which issues from the diseased and *exanthematous* bowel. . . . So many and such striking proof of both the facts here asserted have come before myself, that I have long looked upon them as being as sure as that itch is contagious, and that smallpox may be inoculated."

He continues, "The first case in the series may either be casual and imported, or may be due to the local rekindling, through atmospheric

---

[6] It may be a source of some pride to note that in 1855 (after Snow's first publication, but prior to Budd's) Austin Flint published an admirable study of a water-borne epidemic of typhoid fever with which reference has been made above. This report (which is abstracted in the 1935 edition of Sedgwick's *Principles of Sanitary Science and Public Health*) deals with a small community of forty-three persons in nine families at North Boston, Erie Co., N.Y. On September 21, 1843, a young man suffering from typhoid stopped at the local inn and died there on October 19. Between October 14 and December 7, 25 of the 43 persons in the village came down with the disease. Furthermore, all these twenty-five cases occurred in six families living in the immediate proximity of the inn and in the closest contact with the innkeeper's family using his well and obtaining much of their food from him. Two households some forty rods away, and one family nearby which had a feud with the innkeeper, which precluded any intercourse, escaped. Whether, as Flint believed, the well at the inn was the medium of dissemination is not wholly certain; but he is certainly correct in his conclusion that "contagion offers the only adequate explanation" of the phenomena observed.

or other changes, of poison which had remained as the dormant legacy of some former similar attack. In either case, in the usual cause of things, diarrhoea comes on in the infected subject; and the next thing that happens is that the discharges from the bowels, which are usually at once copious, numerous, and liquid, are thrown into the water closet or privy. In this way the drains, or systems of drains, belonging to the place, become at once saturated with the specific poison in its most concentrated and virulent form. This once occurring, the poison may give the fever to the healthy inmates in one of three ways; either by percolating through the soil into the well which supplies the drinking water; by issuing through defects in the sewer into the air of the inhabited area; or, still more directly, by exhaling from the aperture of some ill-trapped water closet or privy, which is at once the receptacle of the discharges from the sick and the daily resort of the healthy."

The sewer may be looked upon as "*a direct continuation of the diseased intestine*"; and its open exposed surfaces are favorable to "slowly distilling the infection into the soil, or constantly exhaling it in large volumes into the surrounding air." Hence, air contaminated with such exhalations is "*immeasurably more infectious than that which immediately surrounds the fever patients.*" Thus Budd ingeniously harmonises his fundamental concept of contagion with the relative rarity of direct person-to-person transmission. He recognizes a ten to fourteen day incubation period for typhoid fever and this first article concludes with a vigorous plea for the disinfection of excreta and soiled linen (with chlorides of zinc or lime); and describes the successful control, by such means, of an epidemic in a retail store.

Three weeks later, Budd continued with the first of a series of notable papers under the title "On Intestinal Fever: Its Mode of Propagation." In this communication he refers to typhoid fever as "contingent on the powers of an agent so low in the scale of created things, that the mildew which springs up on decaying wood must be considered high in comparison." Later, he says, "If it be true of diseases in general that all prevention must be based on an intimate acquaintance with their causes, it is still more true of that great group of diseases which are the work of definite and specific agents, having not only the power of subsisting within the body, but capable, for limited periods at least, of existing externally to it. For it is clear that in such a case a thing against which we may be powerless, so long as it infects the body itself, may present, on its issue from the body, the conditions of an easy conquest."

Budd recognizes that his belief in the contagiousness of typhoid fever is a view to which "the great weight of medical opinion in this country is directly opposed. Not to speak of minor notabilities, the whole prestige of the Board of Health, and of the London Royal College of Physicians may be cited against it. To make increasing and implacable war against contagion and contagionists seemed with the former, indeed, to be, for some years, the chief purpose of its existence." Budd finds, in his own experience, that physicians in London and other large towns are generally non-contagionists. He puts his finger on the reason for his own success when he points out that "where the question at issue is that of the propagation of disease by human intercourse, country districts, where the population is thin and the lines of intercourse are few and always readily traced, offer opportunities for its settlement which are not to be met with in the crowded haunts of large towns." To illustrate this advantage, he next proceeds to describe his observations on one epidemic of typhoid fever at North Tawton. This was a village of about 1,300 persons, for whom Budd was not only the sole physician but with whom he was intimately acquainted as having been born and brought up in the neighborhood. The grossest conditions of insanitation prevailed in the village, nearly every house or group of houses having a privy with an excavation or open ditch serving as a cesspool, and most had manure heaps as well. Yet the community had for many years enjoyed almost complete immunity from fever.

The polluted conditions of this village "existed for many years without leading to any of the results which it is the fashion to ascribe to them. Much there was, as I can myself testify, that was offensive to the nose, but fever there was none. It could not be said that the atmospheric conditions were wanting, because while this village remained exempt, many neighboring villages had more than once suffered severely from the pest. It could not be said that there were no subjects, for these, as the sequel proved, but too much abounded. Meanwhile, privies and dung heaps continued to exhale ill odours without any specific effect on the public health. Many generations of swine innocently yielded up their lives, but no fever of this or any other sort could be laid to their charge. I ascertained by an inquiry conducted with the most scrupulous care that for fifteen years there had been no severe outbreak of the disorder, that for nearly ten there had been but a single case. For the development of this fever a more specific element was needed than either the swine, the dung heaps, or the privies, were, in the common course of things, able to furnish. In the course of time—as was, indeed, sure to happen—this element was at length added, and it was then found that the conditions which had been without power to *generate* fever, had but too great power in promoting its spread, when once the germ of fever had been introduced. The soil was already prepared; it only needed the seed to bring forth the bitter fruit."

Between July 11 and November 1, 1839, more than eighty of the inhabitants of the village under Dr. Budd's care suffered from typhoid fever; and he promises a full account of the details of this epidemic in a later communication.

In the latter half of 1859, Budd contributed a further series of articles to the *Lancet* on "Intestinal Fever." In the first of these, he gives credit to a number of leading French physicians for recognizing the contagiousness of "intestinal fever" and states, "It is now, indeed, nearly thirty years ago that M. Bretonneau related to the French Academy of Medicine a series of cases, in which the operation of contagion in the propagation of this fever was so plain as to admit neither of question nor doubt." Yet in England Budd finds medical and official opinion (as exemplified by the Royal College of Physicians and the General Board of Health) more vigorously anti-contagionist than ever; and Murchison's new "term 'pythogenic' fever—or fever 'born of putrescence' which Dr. Murchison has coined in order to give point to the opinions he so ably represents— bids fair, for the favour with which it has been received, as well as from the precision with which it expresses the popular view, to supersede, for a time, the many designations by which this disease has hitherto been known amongst us." In the second installment of this communication, Budd returns to an analysis of the North Tawton outbreak. He recites several series of three or four successive cases in the same household as evidence of contagion. Most striking, however, were the histories of three persons who left North Tawton during the epidemic for neighboring villages where each of them set up a new focus of contagion. Two of these persons were sawyers by trade, employed by a timber merchant in North Tawton and living—while there—in a court with a canvas privy and next door to one of the local typhoid cases. Both developed symptoms of the disease and returned to their homes in the village of Morchard. The first died in five weeks, and two weeks after his death his two children came down. The second, while ill at Morchard, was visited by a friend who developed the fever on the tenth day thereafter; and two of the children and the brother of this friend constituted a third crop of cases. There was no fever elsewhere in that part of the country.

A third episode was even more striking. This was the case of a widow (Mrs. L) who felt unwell at North Tawton on August 20, and on the 21st went to the home of her brother (S.) in Chaffcombe. On the 23rd she took to her bed, but ultimately recovered. A few days after her convalescence her sister-in-law (Mrs. S.) fell ill. Mr. S. was the next victim, falling ill on November 4 (the day of his wife's death). Three weeks later, one of the farm apprentices at Chaffcombe was attacked; next a day laborer on the farm; then, the sister of Mr. S.; then another apprentice; and, finally, as a last group, a servant man, a servant girl and a young woman (a daughter of Mrs. L.) who had come to the house to nurse.

This was, however, by no means the end of the story; for two of the victims at Chaffcombe in turn initiated epidemics in *their* native villages.

The servant girl was sent to her home at Loosebeare, four miles away. Before she recovered her father and a farmer across the road who visited frequently in the house came down with the disease; and from this farmer's house it gradually extended to the whole hamlet.

Finally, one of the apprentices stricken down at Chaffcombe (Oliver) was sent to his home, one of two cottages standing together between Bow and North Tawton. He was ill for some time, and finally took to his bed toward the end of December. His mother took the fever; then his sister; then the children of the family next door, every member ultimately becoming infected; then a married sister of Oliver's who had come to nurse the victims and who started another epidemic in her own home at a considerable distance.

Here, then, was an extraordinarily convincing epidemiological study, in which the course of specific person-to-person contagion was traced through five different isolated settlements, like all the other surrounding villages so far as local filth was concerned, and differentiated from those villages which remained free from fever only by contact with the chain of infection initiated in North Tawton.

In a later installment of this series, Budd emphasizes the significance of the power of this fever "to propagate itself and no other." He stresses the "latent" or incubation period of ten days to three weeks; and he adduces evidence, supported by the testimony of Bretonneau, Chomel and Louis, of the immunity produced by a previous attack. The analogy between "intestinal fever" and smallpox in all these respects is emphasized; and as Budd points out, the characteristic of latency inexorably points to the breeding and multiplying of a specific poison within the human body; while the acquisition of immunity must be explained by the fact that one attack so changes the nature of the body that the poison can no longer grow therein.

Later in the same volume of the *Lancet* (1859, II) Budd continues his series of articles "On Intestinal Fever." These communications are largely devoted to a discussion of the differences between typhus and typhoid fever and to the diagnostic value of the intestinal lesions in the latter case. The first of the series, however, contains an interesting citation from an essay presented by Budd in competition for the Thackeray prize in 1839, in which—at that early date—he had pointed out that the two diseases in question propagate themselves specifically and independently, "The form of fever with intestinal ulceration does not communicate the other form."

In his next installment, Budd emphasizes "1st That intestinal fever is an essentially contagious fever, 2nd That the most virulent part of the poison by which the contagion takes effect is cast off by the diseased intestine of the fever patient." He concludes that in rural areas, where common privies are in use, the disease will be clustered closely around an original case; while in a city infection will be spread chiefly by exhalations from the public sewers, so that its incidence will be more endemic and scattered.

In a third installment, Budd cites one case of an epidemic caused by the "tainted air" from a sewer and two others where "poisoned water" was at fault. One of the latter was at Bristol where a row of fifteen small houses obtained their water from a common well. On a certain day in the first week of November 1856 the well (close to the partition wall of a house where there was a case of fever) became suddenly so polluted as to be markedly offensive in taste and smell. About the middle of the month, 8 cases of fever occurred in three houses which used the water of the well, while the family in the fourth house remained in good health. The second outbreak occurred at Clifton in 1847 and the facts were essentially the same. A well supplying thirteen houses became suddenly highly offensive toward the end of September. Early in October, intestinal fever broke out in every one of these thirteen houses while no cases appeared in the twenty-one houses of the same terrace provided with a different water-supply. It happened that one house in each group was used as a girl's school, with about the same number of inmates.

Eleven out of seventeen persons were stricken in the school supplied by the polluted well—none in the other.

In 1860, Budd again returned to the attack, in the columns of the *Lancet*. He presented a series of excellent drawings of the intestinal lesions of typhoid, which he considers as characteristic of this fever as the pustulant eruption is of smallpox. He concludes that "what is cast off by this diseased surface must not only have a contagious power, but must be the chief vehicle of the fever virus." He points out that the discharge from such lesions is a much more probable source of an epidemic than the products of ordinary chemical decomposition, to which Murchison had attributed a recent epidemic at Windsor. "For centuries," he says, "it was as confidently believed that mildew was the actual offspring of damp and decay as it is now believed that intestinal fever is the offspring of common sewage; but when it was discovered that mildew is endowed with powers of self-propagation, sufficient to account in the most natural way for its appearance wherever damp and decay are found, the old and time-honoured faith fell to the ground." Only on the assumption of a contagion, originating from the intestines of the sick and spread through sewer emanations, can the fact be explained that the fever at Windsor was not duplicated at Bristol (where Budd practiced) and in other places where non-specific organic effluvia were just as abundant.

Finally, at the time of his retirement from active practice in 1873, Budd collected all his earlier studies in his classic monograph on *Typhoid Fever*. This work, in large measure, reprints the journal articles of 1856-1860 which have already been reviewed. Presented in collected form, the argument is highly impressive. The first two chapters deal with the contagiousness of the disease, as evidenced by the North Tawton and other local epidemics. The third takes up the nature of the intestinal affection and discusses the pathology of the disease as a "true exanthema of the bowel," with excellent plates. The discharge from the Peyer's patches, Budd (following Rokitansky) emphasizes as the *materies morbi*. Chapter IV deals with the relation of the disease to defective sewerage, and describes a recently-studied epidemic at Kingswood in 1866.

Chapter V deals with the contagious agent of the disease. Here, Budd is primarily concerned with the contention of Murchison that the poison of typhoid "has, when first discharged, no power to propagate the fever at all, but can only acquire this power by going through putrefactive decomposition first." This theory was founded on some famous experiments of Thiersch and Pettenkofer, in which cholera discharges caused illness in mice after putrefaction but not in their fresh state. With this view, Budd is inclined to temporize, admitting that—so far as atmospheric transmission (which he still admits) is concerned—time may be necessary to break up clots and pellets in the stools and liberate finer particles which can be disseminated through the atmosphere. He does contend, however, that this is merely a freeing of powers inherent in the stools and not a creation of any new properties. He maintains that the "specific poison is only reproduced in the living body infected with it"; but that it may retain its powers of potential reproduction for considerable periods outside the body. The dawning recognition of Pasteur's work is manifest in the statement that "There is a growing belief that the specific germs which cause contagious fevers are, in reality, so many living species." In discussing media of transmission, Budd stresses first "the tainted hands of those who wait upon the sick." Next, he mentions bed linen and other fomites and cites the high prevalence of the disease among washerwomen (a phenomenon which the writer can recall in his own early epidemiological studies). Such transmission (free from any influence of sewer-gas, soil or water) "is the act of infection stripped of all extraneous and adventitious conditions, and shown in its naked simplicity." These are, however, merely incidents in the natural history of the disease. "There are two *principal* ways, and two only, in which a poison cast out upon the ground can find its way back again into the living organism. Either through the drinking-water, or by emanations borne upon the air." Under the former head, Budd has the acuteness to note the danger of spread by milk which has been sophisticated by the addition of polluted water.

Chapter vi deals with Disinfectants and Disinfection. Budd recommends boiling of water and the use of such chemicals as chloride of lime and carbolic acid for excreta. Atmospheric disinfection, such as Guyton-Morveau advocated, has disappeared. "The theory is, that the fever is spread by the discharges: in practise it is found that disinfecting the discharges always prevents the fever from spreading."

Chapter vii deals with the pythogenic theory and its inadequacies. Here, Budd recurs to the significant evidence from rural areas where filth is habitually prevalent without fever but where—when specific infection is once introduced—the disease rages with much greater relative severity than in cities. He illustrates the principle that organic putrefaction by itself cannot cause disease by the experience of London during "the Great Stench" in the hot summer months of 1858.

"The occasion," he says, "was no common one. An extreme case, a gigantic scale in the phenomena, and perfect accuracy in the registration of the results—three of the best of all the guarantees against fallacy— were all combined to make the induction sure. For the first time in the history of man, the sewage of nearly three millions of people had been brought to seethe and ferment under a burning sun, in one vast open cloaca lying in their midst.

"The result we all know. Stench so foul, we may well believe, had never before ascended to pollute this lower air. Never before, at least, had a stink risen to the height of an historic event. Even ancient fable failed to furnish figures adequate to convey a conception of its thrice Augean foulness. For many weeks, the atmosphere of Parliamentary Committee-rooms was only rendered barely tolerable by the suspension before every window, of blinds saturated with chloride of lime, and by the lavish use of this and other disinfectants. More than once, in spite of similar precautions, the law-courts were suddenly broken up by an insupportable invasion of the noxious vapour. The river steamers lost their accustomed traffic, and travellers, pressed for time, often made a circuit of many miles rather than cross one of the city bridges.

"For months together, the topic almost monopolised the public prints. Day after day, week after week, the *Times* teemed with letters, filled with complaint, prophetic of calamity, or suggesting remedies. Here and there, a more than commonly passionate appeal showed how intensely the evil was felt by those who were condemned to dwell on the Stygian banks. At home and abroad, the state of the chief river was felt to be a national reproach. 'India is in revolt, and the Thames stinks,' were the two great facts coupled together by a distinguished foreign writer, to mark the climax of a national humiliation.

"Members of Parliament and noble lords, dabblers in sanitary science, vied with professional sanitarians in predicting pestilence." But, alas for the pythogenic theory, when the returns were made up, "the result showed, not only a death-rate below the average, but, *as the leading peculiarity of the season,* a remarkable diminution in the prevalence of fever, diarrhoea and the other forms of disease commonly attributed to putrid emanations."

Against the theory that diseases may be generated by decomposition, Budd emphasizes with convincing force their specificity—as evidenced by clinical observation and confirmed by the remarkable phenomenon of acquired immunity. "What small-pox and measles were in the Arab in the days of Rhazes, they still are in the Londoner, in our own. What they are in the Londoner, they are in the wild Indian of the North American prairie, and in the Negro of the Gold Coast. To all the other contagious fevers, as far as our records go, the same remark applies. In races the most diverse, under climates the most various, age after age, through endless generations of men, these diseases pass down through the human body, perpetuating their own kind, and each maintaining its separate identity by marks as specific as those which distinguish the asp from the adder, or the hemlock from the poppy."

Chapter VIII deals with the question of spontaneous origin and disposes of the doubts cast on the contagion theory by frequent failure to identify the origin of a case by analogy with diseases like smallpox, syphilis and other communicable diseases of men and cattle. Here, too, it is often impossible to trace the chain of infection; yet no one doubts that such a chain exists. Chapter IX is a restatement of the main conclusions, which we have already reviewed; and a vigorous plea for action.

This is indeed one of the great books in the history of epidemiology. Tyndall said of its author, "Dr. William Budd I hold to have been a man of the highest genius. There was no physician in England who, during his lifetime, showed anything like his penetration in the interpretation of zymotic disease. For a number of years he conducted an uphill fight against the whole of his medical colleagues, the only sympathy which he could count upon during that depressing time being that of the venerable Sir Thomas Watson. Over and over again Sir Thomas Watson has spoken to me of William Budd's priceless contributions to medical literature. His doctrines are now everywhere victorious, each succeeding discovery furnishing an illustration of his marvellous prescience."

This statement is, of course, somewhat unfair to John Snow, who preceded Budd in his first publication and who fought as gallantly for the same fundamental point of view. There is glory enough for both to share. To the writer, Snow seems the clearer and more logical thinker and was more completely free than Budd from surviving traces of the concept of atmospheric dissemination. Budd on the other hand was the more eloquent and effective advocate of the two. It was Snow in his studies of the relation of cholera to the Broad Street well and the London water-supplies, who gave the first brilliant demonstration of the effectiveness of the methods of statistical epidemiology. It was Budd, at North Tawton, who made a pioneer contribution to the technique of what my colleague, Dr. John R. Paul, has called clinical epidemiology—the intensive study of the relation of individual cases in the family and its immediate neighborhood.

Between them, these two great English epidemiologists—working in the sixth decade of the nineteenth century and with no knowledge of the work of Pasteur—demonstrated the basic facts with regard to the causation of cholera and typhoid fever; they showed beyond peradventure that these diseases were specific entities; that they were transmitted only by direct transfer of material from an infected human body to a susceptible victim; that the contagious elements were contained in the dejecta from the alimentary canal; that these elements were particulate and not miasmatic in nature; that they enjoyed the biological properties of survival in the environment and continuing reproduction when reintroduced into the human body; and that the passage of these contagious entities from one human being to another was accomplished chiefly by direct contact or fomites and by drinking water. They thus laid the basis for a theoretically sound and practically effective epidemiology of the intestinal infections; and they accomplished this brilliant result by keen observation and sound logical deduction from field experience, with little or no assistance from the germ-theory of disease as that theory was to be elaborated by the bacteriologists. Their accomplishment was perhaps the greatest triumph of pure epidemiology in the history of that science.

CHAPTER XIV

PASTEUR

"Before him, Egyptian darkness; with his advent a light that brightens more and more as the years give us ever fuller knowledge."—OSLER

THE general preoccupation of medicine with miasmatic theories of disease during the eighteenth and early nineteenth centuries should not lead us to believe that the doctrine of *contagia animata* had been wholly forgotten. A few courageous and imaginative scientists kept the torch burning throughout this period.

In the eighteenth century, the chief advocate of contagionist theory was the Austrian physician, Marcus Anton von Plenciz (1705-1786). A trifle over a century later than Kircher, Plenciz published in his *Opera Medico-Physica* an essay on contagion, and two others—on smallpox and scarlet fever—in which the concept of a biological cause of communicable disease is admirably presented. The first and most important of these essays, that on contagious diseases, lists among those maladies which are both epidemic and contagious, malignant, pestilential and petechial fevers, variola, measles, scarlet fever, camp dysentery and the convulsive coughs of infants. Rheumatic and intermittent fevers which are epidemic may also be contagious. Scabies, leprosy, elephantiasis, gout, venereal disease, rabies and phthisis are contagious but not epidemic. Plenciz maintains the independent entity of each of these diseases, which he compares to the specificity of plants and their seeds. To explain the phenomena involved one must postulate specific agents having the power of communicability and multiplication. Miasmatic and malign fermentations cannot meet the specifications. The germs of disease must be "worm-like" "animalculae" which "propagate and multiply" under favorable conditions as flies and other insects do; and he cites Leeuwenhoek to show how numerous such animalculae may be in nature—thus actually identifying the agents of communicable disease with the protozoa and bacteria.

In a second section of this treatise, Plenciz discusses the phenomena of putrefaction. He combats the theory that the microbes present in decomposition are the results rather than the causes of the decomposition; and emphasizes the widespread presence of "vermiculi" in ulcerating wounds, in dysentery stools, in sputum. He suggests that mercury and

Peruvian bark owe their efficacy to their power of destroying micro-organisms; and he confirms the theory of specificity and communicability of infection by the evidence from inoculation against smallpox. He concludes that "in the vegetable world, neither infection nor inoculation can be accomplished without seeds"; that such "seeds can never be evolved except from other seeds" and are not produced *de novo*; and that in contagious diseases the process of inoculation similarly supplies the seeds from which other seeds evolve and multiply. Finally, Plenciz illustrates his theory by a discussion of the etiology of wheat rust.

The same ideas are developed by Plenciz in the second and third treatises of his volume—on smallpox and scarlet fever, respectively. In the first of these essays it is interesting to note that the author considers the phenomenon of protective inoculation to be a result of reduction of virulence by a process of evolutionary modification of the original germ. So, in the case of scarlet fever, he insists that mild and severe forms of the disease are caused by the same material cause, having the power of communicability and self-multiplication. This contribution of Plenciz is remarkable for its clarity and solidity of reasoning, and would deserve a fuller analysis except for the fact that it lay outside of, and did not greatly influence, the general stream of medical thought. After all, the day of armchair reasoning was nearly over. Something more than theory was needed. The really fundamental groundwork for the germ-theory of disease was to be laid by actual experimentation in allied fields; and this experimentation was concerned with three independent but closely related problems.

The first of these three problems whose solution contributed so materially to the groundwork of the germ-theory of disease was that of fermentation. The seventeenth century theory of Willis and Stahl interpreted the process of fermentation as a particular species of internal motion which could be communicated from a fermenting liquid to another liquid capable of undergoing a similar change (in essence, this explanation closely resembled the modern "transmissible lysis" theory of bacteriophage). Lavoisier in 1789 worked out the fundamental nature of alcoholic fermentation, and Gay-Lussac in 1810 (stimulated by Appert's process of preserving food by heat and the subsequent spoilage when the preserved food was opened), concluded that the principle of fermentation was formed by the action of oxygen on the fermentable liquid.

So far, the process had been considered by most of its investigators as purely chemical in nature.

Between 1815 and 1830 the achromatic objective was perfected, and by 1835 really powerful compound microscopes at last became available. This was one of those improvements in instrumental technique which have now and then opened doors to reveal a veritable new world in science. The following decade—as a result of the new microscopes—was characterized by the most spectacular advances in all fields of biology (of which the cell-theory was perhaps the most important). In the study of fermentation, progress was immediate and significant. In 1835 and 1836 Cagniard-Latour, in France, described the yeast plant and its mode of reproduction and attributed the process of fermentation to the action of its living cells (published in full in 1838). Theodor Schwann and F. Kützing in 1837 both independently confirmed these observations in Germany. The leaders of German chemistry (Berzelius, Liebig and Wöhler), however, received these communications with scorn, and Liebig and Wöhler actually published in Liebig's *Annalen* an anonymous, mock-scientific article describing the observation with a wonderful new microscope of yeast cells shaped like stills with streams of sugar going in at one end and alcohol and carbon dioxide going out the other —which has been justly described as the most remarkable contribution which ever appeared in a serious scientific periodical.

At this point, the study of fermentation became intertwined with the second of the three major problems underlying the question of the germ theory of disease—that of spontaneous generation. The drawing of an empirical borderline between the world of the living and that of the non-living was essential to a comprehension of either fermentation or the etiology of communicable disease.

We have seen in an earlier chapter how Redi settled the question of spontaneous generation in the seventeenth century, so far as such higher types of life as insects were concerned. In the eighteenth century the problem was raised in a new form as related to the more minute and primitive forms of organic life. An English Catholic priest, J. T. Needham (1713-1781) published in 1748 the results of experiments on boiled meat juices in sealed flasks, the subsequent development of microorganisms leading him to believe that the spontaneous generation of living organisms had occurred. The Italian Abbé, L. Spallanzani (1729-1799), countered with an admirable series of experiments using flasks with slender necks which were sealed off (while the flasks were immersed in boiling water) so that both the liquid and the air above it were completely protected against contamination from without. Under these conditions, no generation took place.

In the nineteenth century the controversy was again renewed. In view of growing recognition of the necessity of oxygen for the life process, might not Spallanzani's failure to obtain growth have been merely due to the exclusion of oxygen from his sealed flasks? To answer this question, Franz Schulze in 1836 and Theodor Schwann in 1837 made the experiment in flasks which were freely connected with the atmosphere by means of an open, but coiled, tube. In the trap of this inlet sulphuric acid was placed; or the trap was kept red-hot by a flame. As the flask cooled, oxygen bubbled in through the acid or passed in through the heated section; and air thus treated yielded no growth in the flask. Stubborn opponents then claimed that the acidified or calcined air had been so changed that it would no longer support life. Finally, in 1854, H. Schroeder and T. von Dusch, replaced acid or heat in the inlet tube by a filter of cotton wool and still obtained sterile solutions. It seems today that this latter experiment was completely conclusive; but, as we shall note in a succeeding paragraph, the issue continued to be a live one for many years thereafter.

The third line of research which helped to lay a foundation for the future studies of Pasteur was the application, in a few isolated instances, of the youthful science of microbiology to the specific problems of the causation of disease. O. F. Mueller in 1773 had attempted a pioneer classification of the bacteria, and the development of the compound microscope—here, as elsewhere—was followed by rapid advances in the fourth decade of the Nineteen Hundreds. C. G. Ehrenberg's monograph on bacteria and protozoa was published in 1838; but one year earlier than this Agostino Bassi (1773-1856) in Italy demonstrated that a fungus, later named for him, *Botrytis bassiana*, was the cause of a disease of silkworms, called muscardine. In this monograph Bassi boldly advanced the theory that "all infectious diseases are due to parasites or *esseri organici viventi*." Bulloch states that "Bassi can justly be claimed as the real founder of the doctrine of pathogenic microorganisms of vegetable origin."

Two years later, in 1839, a disease of human beings was, for the first time, definitely traced to a parasitic microorganism. This was the work of J. L. Schoenlein (1793-1864) of Bamberg who in 1839 identified the fungus, *Achorion schoenleinii* as the cause of favus of the scalp. This was a communication of only twenty lines in Mueller's *Archiv* but it was of the greatest importance. Here was definite experimental evidence of the parasitic theory of disease—a far more solid basis for that theory than all the brilliant speculations of Kircher or Plenciz.

In 1846 Carl Eichstedt discovered a fungus in the skin-scrapings of patients suffering from pityriasis versicolor, and in 1849 and 1850 Pollender and Rayer and Davaine observed what we now know as the cause of anthrax.[1]

Much of this new research was embodied in 1840 in a notable exposition of the theory of a *contagium vivum* by F. G. J. Henle (1809-1885) which ranks with the contributions of Kircher and Plenciz in the two preceding centuries. Henle studied at Heidelberg and Bonn, taking his doctor's degree in 1832. He came under the powerful influence of Johannes Müller at Berlin and was named professor of anatomy at Zurich in 1840. He moved to Heidelberg (where he taught also physiology and pathology) in 1844, and to Goettingen in 1852. He was one of the outstanding anatomists of his day, and Garrison says that "the histological discoveries of Henle take rank with the anatomical discoveries of Vesalius." His *Handbook of Rational Pathology* is notable for its emphasis on the intimate relationships between pathology and physiology.

Henle's contribution to our field is an essay "Von den Miasmen und Contagien und von den miasmatisch-contagiösen Krankheiten" in his *Pathologische Untersuchungen*, published in 1840. The author recognizes three groups of endemic and epidemic diseases as follows: (1) those which are miasmatic and not, so far as is known, contagious, of which malaria is the sole example; (2) those which arise as miasmatic diseases but are also spread by contagion (such as the contagious exanthemata, smallpox, measles, scarlet fever, typhus, influenza, dysentery, cholera, plague); (3) those which are contagious and not miasmatic (such as syphilis and certain skin diseases). He suggests that the contagious element (given off from the body of the sick and capable of producing the same disease in others) may, in general, be eliminated either in a "fixed" or a "volatile" form. The first is transmitted by material objects only, soiled with pus and the like,[2] the second by volatile

---

[1] We may note that O. W. Holmes (1809-1894) of Boston in 1843 and J. P. Semmelweis (1818-1865) in 1847, demonstrated with reasonably convincing epidemiological evidence the contagiousness of puerperal fever. Both, however, were violently opposed by their obstetrical colleagues and Semmelweis was so persecuted that he ended his days in an insane asylum.

[2] It is interesting that Henle foretold the discovery of the carrier. He says, "Living individuals may also be the carriers of the infectious material which may be attached to them externally without their being themselves affected."

material diffused through the atmosphere from the skin or lungs. Direct contagion is due to the fixed form, miasmatic spread to the volatile form.

The ultimate contagious element, according to Henle, must be organic in nature; and he contends that it is not only organic but consists of individual living units bearing to the human body the relation of a parasitic organism. This element is "the germ or seed" of the disease process, not the disease process itself, just as a thorn which pricks the finger is the cause of the inflammation which may result. Henle bases his argument for the living nature of the infectious element primarily on its self-reproducibility, and supports his view by analogy with fermentation, citing the recent work of Cagniard-Latour and Schwann, to which we have referred above. He explains in some detail the various stages of the disease process on the basis of reaction to a parasitic cause.

Bassi's studies of muscardine in silkworms are reviewed in detail and the presence of similar (but more minute and invisible) parasites is postulated for other communicable maladies. Henle also supports his argument by reference to observations on certain diseases of animals.[3]

On this theory contagion, in the miasmatic-contagious diseases is "as it were, miasma, in the second generation, miasma, which has passed through a first developmental stage in the body of a patient." Henle says, "I will therefore in future, combine miasma and contagion of the miasmatic-contagious diseases under the term 'infective material.' It is always identical for each specific disease and appears as contagion when its origin from a sick person can be directly demonstrated, as miasma, when such a demonstration cannot be made." The relation of filth to certain epidemic diseases is explained by the presence of microorganisms in decaying material. Every disease entity is, however, specific and cannot be generated *de novo*. "Only an apple tree can produce apples."

In a section on the diseases which are contagious but not miasmatic, Henle refers to the mites which had been discovered in certain skin diseases, and to vibrios and infusoria observed in syphilitic discharges by Donné and others and to Schoenlein's discovery of the fungus cause of favus; and discusses rabies in some detail.

In his closing pages, Henle acknowledges that he has been dealing with theories rather than experimental facts. Yet he rightly maintains that theories may be invaluable as guides to experimentation. "Nature," he says, "answers only when she is questioned." The vitally important

---

[3] An interesting monograph could be prepared on the early contributions of veterinary medicine to our knowledge of the etiology of human diseases.

fact was that, in the first half of the nineteenth century, men had begun to ask the right questions. The laboratory bench was replacing the study desk. Real experimental progress had been made in an understanding of the phenomena of fermentation, in the demonstration of the principle of biogenesis and in the proof that at least certain diseases of the skin and scalp were due to parasitic fungi. Thus was the stage set for the entrance of Pasteur upon the scene.

The tomb of Pasteur in the crypt of the Pasteur Institute is the most impressive shrine of science in the world. On the arches of this tomb are inscriptions commemorating nine great discoveries: molecular dissymmetry (1848); fermentation (1857); spontaneous generation (1862); diseases of wine (1863); diseases of silkworms (1865); microorganisms in beer (1871); virulent diseases (1877); preventive vaccinations (1880); and rabies (1885). All but the first and the last two of these discoveries are pertinent to our present thesis.

Louis Pasteur was born at Dôle, December 27, 1822, the son of a veteran of Napoleon's Grand Army who operated a tannery at Dôle and later at Arbois. He studied at Besançon and was admitted to the Ecole Normale in Paris in 1843, taking his doctorate in 1847. He began work in the borderline between chemistry and crystallography, and his first important paper was "on the relations which may exist between crystalline form, chemical composition and the direction of rotary power." He was appointed professor of chemistry at Strassburg in 1849, and in 1853 was made a knight of the Legion of Honor for his success in the conversion of tartaric to racemic acid.

These early studies of Pasteur's on the relation between chemical composition and crystalline form in the asymmetrical tartrates seem remote indeed from the problem of the causation of epidemic pestilences. I often wonder how many medical students notice the isomeric crystals on the cover of the *Journal of Infectious Diseases* and how many of those who notice them grasp their significance. Yet the connection was a very direct one in the evolution of Pasteur's inquiring mind. It was as early as 1855 that he found amyl alcohol in the product of certain industrial fermentations and considered its presence inconsistent with the generally accepted explanation of the process. If fermentation were merely a disintegration of the organic molecules present, it was hard to explain the production of a material having the specific rotating power of amyl alcohol. A synthetic origin seemed rather to be indicated.

In 1854, Pasteur had left Strassburg to become dean of the Faculty of Science at Lille; and the agricultural activities of the region stimulated his interest in the problem of fermentation. In 1856 he was consulted in regard to difficulties in the manufacture of alcohol from beet-roots; and in August 1857 he presented before the Scientific Society of Lille his first important contribution in this field. It dealt with the lactic fermentation and concluded that "fermentation displays itself as a correlative of the life, of the organization of globules, not of the death or the putrefaction of these globules, any more than it appears as a phenomenon of contact or of a transformation of sugar accomplished in the presence of a ferment to which it gives nothing and from which it takes nothing."

Later in this year (1857) Pasteur returned to the Ecole Normale where he completed important studies on the alcoholic fermentation, summarized in an extensive monograph in 1860. His most important experimental contribution was the development of fermentation in a synthetic medium of sugar, ammonia and mineral salts inoculated with yeast cells which demonstrated the correlation between cell growth and formation of alcohol in the absence of any preexisting complex organic material. In 1860, the transformation of Pasteur from chemist to biologist was recognized by award of the Prize for Experimental Physiology of the Academy of Sciences, and in 1862 he was admitted to the ranks of the Academy itself (although in the mineralogical section).

Between 1862 and 1864 Pasteur extended his field widely and rapidly. He described the *Mycoderma aceti* and studied its relation to the process of vinegar-making, and in 1866 published his *Etudes sur le vin*. In this classic monograph he not only demonstrated that the various types of spoilage of wine were related to the development of particular types of specific bacteria (which he figured ana described) but also demonstrated how effectively such abnormal fermentations could be controlled by heating (a process to which the term pasteurization was later applied).

Between 1866 and 1870, Pasteur's work on fermentation was interrupted by his preoccupation with the diseases of silkworms which we shall consider in a later paragraph. In 1871 he began a new series of investigations on the abnormal fermentations which occurred in the process of brewing, summarized in 1873 in *Etudes sur la bière*. By the middle of the seventh decade of the nineteenth century, however, he had made his first major contribution to biological science, through the demonstration that the processes of fermentation were due to the activity of living microbes and that each particular kind of fermentation was the work of a specific microbe; and he had done this, not by any single brilliantly conceived *experimentium crucis* but by the far more effective evidence of a vast mass of observations in allied but diverse fields. The weight of the demonstration of the role of different specific microorganisms in lactic, alcoholic and acetic fermentations, and in the diverse abnormal decompositions of wine and beer, was irresistible.

With Pasteur, as in the case of his predecessors, the problem of fermentation was intimately related to that of spontaneous generation. As we have seen, Schulze, Schwann and Schroeder and von Dusch had really settled this question by 1854; but the conservative scientific world was not convinced and it remained for Pasteur to settle the problem once and for all.

There were several reasons why the conclusions of Schroeder and von Dusch—impressive as they seem to us—were not universally accepted. The whole conception of a world of unrecognized microbes in air and water was unfamiliar and difficult to grasp. Above all, however, there were uncertain factors in technique which made it inevitable that conflicting results should be obtained. Against a "crucial experiment" proving biogenesis could be set another "crucial experiment" demonstrating the opposite conclusion.

In 1858, F.-A. Pouchet, director of the Natural History Museum at Rouen, sent a note to the Academy of Sciences in which he claimed to have demonstrated that "animals and plants could be generated in a medium absolutely free from atmospheric air, and, in which, therefore, no germ of organic bodies could have been brought by air." Pasteur at once threw himself into the fray and began a series of brilliant studies, presented before the Academy in 1860 and summarized in an extensive monograph in 1862. The earlier work had been largely negative, resting on the absence of decomposition in properly protected infusions. Pasteur attacked the problem from a positive standpoint, demonstrating the actual agents of the fermentative process. He replaced the filter of Schroeder and von Dusch by one of gun-cotton and on dissolving the filtering material showed under the microscope the particulate material which it contained. In an ingenious series of experiments, he demonstrated how growth could be started in a sterile flask by introducing a fragment of filtering material through which air had passed, visible mold development often taking place on the surface of the fragment.

One of the prime arguments of the "heterogenists" was the impossibility of the presence of germs in the air in sufficient numbers to cause fermentation. Pouchet said, "Such a crowd of them would produce a thick mist as dense as iron." Could the distribution of germs in the air be irregular, denser in some places than in others? "Then there would be sterile zones and fecund zones, a most convenient hypothesis, indeed!" Pasteur attacked this problem by the use of swan-neck flasks containing fermentable solutions, sterilized and the neck sealed while the flask and the air in it were hot. When the neck of such a flask was broken, air rushed in and the neck was again sealed. By this procedure a roughly quantitative analysis could be made of the germ content of the air. Flasks opened in Paris streets all spoiled, while of ten flasks opened in a cellar only one showed alteration. There *were* sterile zones and fecund zones.

The battlefield now shifted to the high mountains. Pasteur took his flasks to the Montanvert above Chamonix—and only one of twenty was decomposed. Pouchet was, however, similarly occupied. In the summer of 1863, with his assistants, Joly and Musset, he went up on the Maladetta glaciers of the Pyrenees (Joly nearly losing his life on a precipice) and their flasks all showed decomposition. A Commission of the Academy was appointed to judge between the rival disputants; but Pouchet and his associates temporized and finally in the spring of 1864 they yielded without further tests.

The curious thing is that if they had persisted they would—for the time being—have been victorious. In their studies, they had used a hay infusion which contained spores which resist the temperatures then employed in sterilization while Pasteur used yeast water which rarely contains such spores. These facts were then, of course, unknown; and if the heterogenists had not lost their nerve the theory of biogenesis might have been set back for years.

It was more than a decade later that the problem was finally settled. In 1873, a young English neurologist, H. C. Bastian raised the issue again. He heated sealed flasks of urine to 50° C. and demonstrated the development of swarms of bacteria. By this time, however, Pasteur was ready for a crucial test. He had discovered the resting spore stage of the bacteria and by 1876 he and his associate, C. Chamberland, showed that in such experiments as those of Pouchet it was resistant spores introduced in the water or the urine which accounted for the subsequent growth. By heating to 115°-120° C., Chamberland destroyed these spores and sterility could be universally maintained. Thus was the long battle of Abiogenesis vs. Biogenesis at last brought to a close.

In the interest of logical analysis, the studies on fermentation and spontaneous generation conducted by Pasteur throughout his life have been briefly reviewed. Their major conclusions had, however, been reached by the early 'sixties. We must now digress from the tracing of his investigations to the application of these early results in the field of human diseases which was made at this time by Lister.

Pasteur had very early realized the possible significance of his conclusions in the field of medicine. In his description of the studies at Chamonix, presented to the Academy on November 5, 1860,[4] he says, "I have by no means completed these studies. What would be most desirable, would be to carry them far enough to prepare the way for a serious research on the origin of various diseases." Yet, at this stage, Pasteur himself had progressed from chemistry to microbiology but not yet to medicine. His researches were brought to their first fruition in this field by a young British surgeon.

Joseph Lister (1827-1912) was the son of a Quaker wine merchant of London (who was an amateur microscopist and made important contributions to the perfection of the achromatic objective). He graduated in medicine at the University of London in 1852 and went to Edinburgh to follow surgery under Syme, whose daughter he married. In 1860, he became professor of surgery at Glasgow and in 1869 succeeded Syme at Edinburgh. In 1877 he returned to London to take the chair of surgery at King's College, retiring in 1896. He was president of the Royal Society for five years, received a baronetcy in 1883 and was elevated to the peerage in 1897.

Lord Lister made many important contributions to surgical science, but his chief title to fame was the development of antiseptic surgery during his incumbency at Glasgow.

Early in his hospital experience, Lister had been impressed—as were all surgeons of his day—with the appalling mortality from various forms of wound infection. In his own statistics of amputation he reported 45 per cent of fatalities and he came to have grave doubts of the current theory of "laudable pus." The resemblance between hospital gangrene and putrefaction had been obvious since the days of Fracastorius, and when Lister heard of Pasteur's studies he sought to apply the concept of the germ theory in his own field. This was his inspiration;

4 Not "March 5, 1880," as Vallery-Radot cites the date.

and it was a real stroke of genius for a surgeon of those days to realize the possible connection between his art and the researches of a French student of fermentation.

Sterilization by heat would obviously be inappropriate for the treatment of wounds, and Lister therefore sought for a chemical disinfectant and, fortunately, hit upon carbolic acid which had been employed for the disinfection of sewage at Carlisle (another example of his catholic knowledge and imagination). On August 12, 1865, he employed this disinfectant in a case of compound fracture with complete success and two years later published his first communication on the subject.

In this paper (published in the *Lancet* for 1867) he says, "Turning now to the question how the atmosphere produces decomposition of organic substances, we find that a flood of light has been thrown upon this most important subject by the philosophic researches of M. Pasteur, who has demonstrated by thoroughly convincing evidence that it is not to its oxygen or to any of its gaseous constituents that the air owes this property, but to minute particles suspended in it, which are the germs of various low forms of life long since revealed by the microscope, and regarded as merely accidental concomitants of putrescence, but now shown by Pasteur to be its essential cause."[5] Lister then describes eleven cases of operations conducted with the aid of carbolic acid. In a second paper, published during the same year, he reviews some of the more general results of the new procedure. He says, "I have felt ashamed when recording the results of my practice, to have so often to allude to hospital gangrene or pyaemia. It was interesting, though melancholy, to observe that, whenever all, or nearly all, the beds contained cases with open sores, these grievous complications were pretty sure to show themselves; so that I came to welcome simple fractures, though in themselves of little interest either for myself or the students, because their presence diminished the proportion of open sores among the patients. But since the antiseptic treatment has been brought into full operation, and wounds and abscesses no longer poison the atmosphere with putrid exhalations, my wards, though in other respects under precisely the same circumstances as before, have completely changed their character; so that during the last nine months not a single instance of pyaemia, hospital gangrene, or erysipelas has occurred in them."

[5] Lister's recognition of Pasteur's works was always most generous. His inaugural address at Edinburgh (on the "Causation of Putrefaction and Fermentation") was largely devoted to the work of Cagniard-Latour and Pasteur. At Pasteur's jubilee, in 1892, he paid to him a tribute which did equal credit to both participants.

Three years later (in 1870) he presented statistics which indicated that for two years preceding the antiseptic period 16 fatalities occurred in 35 amputations; while in 1867-1869, only 6 deaths occurred in 40 cases.

Thus was the germ theory first brilliantly applied to the control of diseases of human beings.

There were other applications to veterinary and medical science in this period, whose significance we can now realize. C. Davaine between 1860 and 1865 showed that anthrax could be transmitted by the blood of an infected animal if that blood contained sufficient numbers of anthrax bacilli. J.-A. Villemin (1827-1892) demonstrated the inoculability of tubercle between 1861 and 1868. O. Obermeier (1843-1873) was studying the spirochete of relapsing fever from 1868 to the time of his death. Yet these isolated observations failed to produce any important effect upon medical thinking. Here again, as in the case of fermentation and biogenesis, it remained for the infinite patience of Pasteur to amass a weight of evidence sufficient to break down the inertia of tradition.

It was in the year of Lister's first antiseptic operation that Pasteur was led from the field of organic decomposition to that of disease causation, in what seems to us a somewhat unusual experimental animal—the silkworm.[6]

For about twenty years the important silk industry of France had been in serious difficulty. In the words of Lady Claud Hamilton's translation of Vallery-Radot's life of Pasteur, "The life of the population of certain departments in the South of France hangs on the existence of silkworms. In each house there is nothing to be seen but hurdles, over which the worms crawl. They are placed even in the kitchens, and often in well-to-do families they occupy the best rooms. In the largest cultivations, regular stages of these hurdles are raised one above the other, in immense sheds, under roofs of disjointed tiles, where thousands and thousands of silkworms crawl upon the litters, which they have the instinct never to leave. Great or small, the silkworm-rearing establishments exist everywhere. When people accost each other, instead of saying 'How are you?' they say 'How are the silkworms?' In the night they get up to feed them or to keep up around them a suitable temperature. And then what anxiety is felt at the least change of weather! Will not the mulberry leaves be wet? Will the worms digest well? Digestion is a matter of great importance to the health of the worms, which do nothing all their lives but eat! Their appetites become especially insatiable during the

6 Yet it was in the silkworm that Bassi had discovered the fungus agent of muscardine.

last days of rearing. All the world is then astir, day and night. Sacks of leaves are incessantly brought in and spread out on the litters. Sometimes the noise of the worms munching these leaves resembles that of rain falling upon thick bushes. With what impatience is the moment waited for when the worms arrive at the last moulting! Their bodies swollen with silk, they mount upon the brambles prepared for them, where they shut themselves up in their golden prisons and become chrysalides. What days of rejoicing are those in which the cocoons are gathered; when, to use the words of Olivier de Serres, the silk harvest is garnered in! . . .

"In the epidemic which ravaged the silkworm nurseries in 1849, the symptoms were numerous and changeable. Sometimes the disease exhibited itself immediately. Many of the eggs were sterile, or the worms died during the first days of their existence. Often the hatching was excellent, and the worms arrived at their first moulting, but that moulting was a failure. A great number of the worms, taking little nourishment at each repast, remained smaller than the others, having a rather shiny appearance and a blackish tint. Instead of all the worms going through the phases of this first moulting together, as is usually the case in a batch of silkworms, they began to present a marked inequality, which displayed itself more and more at each successive moulting. Instead of the worms swarming on the tables, as if their number was uniformly augmenting, empty spaces were everywhere seen; every morning corpses were collected on the litters."

By 1861 the revenue of the silk industry had been cut down from 130 million to 8 million francs; and in 1865 the cultivators made an urgent appeal to the government for aid. J. B. Dumas, as senator, had been asked to prepare a report and called upon Pasteur to study the problem. Pasteur pleaded his ignorance of the field; "Remember, if you please, that I have never even touched a silkworm." "So much the better," replied Dumas, "For ideas, you will have only those which come to you as a result of your own observations." So Pasteur dropped his researches on fermentation and set up at a laboratory at Alais where for five years he was to labor in a new field.

Earlier observers, particularly M. Osimo, had observed great numbers of characteristic corpuscles in diseased eggs and worms and had suggested in 1859 the selection of eggs free from such corpuscles as a method of control. Other students of the subject had, however, denied these conclusions, which were unsubstantiated by any convincing evidence. Pasteur, by the summer of 1865 accepted as sound the diagnostic value of the corpuscles and the process of selection of sound eggs by the microscopic examination of the parent moths. It is of interest to note, however, that at this time, he considered the corpuscles as merely pathological manifestations of the disease, not as its causative agents.

The problem was enormously complicated—by variations in resistance of various strains of worms, by the difficulty of securing stocks wholly free from infection, by the fact that worms containing so few corpuscles that they could not be detected, and themselves developing quite normally, might give rise to highly infected pupae and adults, and, above all, by the fact that two different diseases were rampant among them, pébrine (the corpuscular disease) and flâcherie (an independent communicable malady, greatly influenced by hereditary and environmental factors). Thus, in his early experiments, Pasteur was confronted with extremely puzzling phenomena, the presence of corpuscles in pupae from worms which had developed normally and the absence of corpuscles in worms which were obviously sick (flâcherie).

The summer of 1866 was devoted to breeding experiments, conducted with Pasteur's inimitable care; but the problem remained obscure. In January, 1867, he still doubted the parasitic nature of pébrine. That this should be the case after eighteen months of study, is a vivid indication of the fact that—in spite of Kircher and Plenciz and Henle—the concept of a *contagium vivum* seemed still a new and strange one. In the course of this year (1867), however, the major difficulties were overcome. Pasteur, now professor at the Sorbonne, recognized the difference between pébrine and flâcherie and he obtained stocks of eggs free from the former disease. Crucial experiments demonstrated that the corpuscles were indeed the cause of pébrine and that it could be communicated to sound stock by injection or by the feeding of contaminated leaves. By 1868 the problem was essentially solved.

In October 1868 Pasteur suffered a cerebral hemorrhage which paralyzed his left side; but within a week he was dictating a communication to the Academy, and by January 1869 he was again at Alais. By 1870 he published a complete résumé of all the work in his "Etudes sur les Maladies des Vers à Soie." He had demonstrated conclusively that the corpuscles were the active agents in pébrine, that they were transmitted from the eggs through the larva and pupa to the adult and that by microscopic examination of the moth one could determine whether the eggs of the next generation were infected or sound. Flâcherie, on the other hand, was due to other parasitic microorganisms widely distributed in nature; and for its control required not only the selection of uninfected stock but also the maintenance of vital resistance by favorable conditions for the worms under cultivation.

For the second time—as in the case of wine-making—Pasteur had saved one of the great industries of France.

In 1870 came one of the greatest tragedies of Pasteur's life, the Franco-Prussian War. As usual, with a Prussian raid, the war was directed against science as well as against humanity. In the laboratory of Regnault, the celebrated physicist, not a window was broken, not a lock forced; but a Prussian, evidently an expert had been there. In the words of Dumas, "Nothing seemed changed in that abode of science, and yet everything was destroyed; the glass tubes of barometers, thermometers, etc. were broken; scales and other similar instruments had been carefully knocked out of shape with a hammer." In a corner was a heap of ashes, the notes and manuscripts of Regnault's work for the last ten years.

With the close of the war, Pasteur devoted himself passionately to the rehabilitation of his country; and his first service was in the study of improvements in the national brewing industry, completed in 1873. Between that date and 1876, he was largely preoccupied with the final controversy (with Bastian) on biogenesis. In 1873, however, he was elected to the Academy of Medicine and began more and more clearly to perceive what the science of microbiology might mean to the healing art. As Garrison says, "Pasteur was virtually transformed from a chemist to a medical man."

It was two centuries since Robert Boyle had predicted that he who could probe to the bottom the nature of ferments and fermentation would probably be capable of explaining certain problems of disease. Yet there was still strong opposition—even to the idea of individual disease entities, which was obviously basic to a germ theory. Vallery-Radot cites the vehement reaction aroused by Villemin when he announced the inoculability of tuberculosis, "He was treated almost as a perturber of medical order. Dr. Pidoux, an ideal representative of traditional medicine, with his gold-buttoned blue coat and his reputation equally great in Paris and at the Eaux-Bonnes, declared that specificity was a fatal thought." "Applied to chronic diseases," said Pidoux, "these doctrines condemn us to the research of specific remedies or vaccines and all progress is arrested. . . . Specificity immobilizes medicine."

By 1873, however, when Pasteur was admitted to the Academy of

Medicine, A. Guérin was using the Lister methods of antiseptic surgery in Paris; and Davaine's earlier thesis that his bacteridium was "the cause and the only cause of anthrax" was beginning to gain adherents. In 1876, came the brilliant experiments of Koch to which reference will be made in a later paragraph. With this stimulus Pasteur entered upon a feverishly active period of medical experimentation. In April 1877 he presented to the Academy of Sciences a convincing report on the cultivation of the anthrax bacillus *in vitro* through many transfers and the production of the disease by these cultures (but not by their filtrates from which the bacilli had been removed). In July 1877 he (with Joubert) described the germ of malignant edema. In April 1878 he presented (with Joubert and Chamberland) a comprehensive review of "La Théorie des Germes et ses Applications à la Médicine et à la Chirurgie." In 1879 he discussed the cause of puerperal fever with Gallic sense of drama saying, as he drew a streptococcus on the blackboard: "Dr. Hervieux said at the close of his lecture, after having learnedly challenged the applications which have been made of the germ theory to puerperal fever, 'I shall not live long enough to see the vibrio which produces that fever.' Well, if the Academy will permit, I will draw under his eyes the dangerous microbe to which I attribute the existence of that fever." In May 1880 he described the staphylococcus as the cause of furunculosis.

With Pasteur's last and greatest work, the discovery of the principles of acquired immunity and the development of practical methods of producing such immunity by artificial means, we are not concerned in the present discussion. This work, begun with chicken cholera in 1880, was carried on with anthrax, rabies and diphtheria to the end of his life. In this phase of his career he was showered with honors, of which his election to the Académie Francaise in 1882 was one of the greatest. The Pasteur Institute was erected for him in 1888, and he died in 1895.

We must turn now to the third of the great trio who in the fifteen years between 1867 and 1882 contributed in their various ways to the creation of the germ theory of disease.

Robert Koch (1843-1910) was born at Klausthal in Hanover and took his medical degree in 1866 at Göttingen where he was greatly influenced by Henle. With this inspiration and with Pasteur's study of fermentation in the background, it was natural that young Koch should have been keenly interested in the parasitic theory of disease. What was more surprising was that, after serving in the war of 1870 and receiving appointment as a district physician in the rural area of Wollstein, he should have had the courage and initiative to make this interest bear fruit. In the midst of the urgent demands of country practice, and with no stimulus from any professional colleagues, he labored intensively with his microscope on the cause of anthrax which, in an agricultural district, was a problem of major importance. In 1876 he came up to the University of Breslau on the invitation of the botanist Ferdinand Cohn to demonstrate the discoveries he had made. W. H. Welch, one of the fathers of American bacteriology, was a student under Cohnheim; and all of us remember how he recalled the students waiting while Cohn, Weigert, Cohnheim and other members of the faculty were closeted with an unknown young country doctor and how Cohnheim suddenly burst into the laboratory, crying out, "This is the greatest discovery ever made in bacteriology."[7]

In the same year (1876) Cohn published in his Beiträge Koch's first classic contribution, "Die Aetiologie der Milzbrand-Krankheit, begründet auf die Entwicklungsgeschichte des Bacillus Anthracis." In this paper, Koch worked out the full life history of the organism and demonstrated the significance of the spore stage (whose resistance to heat had caused many of the contradictory results obtained by earlier observers). He cultivated the organism *in vitro* in the aqueous humor of the ox's eye and showed that this pure culture, containing living anthrax bacilli (or their spores) could cause the disease; and he predicted that similar studies would reveal the secret of cholera and typhoid fever. His results—as we have seen above—were promptly confirmed by Pasteur.

In the next year (1877) Koch began to develop the practical techniques of bacteriology in a systematic form suitable for general use—a task which had never interested Pasteur and whose accomplishment was to make Germany the mecca for young students from all countries of the world. In this paper he developed in particular the application of the anilin dyes which C. Weigert had used for the staining of bacteria in 1871, and the possibilities of photo-micrography. In 1878, he published a notable memoir on traumatic infections, in which the causes of six different kinds of surgical infections were described in detail.

In 1880, as a result of his early contributions, Koch was given a laboratory in the Imperial Department of Health, with F. Loeffler and G.

[7] In the admirable life of Welch by S. Flexner and J. T. Flexner (1941) it is pointed out that Welch was actually not at Breslau until 1878, and that in his reminiscences he telescoped a second visit of Koch's to Breslau in that year with the original demonstration.

Gaffky as his assistants. In 1881, he published a second major paper on methods, in which he described the solid-culture method of cultivating bacteria, which was to prove of such inestimable value.[8] He worked out various practical methods of disinfection in the same year. In 1882, came the classic monograph on tuberculosis, to which further reference must be made in a succeeding paragraph. In 1883, Koch as the head of a German Cholera Commission visited Egypt and India and discovered the cholera vibrio. In 1885 he was appointed professor of hygiene and bacteriology at the University of Berlin, and in 1891 the Institute for Infectious Diseases was established under his direction. He received the Nobel Prize in 1895, and in 1896 visited Africa again at the head of a Commission on Sleeping Sickness. He died in 1910.

The high point of Koch's scientific career was his communication on tuberculosis presented before the Physiological Society of Berlin on March 24, 1882. This paper has always seemed to the writer the most outstanding single contribution in the history of bacteriology—perhaps equalled only by William Harvey in any medical field. The paper includes demonstration of three major facts: (1) the presence of the tubercle bacillus (as proved by staining) in tubercular lesions of various organs of men and animals; (2) the cultivation of the organism in pure culture on blood serum; and (3) the production of tuberculosis at will by its inoculation into guinea pigs.

Here was a disease which was not even recognized as a specific entity[9] and of whose causation there was—in spite of Villemin's experiments— no accepted theory. Before the presentation of this paper, nothing was definitely known about the etiology of tuberculosis; after its presentation, the whole picture was clear. In a memoir which occupies seventeen pages in Koch's collected works, there is not a single error, except the interpretation of certain structures in the cell as spores. Furthermore it contains practically everything we now know about the bacteriology of the tubercle bacillus except the difference between the human and bovine types and the recent knowledge of the chemistry of the tubercle bacillus (perhaps also its filtrable stage, if such a stage really exists).

If one may imagine initiating a class in bacteriology into the technique of the science by asking them to make pure cultures of the tubercle

8 When Koch demonstrated this procedure at an International Medical Congress in London, Pasteur rushed forward with the exclamation, "C'est un grand progrès."

9 Of the two leading medical schools of New York City at this time, one taught that tuberculosis was a single disease, the other that the development of tubercles was merely a symptom of various diseases.

bacillus, one gains some conception of the difficulty of the task accomplished by Koch in 1882.

The influence of this paper was as phenomenal as its quality. Pasteur, up to 1877, had worked with no animal host higher than the silkworm; and the studies of Davaine, Koch and Pasteur on anthrax had related to a malady which—while it did affect man—was primarily of veterinary interest. In tuberculosis, however, Koch was dealing with perhaps the greatest plague affecting the human race at that time. His elegant technique applied to such a central problem was electrifying in its effect. Garrison lists the observation before 1882 of the causative organisms of leprosy (A. Hansen), gonorrhea (A. Neisser), typhoid fever (C. J. Eberth) and lobar pneumonia (Pasteur and G. M. Sternberg). Between 1882 and 1889, the microbic causes of glanders, erysipelas, diphtheria, tetanus, infection with *Escherichia coli*, malta fever, cerebro-spinal meningitis and chancroid were discovered; in the next decade, those of influenza, aerogenes infection, plague and dysentery.

The three great leaders, Pasteur, Lister and Koch, had between them ushered in the Golden Age of Bacteriology and had definitely and finally established the parasitic theory of communicable disease.

CHAPTER XV

PETTENKOFER—THE LAST STAND

"His name will always be inseparably connected with this most important contribution [the ground-water theory] to epidemiological science."—VOIT

IT WOULD be ungenerous to the lost cause of the miasmatists to omit mention of their last great advocate, who made a gallant effort to uphold the banner—all through the period of Snow and Budd, and even long after the discoveries of Pasteur. This Leonidas was the distinguished German hygienist, Max von Pettenkofer.

Quite aside from his theory of the causation of cholera—with which we are concerned in the present chapter—Pettenkofer was one of the most outstanding figures in nineteenth century medicine and was the father of modern experimental research in the field of hygiene.

He was born at Lichtenheim in 1818, fifteen years younger than Liebig, three years older than Virchow, and four years older than Pasteur. He was adopted by his uncle, an apothecary in Munich and, after a brief period of revolt in which he ran away and became an actor, took his degree in medicine at Munich in 1843. His early research was in pharmacology, and he did graduate work at Würzburg and with Liebig at Giessen, being associated with him in the isolation of creatinin. He served as chemist in the mint in 1845 and won the favor of King Ludwig by preparing a successful imitation of the ancient Pompeian porphyry glass. In 1847 he was appointed professor of medical chemistry in the University, with a yearly stipend of 700 gulden in gold and compensation in kind of two measures of wheat and seven measures of rye. He shifted his interest from physiological chemistry to the hygiene of food, clothing, air, water and sewage—then a virgin field. In 1851, King Max II sought advice from him as to the merits of direct and indirect heating, and thus confirmed him in his new interests. In 1852 the King persuaded Liebig to come to Munich, and in 1853 Pettenkofer was appointed to the Medical Faculty. During the next ten years, he initiated pioneer work on the hygiene of nutrition and air-conditioning which has been basic in all future progress in these fields. In 1865, at Pettenkofer's urgency the subject of hygiene was recognized as an independent field in the Bavarian universities, and Pettenkofer was, of course, the first to bear the title of professor of hygiene at Munich. In nutrition, Pettenkofer trained Voit (1831-1908), who in turn trained Rubner, so that the line of intellectual filiation was complete. In the field of air-conditioning he had no equally brilliant pupil, and much of the work done at Munich (except the use of CO_2 as a measure of atmospheric vitiation) was temporarily forgotten; but it has been rediscovered during the past twenty years and forms the foundation of many recent advances. In 1872, Pettenkofer was called to Vienna, and in order to hold him in Munich the University provided him with a Hygienic Institute, the first important institution of its kind in the world. He was ennobled in 1883.

Pettenkofer's interest in epidemiology was aroused by the cholera epidemic of 1854, the same which stimulated the work of Snow, and on the basis of his studies of cholera developed the famous "ground-water theory." Under Pettenkofer's influence a new water supply and a new system of drainage were introduced at Munich.

In 1892, at the age of seventy-four, Pettenkofer and a group of his pupils swallowed virulent cultures of the "comma bacillus" to prove that this organism could not cause cholera without the other attendant circumstances which he considered necessary. The master escaped, and although two of the pupils developed what were perhaps mild cases of the disease, the Munich group claimed a victory. In 1901, old and lonely, Pettenkofer committed suicide.

Pettenkofer's first important contribution to epidemiology was his *Investigations and Observations on the Method of Spread of Cholera* (1855), and, in this volume the main fundamentals of his etiological viewpoint are already well developed. This is a serious and perceptive epidemiological study of the 1854 epidemic in Bavaria prepared in connection with the studies of an official Commission on the Scientific Investigation of Indian Cholera. Epidemics at Munich and nine other localities are reviewed and, for Munich, the course of the epidemic is analyzed in detail by location and date of onset. A report by Jameson on cholera in India and the 1852 report on cholera in London are extensively cited and extracts reprinted in appendices.

In the concluding chapter of this volume, Pettenkofer poses the fundamental problem with regard to the epidemiology of cholera in these words: "This disease, in its spread, follows neither the laws of the purely contagious, nor those of the purely epidemic-miasmatic diseases." He points out that the non-contagionists may properly say that, "If the disease be contagious, why are not doctors and attendants attacked to a greater degree than the other inhabitants of a community who have not been in contact with the sick?" They also inquire, "How does a cholera epidemic arise in a locality which has in no way been exposed to cholera cases?" On the other hand, the contagionists reply by asking: "How does it come about that cholera in its spread so notably follows the routes of human travel? Through India, through Russia, through the whole of Europe? Why does this spread correspond so regularly with the curve, not only of caravans and military forces, but also of ships and railroads? Why does it affect first the harbors and market-towns on islands, and only later, the interior? Why does the plague break out on islands which have been visited by vessels from cholera-infected regions and not on those which have received no such visits?"

From experience in India and elsewhere, as well as from his own researches, Pettenkofer fully accepts the reality of a contagious factor in the spread of cholera, and—as fully as Snow or Budd—identifies this factor with excretal discharges; but he insists that a certain condition of the soil is essential for the dissemination of the disease.

He is convinced that the infectious element is without power to produce an epidemic on high, dry, rocky soil, citing the experience of Jameson in India and his own in Bavaria. He presents evidence that it is not altitude *per se* but some characteristic of damp, porous and polluted soil which is associated with local epidemics; and he concludes that such soil must influence the development of the poison of the disease, rather than the vital resistance of the human body. The conception that a terrain of this type exhales a miasma into the atmosphere is confirmed by the observations of Schönbein indicating the disappearance of ozone from the air during a cholera epidemic. "The cholera germ-bearing excrements which penetrate into porous and otherwise suitable layers of the soil, by the fine subdivision which they experience modify the existing processes of decay and decomposition in the soil in such a way that in addition to the normal gases of putrefaction a specific Cholera-Miasm is developed, which is then spread along with other exhalations into the houses." This process can only occur in the deeper layers of the soil, protected against winter frost and the drying effect of summer heat. The miasma is readily diluted and dissipated by moving air, and long exposure such as occurs in the case of a badly-ventilated room is necessary to produce serious effects. The disease is therefore generally acquired in the dwelling and particularly during the hours of sleep. When the germs of cholera are introduced to a given locality from outside, the possibility of the development of an epidemic depends on the character of the soil. If the soil be favorable for the evolution of miasma, some individuals will "fall sick or be at least so affected[1] that their excremental discharges will in turn become bearers of the germ or ferment [of cholera]"; and further development of miasma will follow in the soil.

An epidemic initiated in this way finally dies out, "partly through its own inherent tendencies, partly because after a time the saturated population of the area loses the power of reproducing the germs. I postulate the course of this process in the soil as like the course of the fermentation of a great mass of must or beer-wort, whose fermentation, when it has once begun, proceeds rapidly to a certain height and then slowly diminishes."

Pettenkofer then proceeds to demolish the theory of the spread of cholera "by contagion in the narrow sense of the word." "What has all the fumigation and disinfection of clothing and merchandise at the Cholera Quarantine Stations accomplished except to give the clothing a sickly smell and to damage the merchandize? How does it happen that the first cholera cases in an area are so often persons who have had no contact either with the sick or with visitors? Those persons who dedicate their powers with earnest endeavor exclusively to the care of the sick are in no greater danger than those who keep carefully shut up in their own chambers."

Pettenkofer minimizes the direct influence of obvious meteorological factors in the spread of cholera; and attributes its generally greater summer prevalence to the greater amount of travel in summer and to the fact that, at this season, "the processes of decomposition in the soil go on at such a depth that warm and moist air at the surface of the earth will develop miasma to the greatest extent."

In water-supply as an agent (which Snow at this very time was proving of such importance), Pettenkofer takes no stock whatever. He says, "I believe that in my report on Munich, I have disposed, once and for all, of the spread by drinking water" (although, in another connection he has wisely said that "observations made by a single man in a single locality" are insufficient to prove or disprove a theory).

A very clear restatement of Pettenkofer's theory is given in the following sentences. "Cholera is produced by the development of a gas through the decomposition of liquid excremental discharges (arising from either urine or feces) in moist, porous layers of the soil (or some equivalent material). The discharge in question must come from human beings

---

[1] Here, as in other passages, Pettenkofer suggests the existence of the well carrier.

who have suffered in greater or less degree from symptoms of cholera or perhaps from those who have merely come from places where cholera is epidemic."

The possibility of control of the disease by disinfection is then discussed. Pettenkofer believes that little can be accomplished after an epidemic has actually developed but that "prophylactic disinfection is of great value." The adoption of procedures which will "minimize not only the pollution and impregnation of the soil with the excrement of men and animals but also the decomposition of such materials until they have been entirely removed from the neighborhood of human dwellings" is the essential aim. The attainment of this end should control not only cholera but other epidemic diseases—particularly "typhus."

In considering Pettenkofer's theory, one is forcibly reminded of the monograph of Richard Mead on plague, published a little over a century before. Both attempted to resolve the problem of Contagia vs. Miasma by a combination of both factors—essentially a sound and scientific recognition of the real complexity of the problem in hand. On the whole, however, Mead stressed the contagious factor, Pettenkofer, the miasmatic factor. In the German hygienist's theory—as in the cruder conceptions of Chadwick—there was enough truth to work. The emphasis placed by him on the control of soil pollution led him to the vigorous advocacy of sewerage and thus to the effective reduction of intestinal diseases in Munich and elsewhere.

In this first report of 1855, Pettenkofer had not fully developed the "ground-water" explanation of the soil-factor in cholera epidemiology which dominated his later work. The idea came to him in the course of an extensive survey of cholera incidence in various parts of Bavaria in relation to possible contagion along routes of travel and possible relationships to terrain. This study indicated that in elevated regions—in spite of much movement of population—local epidemics were rare while in lower regions they were common. In reviewing this work in 1873, Pettenkofer says, "Considerations of this kind gave me the idea that this striking incidence of cholera in certain river valleys was to be ascribed not to the circumstance that the rivers were routes of travel but to the fact that they were regions of natural soil drainage; and this led to a consideration of the changing moisture relations of the soil. I began studies of the movements of the ground-water in Munich in March, 1856."

This conception of the influence of ground-water level fitted in **very** aptly with Pettenkofer's fundamental conception of miasmata from the soil as the basic cause of epidemics. The generally lower level of the ground-water in summer increases the area of soil in which the miasm can be generated and accounts for the normal seasonal curve of the disease. The problem was not visualized, however, as merely one of ground water level. In his retrospect of 1873, Pettenkofer says: "The essential factor, in my view, is a certain alternation of humidity and dryness and I believe that two conditions—a previous moistness and a subsequent drying—play an essential part in the process. If the soil remains always equally wet or always equally dry, the process cannot go forward, since in one case a certain degree of moisture, in the other, a certain degree of dryness, is missing. I have always, therefore, laid great emphasis on variations. The ground-water level is, for me, only an index of the variations in moisture content of the porous layers of soil above the water-table." The fall of ground-water leaves a layer of moist soil in which the "germination" of cholera takes place.

The first volume of the *Zeitschrift für Biologie* (edited by the Munich group) for 1865 contains three important papers in which the ground-water theory is fully outlined. The first two are by L. Buhl and L. Seidel and deal with typhoid fever; the third is by Pettenkofer, himself, and relates to cholera. In all three, evidence is presented to show that variations in the incidence of these diseases, from month to month and from year to year, are related to the ground-water level in such a way that a falling ground level is associated with increased incidence of disease.

In his own paper, Pettenkofer outlined the five conditions necessary for an epidemic of cholera as follows:

"1. Human habitation on soil layers permeable down to a certain depth (above the ground-water level) to water and air.

"2. A considerable secular variation in the moisture content of this soil layer, which, in alluvial soils, manifests itself most simply and reliably in the changing level of the ground-water, the period of falling back after an unusual rise constituting the period of danger.

"3. The presence of organic matter, particularly that arising from excrement in the suitable soil.

"4. The specific germs disseminated by human intercourse, the specific cause of cholera, of which the chief medium is the intestinal excrement of patients suffering from choleraic diarrhea, and perhaps also of well persons coming from cholera-infected localities.

"5. A disposition to contract cholera on the part of the individuals concerned."

In both his 1855 and his 1865 discussions, Pettenkofer thus maintained what he later called a "compromise" position, between the Indian view that cholera epidemics were due to the properties of the localities concerned and the conception generally developing in Europe that they were related to the presence of infected individuals. Later, he moved gradually toward the "localist" and away from the "contagionist" pole of the argument. His experience with the German epidemic of 1866, and the failure of disinfection to control its spread, led him to doubt the specificity of the excreta of the sick as the primary cause of cholera. In 1868, he made a special trip to Lyons on the one hand, and to Malta and Gibraltar on the other, to study the importance of "local" factors. Lyons, in spite of highly insanitary conditions and much intercourse with infected regions, had for years enjoyed an extraordinary immunity from cholera. This fact, Pettenkofer concluded, was due to two factors. The upper part of the city owed its permanent freedom from cholera to its situation on granite rock, the lower part of the city, to its generally high ground-water level. When this ground-water level was abnormally reduced during the very dry year of 1854, this section did develop an epidemic. At Malta and Gibraltar, on the other hand, he found that the consistently high cholera incidence could be explained by the nature of the soil which—in spite of the generally rocky terrain below—was actually porous and water-bearing.

In the same year, 1868, Pettenkofer met Douglas Cunningham and Timothy Lewis, who had been sent out by the British government to study cholera in India under James Cunningham, sanitary commissioner in Calcutta, and was greatly impressed with the attitude of these investigators, which was strongly on the miasmatic side.

In 1869, he contributed to the *Zeitschrift für Biologie* an extensive monograph on "Soil and Groundwater in Relation to Cholera and Typhoid Fever," which was designed particularly to meet the scepticism of Virchow with regard to the theories of the Munich school. He reiterates the necessity for both the "x-factor," dependent on human intercourse and the "y-factor" derived from the soil as essential for the production of an epidemic. He quotes a study by Macpherson in India as proving that the peak of cholera in its native land occurs not in the hot moist months but in the later hot dry months (when the ground-water level is falling). He stresses the results of Buhl and Seidel on typhoid.

There follows a long discussion of various types of soil in relation to their power of generating the y-factor (in which the Malta and Gibraltar data figure largely). Pettenkofer denies Virchow's conclusion that the freedom of Würzburg from cholera is due to the purity of its water-supply rather than to the character of its soil. He analyzes the English evidence with regard to the recent cholera epidemics in London (as presented by John Snow and Radcliffe) and cites against the drinking-water theory the contentions of Letheby and other English miasmatists. Instances are cited in which cholera epidemics were clearly not related to water supply, and the more intensive localization in certain houses is advanced as evidence against water transmission. Letheby, for instance, suggests that if alcohol or arsenic were mixed with the water supply of a certain district and distributed to the public on a certain day, the effects of the poison should be manifest all over the district at the same time and in no other district; yet no such sharp distinction is observed. The apparent coincidence between one local London supply and cholera incidence is explained as due to the distribution of that supply in low-lying areas of the city.[2] An epidemic at Southampton, attributed by Parkes to infection from a steamship, the *Poonah*, is reviewed and similarly explained. Pettenkofer scoffs at the multiple explanations of the contagionists, sometimes direct infection from the sick to the well, sometimes drinking water, then sewers and privy-pits, while his own theory remains the same, at London, Southampton and everywhere else. "If, as Virchow maintains, privies or even human intestines sufficed for the increase of the cholera poison and the development of cholera cases, it would be impossible for cholera epidemics to be limited by time and place as is actually the case. I cannot believe that the inhabitants of Lyons or Würzburg have intestines or privies any different from those of Marseilles, Paris and Rothenfels."

Pettenkofer here emphasizes three factors in the spread of cholera, the influence of human intercourse, the influence of place and the influence of time. The first of these three factors may be related to a fungus or a vibrio—no one can tell. In any case, its efficacy depends on the other concomitant circumstances of local and secular factors, since the advent of a cholera case sometimes produces new cases at once, sometimes after long delay, sometimes not at all. Long passages are devoted to rebuttal of specific cases cited by the opponents of the ground-water theory. Then

[2] This conclusion is obviously unfair since the different water supplies of London were, in many areas, delivered from parallel pipes in the same streets.

follows an interesting theoretical analysis of Pettenkofer's three factors. The "specific cause of cholera" (the factor related to human intercourse) is probably "organized in nature, of such fineness and smallness that it has so far escaped detection, similar to the germs of fermentation carried by the air which we detect by the results of their activity and observe as yeast cells in their later development on a suitable medium." The germs of cholera are not, however, spread directly through the atmosphere, since cholera cases often fail to produce other cases in the neighborhood and since, on the other hand, the disease may spread against prevailing winds. Pasteur's studies on the microbic content of city and mountain air are cited as indicating the limited range of dissemination of atmospheric germs. If "the specific cause of cholera is considered a sort of fungus spore and the cholera process something like a sort of fermentation," we must seek for a medium in which this specific cause develops. Such a medium, comparable to the cider in which yeast grows is—for the cholera germ—the suitable soil. Neither the cholera germ nor the cholera medium alone can produce the disease; both must be present. To believe that the germ alone can cause cholera is like thinking that swallowing yeast cells can cause intoxication! The nitrogenous organic matter in the soil is essential for the generation of the cholera poison, as the sugar in fruit juices is necessary for the production of alcohol. The combination of the germ and the factor from the soil which it ferments may take place in the soil itself, in the air of the dwelling or perhaps the human body may serve as the "fermenting vat" in which the reaction takes place.

A few of the conclusions from the end of this paper may be cited as concise statements of the Pettenkofer doctrine.

"One may designate the specific germ of the cholera of India as x, the substrate which must be provided for that germ by place and time as y and the product arising from these two, the true cholera poison as z.

"Neither x nor y can produce cases of Asiatic cholera, but only z.

"The specific nature (quality) of z is determined by the specific germ x; its amount (quantity) by the amount of y.

"The nature of x, y and z is so far unknown but one may assume, with a scientific probability bordering on certainty that all three are of organic nature and that x, at least, is an organized body or germ."

"The facts warrant the assumption that x may survive for a time and perhaps even increase considerably in the human body, for instance in the intestine; but the human body in a case of cholera is only the scene of the operation of z and by itself can produce no more z without the combination of x and y.[3]

"Materials from the soil, even from great depths, can reach human beings in two ways, by the soil water and by the soil air. The latter seems, in the case of cholera to be most important.

"The formation of y is favored by: 1. A soil which is permeable for water and air to a depth of several feet, such as an alluvial soil. 2. A period of marked variation in ground-water level. 3. The presence in the soil layer affected by varying ground-water level of organic and mineral substances suitable for the generation of y. 4. A soil temperature favorable to the organic processes involved."

Here, as elsewhere, the etiology of cholera in India, and the views of the Anglo-Indian authorities loom large in Pettenkofer's thinking. He published in 1871 a book on the *Mode of Spread of Cholera in India*[4] and accepted the conclusions of James Cunningham (Tenth Annual Report of the Sanitary Commissioner with the Government of India, 1873): "That if human intercourse plays any part in the dissemination of cholera, it must be a very secondary part"; "That the facts of individual outbreaks, and especially the remarkable immunity of attendants, are altogether opposed to the doctrine that the disease is spread by communication with the sick"; "That there is no evidence to show that a person affected with cholera multiplies within himself any specific poison, or that he disseminates any such poison either by means of the intestinal or any other discharges"; "That the cholera in India appears to be due to certain conditions of air and soil, or of both combined"; "That the great danger arises from exposure to these conditions and not from exposures to any emanations from the sick"; "That even if the contagious character of cholera could be proved beyond all manner of doubt, any general system of quarantine sufficiently strict to be effectual is impracticable and must do much more harm than good"; "That the great safeguards against cholera are sanitary improvements—the improvement of drainage, of water-supply, of dwellings, of every thing in short, which can contribute to health. Of water-supply, it may be remarked, not that it may be safe only against cholera evacuations and the

---

[3] But a certain quantity of z brought into a locality by human beings may cause a few cases in susceptible individuals without presence of y.

[4] The development of Pettenkofer's thinking is well reviewed in his 1875 monograph on "Artificial Prophylaxis against Cholera," to which reference will be made in a subsequent paragraph.

results, which have been theoretically attributed to them, but that it may be safe against every form of impurity."[5]

In 1875 Pettenkofer published another monograph on "Artificial Prophylaxis against Cholera," which was a critique of a report by a certain Dr. Frank on the Munich epidemic of 1873-1874. He objects to Frank's recommendation of special isolation hospitals for cholera, and criticizes severely the plan of evacuating and closing individual infected dwellings. When he comes to Frank's recommendation of disinfection of excreta as a means of prophylaxis, Pettenkofer really takes the bit between his teeth. The whole procedure, he says, is the corollary of his own "unfortunate compromise" of 1855[6] between the possible influences of human intercourse and local factors. "We know nothing of the infectious material of cholera nor can its localization in the excremental discharges of the sick—irrespective of the factor of cholera-locality—be established. All one can say is that this element must have a place in some object associated with human travel." That this "object" was the excrement of cholera patients seemed a natural assumption; but Pettenkofer believes that experience has now shown the disinfection of excreta to be actually ineffective in the control of epidemics. He cites Sir John Simon (at the 1867 Cholera Conference) as supporting the view that emphasis on disinfection merely diverts attention from the really important tasks of sanitation. Pettenkofer, himself, concludes that "the time has now arrived and the necessary amount and quality of evidence has been accumulated to overthrow completely any belief in the efficacy of the disinfection of the excreta of cholera patients." That the infectious material of cholera is really present in the stools is disproved by the lack of spread among doctors and attendants, and Pettenkofer has now even abandoned his earlier belief that cholera stools may acquire the power of spreading the disease after their decomposition. His evidence is, as usual, quite logical on the assumption of contagion as a process of disseminating gases and could be answered only by a theory of particulate contagious elements. Attempts to infect animals by means of cholera stools had, of course, failed. Pettenkofer finally concludes that "disinfec-

---

[5] It should be noted that in India at this period—with the widespread prevalence of infection—it is quite probable that general sanitation was a more practical method of control than quarantine. Yet it was most unfortunate that Pettenkofer's English acquaintanceship did not include Snow and Budd, as well as the Cunninghams.

[6] At this stage Pettenkofer laid a heavier stress on local factors than at any other period. He was almost what he later called an "autochthonist." In the 'eighties, the "x-factor" became again important in his thinking.

tion is a measure of cleanliness which it is very well to recommend but I can see no ground for relying on it alone and carrying it out generally by compulsion." Compulsory disinfection could be justified only "so long as it could be believed that disinfection had a specific effect on the infectious material in the stools," which Pettenkofer considers an untenable contention. The one effective method of controlling cholera is sanitation. "Sewerage and water-supply, these two well-proven methods so operate that the soil of a city is much less polluted by the discharges of human households and that the variation in the moisture content of the soil layers is greatly reduced."

In 1875, there was still much to be said for this line of reasoning; but the remarkable thing is that the Munich group continued to fight for their lost cause so long after the full demonstration of the germ theory of disease. In 1883, the "comma bacillus" was isolated by Koch; and Pettenkofer at once accepted this organism as his own "x-factor." He did not, however, modify his views as to the relative importance of infectious and local factors, and in 1884 contributed a series of letters to the *Lancet* vigorously attacking Snow's explanation of the Broad Street outbreak.

In 1886 and 1887, Pettenkofer published in the *Archiv für Hygiene* (which had now replaced the *Zeitschrift für Biologie* as organ of the Munich laboratory) a notable series of articles in which his theories were outlined in still greater detail. These essays were stimulated by the outbreaks of 1883-1885. Pettenkofer recognizes two major schools of thought, the "Autochthonists" who emphasize telluric, atmospheric and individual factors as the cause of cholera and the "Ephodists" who attribute the prevalence of the disease to a specific germ brought in from outside. The Ephodists are further subdivided into the "Contagionists" who hold that the germ alone is the sufficient cause and the "Localists" who consider the disease as caused by interaction between the imported germ and some property of a cholera-susceptible area.

In support of the autochthonist theory, he cites evidence presented by Jules Guérin in France and by James Cunningham in India, indicating that the development of cholera cases does not follow closely the lines of travel between one community and another or the neighborhood associations within a given community. On the other hand, however, Pettenkofer cites experience which shows that localities favorable to cholera may be free from the disease for long periods and that an epidemic may break out only when infection is introduced from outside. He fully accepts the results of laboratory research, saying, "Since bacteriology, in recent times, has succeeded in demonstrating with certainty in a number of infectious diseases (anthrax, typhoid, tuberculosis, erysipelas, glanders, etc.) that certain microorganisms are the causative agents, and since other infectious diseases, in which such a proof has not yet been provided or has not yet been fully demonstrated are of wholly analogous character, one is forced to conclude by analogy that in all infectious diseases microorganisms (generally bacteria) must be accepted as the cause." He disposes of the extreme autochthonist position by concluding that in Europe at least a fresh importation of infection is essential for the production of each epidemic.

Pettenkofer then proceeds to an analysis of the contentions of the "Contagionists." He first analyzes an impressive body of evidence with regard to the incidence of cholera among doctors, nurses and other hospital personnel and concludes "the well-established fact that physicians and attendants on cholera cases are no more frequently infected than persons who have had no contact with the sick can only be explained on the assumption that the cholera patients produce no effective infectious material and that, in the rare cases when they do produce infection, some other factor—namely, the ectogenous infectious element arising from a cholera-locality must have been added to the elements derived from the patients themselves." Next follow citations of cases where elaborate precautions for the disinfection of excreta had failed to control epidemics and of others where gross carelessness in the disposition of cholera excrement was not followed by new cases. The stress laid by contagionists upon epidemics in hospitals and barracks is countered by data showing the wide difference in the results of infection in different institutional groups. Thus, in seven barracks at Munich, all having cholera cases, the incidence rate per 1,000 varied from 2 to 42. Finally, he analyzes evidence with regard to the spread of cholera by the laundering of the linen of cholera patients, using the same arguments—that soiled linen often fails to infect those who handle it and that many cases arise without exposure to such linen.

In a second instalment of his monograph (Vol. v of the *Archiv*) Pettenkofer elaborates the theory of the "Localist" school to which he belongs. First, he emphasizes the differences in cholera incidence over considerable periods of time between various regions in India and in Germany. "Cholera cases are present in every district and, according to the Contagionist viewpoint, a single cholera patient, coming from India to Europe, may infect a whole region of the earth; why then do epidemics develop only in certain places and at certain times?" Further-more, the disease is not only localized in certain areas but in particular localities and parts of localities within those areas. River valleys in Germany are specially affected; but not all river valleys, or all parts of the same valley. "Why does the cholera poison, discharged by the sick, flow, in France, along the river Tille only from Villey to Crecy, or in Bavaria along the Danube only from Ingolstadt to Regensburg and along the Isar only from Munich to Landshut and no further?"

Even in a single locality, the disease is localized in certain groups of houses, particularly those in depressions and other low-lying areas; and Pettenkofer cites the interesting case of an area in Munich, "the Hollow," where cholera had raged in early epidemics but was minimal in 1873-1874, as a result of drainage. (We should today consider this as evidence of control of excremental pollution, but to Pettenkofer it meant a drying of the soil.)

In regard to the fundamental influence of terrain, William Farr in discussing the 1848-1849 London epidemic had worked out a formula relating altitude and cholera mortality with the following striking results which Pettenkofer cites.

ELEVATION ABOVE SEA LEVEL	CHOLERA DEATHS PER 10,000	
	Computed	*Actual*
0	177	174
10	102	99
30	65	35
50	34	34
70	27	27
90	22	22
100	17	20
350	7	6

Sanitary improvements obscured this basic relationship in later outbreaks in London; but Pettenkofer notes a similar statistical coincidence at Gibraltar. Sometimes, however, the lowest, dampest and most insanitary areas escape. "It appears that a certain degree of moisture and pollution may actually protect against cholera, just as a certain concentration of a sugar solution may limit fermentation." He closes this essay with a consideration of local variations in cholera incidence with regard to the character of the soil, particularly its porosity, buttressing his arguments by the results of his personal studies in Austria, Malta and Gibraltar.

In the next year, Pettenkofer continued with four more instalments of his discussion (occupying 315 of the 501 pages in Vol. vi of the *Archiv*). The first of the articles continues the discussion of localization and concludes (on the basis particularly of a Würzburg hospital epidemic) that the occurrence of epidemics in particular buildings cannot be explained on the basis of contagion and, therefore, must have a local basis.

Pettenkofer then proceeds to discuss the seasonal prevalence of cholera but with somewhat unconvincing results. He dismisses temperature as not directly important and fails to establish very conclusive relationship to rainfall. A diagram of the 1873-1874 cholera year in Munich shows an August epidemic following a high but falling ground-water and a second peak in December with very low ground-water. It is no wonder that a simple explanation was lacking. Only a quarter of a century later was it clearly shown that summer peaks of intestinal disease are commonly due to spread by contact—flies and the like—while winter epidemics result from large-scale pollution of public water supplies.

Pettenkofer cites a number of epidemics attributed by other investigators to contagion (including one report by Charrin of infection brought to an island where no cholera had existed—as beautiful as any of Snow's or Budd's studies). He discredits such evidence on the usual grounds; (a) that not all outbreaks can be so traced to contact; and (b) that contact does not always produce an epidemic. Why, he asks, in Charrin's epidemic did not the last case which occurred continue the chain?

Next, individual disposition is discussed at length, and it is suggested that a mild diarrheal attack may have a dehydrating effect which will increase resistance to true cholera.

The following section deals with localities immune (or nearly immune) against cholera. Lyons, as usual in Pettenkofer's thinking, looms large here; and he believes that the constantly moist condition of the soil is the chief reason for immunity.

The third instalment in this volume deals with "Theories of Cholera," disposing of the autochthonists in a few well-chosen words and then developing the author's own view of the superiority of the localist as compared with the contagionist theory. Pettenkofer grants smallpox (except for extraordinary epidemics) to the contagionists. For yellow fever, on the other hand, contagion offers no adequate explanation. The contagionist theory of cholera, advocated by Koch and Flügge, he cannot, of course, accept. He is much more charitably disposed toward

Nägeli's views. The distinguished veteran Swiss botanist had maintained that in typhoid fever, cholera and yellow fever two essential factors must combine to produce infection, one coming from the sick person, one from the soil; and that the latter factor can not be provided by every soil or even by a dangerous soil at all times, so that its presence is governed by both space and time. With regard to the role of the soil in this process, Nägeli recognizes two—and only two—possibilities. "The infectious germ coming from the sick, before it can produce infection, goes through a stage of its development in a soil liable to decomposition." This, he calls the monoblastic theory. Or, "such a soil brings about in the inhabitants a [miasmatic] infection, without which the [contagious] germs arising from the sick are unable to develop." This is the "diblastic theory," which Nägeli is inclined to favor. Pettenkofer compares his own theory with Nägeli's as follows: "X is, for Nägeli, as for me, the transportable specific cholera germ which in itself can not produce infection, but which, according to Nägeli comes only from cholera patients which I assume may be spread by human travel in general, both by the sick and the well coming from a cholera locality. Y is for Nägeli the unknown soil fungus which must enter the human organism at the same time as x or before in order to produce the individual predisposition which is essential if the introduction of x is to produce a case of cholera. For me, y is the sum of all the local and secular conditions, some known and some unknown, which are essential in order that the cholera germ x, spread by human intercourse, may experience such a quantitative increase or may reach such a degree of virulence that it becomes capable of producing infection, when x becomes z. Nägeli understands by z the actual case of cholera which he similarly conceives as the sum of x and y."

The possible nature of the "y-factor" is made more concrete in the following passage where Pettenkofer says of the soil characteristics which favor cholera epidemics: "There are two possibilities. It is possible that under these circumstances, at a certain place and time, there is produced a substrate [a chemically and physically suitable culture medium] favorable to the cholera germ spread by human intercourse; or there may be present an organized host on or in which the infectious form of the cholera germ develops and from which it passes to man."

Pettenkofer cannot accept the conception of infection by means of drinking water, a conception, he says, "which prevails almost universally in England, which is beginning to increase rapidly in France and has a number of adherents in Germany and other countries." While he acknowledges that he cannot completely confute this theory by epidemiological experience, he hopes it may be overthrown by bacteriological evidence. He cites the difficulty of isolating typhoid bacilli from suspected drinking water and the results of experiments by Kraus showing how rapidly the comma bacillus dies out in unsterilized water in the laboratory. In regard to his own theory, he looks to bacteriology for future researches which will reveal the true nature of the "y-factor" in the soil and its relation to the "x-factor," the comma bacillus.

The last two instalments of this ponderous monograph (at the end of Vol. VI and the beginning of Vol. VII of the *Archiv*) deal with practical methods of control of cholera. Pettenkofer still minimizes the value of quarantine, citing numerous cases of its failure in various Mediterranean countries; and supports his thesis by an ingenious analogy with the enforcement of customs regulations. He points out that while customs control cuts down the volume of imported goods, there is always a certain amount of smuggling. In the case of contraband goods, this is not important because the amount of smuggling is relatively small. In the case of quarantine, however, the inevitable occasional failure is fatal to the whole scheme because the few germs which pass the barrier have infinite power of multiplication. Protection must be sought "not at the frontiers but within the country itself." He supports his view by analysis of cases which fail to show close correspondence of cholera epidemics with pilgrimages in India and with military campaigns in Europe. He denies that the detection by bacteriological methods of the early cholera case can have any practical value as a control measure, since germs may be brought in by various materials and objects as well as by human beings, and even if all avenues of travel could be made "germ tight" the first patient would have disseminated his infectious material before he could be detected. "It may be demonstrated that the isolation of cholera cases after the outbreak of an epidemic is equally useless; and so is the special cholera hospital." "It is obvious that I consider the disinfection of the excreta of cholera patients to be as ineffective as the isolation of cholera patients."

A "flight from cholera" to a locality free from the disease is, on the other hand, justified both by contagionist and localist theory, and Pettenkofer, of course, considers that such migration creates no substantial hazard to the localities to which the refugees may go. Markets, festivals and gatherings of various kinds constitute no danger unless they are held at a locality where the local soil factor is powerful. The closing of schools and even the exclusion from schools in cholera-localities of children from areas free from cholera, he considers of doubtful value. On the other hand, he cites evidence to show that those who handle the bodies of persons who have died of cholera have sometimes shown a high incidence of the disease. This is not due to infection, however, but to the effect of the "cholera locality." Visits to the places where people are suffering from cholera should therefore be restricted.

In general, Pettenkofer deprecates all measures designed to limit the spread of cholera germs from person to person, denies the spread of the disease by drinking water and, in the end, pins his faith on the control of the soil factor by drainage and sanitation—in essential accord with the English school of sanitarians prior to 1850. "On these measures alone must rest our actual cholera prophylaxis. Those areas which Nature has not rendered cholera-immune must be made immune by the hygienic art."

It is probable that, for a quarter of a century, no one but the writer has actually waded through the many hundreds of pages of the Pettenkoferian writings; and the completion of the task is one that is accompanied with some relief. The monographs which have been reviewed are prolix and repetitious. They are largely made up of special cases cited to prove a point and largely devoid of any convincing objective evidence. It is a relief to turn to the group of Pettenkofer's pupils, Buhl, Seidel and Soyka, who worked (on typhoid fever) in a very different spirit. Here are actual statistical analyses which can be evaluated and criticized; in ten pages of these studies there is more concrete scientific evidence (whether convincing or not) than in a hundred pages of Pettenkofer's disquisitions on cholera.

We may take the Soyka paper (published in 1887 in the *Archiv*) as an example of the real evidence in favor of the ground-water theory. The first half of this study deals with the seasonal cycle and includes tables and diagrams showing the relation of typhoid incidence to ground-water level in four German cities. For Berlin, Frankfurt-on-Main and Bremen, the seasonal curves for typhoid and ground-water show an almost perfect mirror relation. The peak of typhoid and the minimum ground-water level appear in October; the minimum of typhoid and the highest ground water in March or April. Munich shows a somewhat different picture. Here the highest ground-water level is in July, the lowest in November, while the typhoid peak is in February, its trough in October. There is again a general mirror relationship, but the shifted typhoid curve is about three months to the right on the graph, as if the influence displayed in the other three cities were delayed for that period. Soyka attributes this to the fact that the actual variations in ground-water at Munich were relatively slight. The curves for Berlin, Frankfurt and Bremen represent the normal seasonal curve of typhoid which we today attribute primarily to the influence of season upon opportunities for transmission (vacations, flies, use of green vegetables and soft drinks) and to the influence of temperature upon the resistance of the human host. It cannot be denied, however, that the coincidence of a quite unusual seasonal ground-water curve in the case of Munich, with an equally unusual typhoid curve, is a striking argument for the ground-water theory.

The second part of Soyka's paper deals with the variations of typhoid and ground-water from year to year. For the same four cities, Soyka presents graphs which bring out the following facts. In Berlin, two out of three epidemics occurred in years of very low ground-water, the third in a year of rapidly falling ground-water. In Frankfurt, one epidemic occurred in the year of lowest ground-water. In Bremen, one epidemic occurred in a period of falling ground-water, the other in a period of high ground-water. In Munich, four epidemics occurred in periods of low ground-water and two in years of falling ground-water, but only two in years of high ground-water.

Soyka concludes as follows;

"1. There is a time-relationship of typhoid fever during the course of the year which reveals a definite rhythm which does not consistently correspond with the rhythm of ordinary seasonal phenomena.

"2. This rhythm does, on the other hand, consistently correspond, in the localities studied, with variations in the ground-water level, in such a way that the rhythm of typhoid fever incidence is, in general, the mirror-image of the rhythm of variations in ground-water level.

"3. The relation between typhoid fever and the climatic conditions related to the ground-water manifests itself also in comparing different years in such a way that

"a. every major typhoid epidemic corresponds to a low level of ground-water and

"b. every particularly high state of the ground water corresponds to a low incidence of typhoid."

This is a type of objective evidence which is far more convincing than anything to be found in Pettenkofer's own writings. It is evidence which, on the face of it, gave strong support to the ground-water theory. It remains more or less inexplicable today when that theory has become untenable. We have a comparable case in the paper published by Sedgwick and MacNutt in 1908 which seemed to demonstrate that "for every death from typhoid fever avoided by the purification of public water supplies two or three deaths are avoided from other causes"—a contention negated by wider analysis of statistics. In both cases it appears that the data used happened by chance to suggest very strongly a conclusion not borne out by wider sampling.

The 1886-1887 monograph represents Pettenkofer's last major contribution to this subject. He had several times, however, played with the idea of experiments on the human subject. After the great epidemic of cholera at Hamburg in 1892, and Koch's demonstration of the relation of that epidemic to water-supply, Pettenkofer was spurred on to the *experimentium crucis* of drinking a rich culture of the "comma bacillus." The negative results of this experiment (in his own case and that of Emmerich, the first pupil to follow his example) were reported in the *Münchener Medicinische Wochenschrift* for 1892 with a long argument demonstrating that the "x-factor" alone is powerless without the "y-factor."

Meanwhile, however, positive evidence was accumulating from many sides which emphasized so strongly the importance of the germ factor that even such a dramatic bit of negative experience could no longer stem the tide. The Hamburg epidemic and several subsequent cholera outbreaks in Germany were worked out by Koch with consummate skill. In reporting these results, Koch rubbed salt on the wound by stating that "should Von Pettenkofer nevertheless persist in his attitude of opposition, I should understand that, not indeed from the scientific but from the human point of view. It must be extremely difficult for him, bound up and grown old with the opinions advocated by him during a long series of years with the greatest expenditure of genius and sagacity, to sever himself from them, at least in part."

The long battle between Berlin, with its Marshal Koch and the *Zeitschrift für Hygiene* for ammunition and Munich with its Marshal von Pettenkofer and his *Archiv für Hygiene* was nearly over. By the turn of the century, the influence of the ground-water theory had almost disappeared—outside of Bavaria.

At Munich, however, the Pettenkofer philosophy died hard. In the first decade of the twentieth century Rudolf Emmerich and a group of his associates at Munich published a series of weighty volumes to commemorate the half-century anniversary of the founding of the Localist School. The first, by Emmerich and Wolter of Hamburg is devoted to a recent epidemic of typhoid at Gelsenkirchen, which had been attributed by Koch to the public water supply. Emmerich, of course, denies this conclusion on the ground that evidence of unusual pollution of the particular water supply was inconclusive, while, on the other hand, ground-water conditions and soil pollution in the area favored an epidemic (on the localist theory). Supporting evidence for the latter theory is presented in the form of secular curves of typhoid and ground-water level for various communities—in which the usual seasonal cycle is the major factor. The first argument cited above—the lack of conclusive demonstration of the particular mode of infection[7]—is typical of one of the important psychological characteristics of the Munich thinkers. They sought always for broad and universal relationships and never recognized as Koch did, and as we do today, that the spread of disease, being due to transfer of particulate germs, is often governed by chance concatenations of circumstances which cannot always be disentangled.

A second volume in this jubilee series, by Wolter, expounds in more general terms the epidemiology of typhoid and cholera, as conceived by Koch and Pettenkofer, respectively. The conclusion advanced by Koch in 1902 that the causative agents of cholera, typhoid and malaria are obligate human parasites which, outside the body, in soil as in water, soon die out and disappear, would appear to have clarified and sharpened the issue between Munich and Berlin. Wolter, however, saw in this conclusion of Koch's a last chance to harmonize the two viewpoints on the basis of the following hypothesis:

"The soil exerts its undoubted established influence on the development of typhoid through the medium of the ground-air, particularly the gases from the soil, in such fashion that the primary effect is an intoxication of the blood and body tissues from the ground-air inspired through the lungs while the secondary effect is the development of disease-producing bacilli of the typhoid group from other bacteria present in the human body."

The bulk of this voluminous communication is devoted to analysis of

[7] Koch, of course, believed that he had furnished such a demonstration and confirmed it by evidence of gross pollution in the water itself.

individual epidemics to show their coincidence with local soil conditions. The London epidemic of 1854 and the Hamburg epidemic of 1892, among others, are attributed to this cause, the relation to water supply being purely incidental. "The localistic doctrine of Max von Pettenkofer is the Ariadne thread which—in the labyrinth of hypotheses and theories which surround the problem of typhoid and cholera—will protect us against false roads and lead us to the recognition of the true causes of epidemics."

A third volume in the series, by Emmerich and five of his colleagues, is less eirenic in tone. It gives us in its preface a parallel-column statement which is worth citing as showing the final credo of the localists.

Pettenkofer's Cholera Theory	*Koch's Cholera Theory*
1. The Koch cholera vibrio is the cause of Cholera Indica.	1. Same.
2. Fatal cholera is not contagious; that is, it is not communicated directly from one person to another by the dejecta and no epidemics can arise from the dissemination of the dejecta since Emmerich has shown that these dejecta have partially lost their property of forming poisons in their passage through the intestine.	2. Cholera is contagious and even fatal cholera may be spread directly from person to person through the cholera vibrios present in the dejecta so that through contact a series of cases and an epidemic may arise.
3. The cholera vibrios may undergo an ectogenous development in porous polluted soil during periods of falling ground-water and the non-toxic cholera organisms of the dejecta acquire again in suitable soil their full toxicity and only by such bacteria from soil can epidemics be caused.	3. Since typhoid and cholera bacteria are obligate parasites, capable of development only in the human body, the soil plays no important role in cholera. The cholera organism and susceptible human beings suffice to produce an epidemic.
4. The propagation of cholera depends chiefly on the properties of the soil. Certain soils are porous and favorable to cholera (sand, gravel, etc.) while other soils are cholera-immune (rocky or clay soils).	4. The propagation of cholera, with regard to the predisposition of immunity of certain localities, is not determined by the soil but is conditioned by certain social characteristics (economic prosperity, concentration of dwellings, habits and customs, particularly cleanliness in respect to food and drink).
5. Cholera shows a pronounced seasonal rhythm, of such a nature that in Prussia, between 1848 and 1859, only 50	5. The seasonal rhythm of cholera and its increase in summer and fall depend on the fact that, in the warm

cholera deaths occurred in the first half of April, while in the first half of September there were 31,048 or 620 times as many. This can only be caused by external conditions (such as rainfall, dryness, temperature, relative humidity and, also, according to Emmerich, the status of the capillary upward flow of liquid in the soil).

6. Serious cholera epidemics occur in periods of soil dryness with falling ground-water. No epidemics can occur in rainy periods. Heavy rains with rising ground-water cause the cessation of cholera epidemics. Epidemics may, however, be brought to a close by other causes, particularly by the development of soil immunity through accumulation of the decomposition products of the cholera bacillus in the surface layers of the soil.

7. Drinking water plays no part in the causation of cholera epidemics.

8. The best means of prophylaxis against cholera is the control of the local disposition of porous soils by sewerage, water supply, etc. as well as by paving or asphalting of streets and yards. The isolation of the so-called "first case" has little value since an epidemic will occur just the same if the time and place disposition be present, since it is impossible to control all cholera vibrios in time.

season of the year, people drink more water, consume more ice and fruit and that they are predisposed to cholera by intestinal upsets and in general are in a reduced state of health.

6. The origin of cholera epidemics in dry periods is attributed to the fact that through the low state of the rivers and the sinking of ground-water in wells, the dissemination of the cholera germ is promoted through the fact that pollution reaching the water is less diluted and, in the rivers, less rapidly carried away.

7. Explosive cholera epidemics are caused by drinking water. (This entirely hypothetical assertion is incorrect, since the explosive outbreak can also be caused by the sudden development of a suitable condition of the surface layers of the soil at many points in a local area.)

8. The best control measure for cholera is the detection of the first case by bacteriological examination of stools, etc. and by the isolation and rendering harmless of such a case.

The seven hundred and fifty pages of this monograph are devoted to the elaboration of the Pettenkofer theory as outlined above and to the support of this theory by recent bacteriological and chemical research. It discusses the toxic action of the cholera vibrio and its relation to the production of nitrites in the intestines; cites experiments in which ingestion of the "comma bacillus" had failed to produce the disease; reports studies of the viability of the organism in various soils; and includes the usual analysis of individual outbreaks.

A fourth volume of the jubilee series, by R. J. Beck of Mengen, dealt with the relation of typhoid to drinking water and analyzed twelve epidemics of typhoid fever attributed to water supply, claiming, as usual, that soil conditions were really at work. It is interesting to note that the Lausen epidemic of 1872—one of the most conclusive studies in the history of epidemiology—is among those thus disposed of. A fifth volume, by Wolter, deals with epidemics which occurred during the war of 1870-1871; and a sixth by H. Gleitsmann with the causation of dysentery, both along the usual lines.

Greenwood in his *Epidemics and Crowd-Diseases* says, "Pettenkofer was probably the only man in the nineteenth century in an important teaching post really to modernize—that is, to translate into modern notation, and test upon data and by methods not available to Hippocrates—the Hippocratic plan of research exemplified in the tractate on Airs, Waters, and Places. In doing this he threw a great deal of light upon some factors of epidemicity of typhoid fever and of cholera. His teaching, sometimes called the Buhl or the Pettenkofer-Buhl 'law,' of the relation between changes in the level of the sub-soil water and changes of prevalence of the typhoid group of illnesses was very valuable. One will find that the important writers on epidemiology who were active *before* the bacteriological school had become psychologically omnipotent, such writers as Haeser and Hirsch, speak of this work with the greatest respect. Now, except to a small group of mainly south German writers, Pettenkofer and his teaching are as obsolete as Galen. This is not because anybody has refuted Pettenkofer's arguments, which like those of most mortals are partly good and partly bad, but because nobody any longer was interested in the *kind* of argument which appealed to Pettenkofer."

Stanhope Bayne-Jones in his presidential address before the Society of American Bacteriologists in 1930 drew a pertinent comparison between the influence upon medical thinking of Claude Bernard and Pasteur. Bernard recognized the vast complexity of the factors which influence the human body and its *"milieu intérieur,"* Pasteur was preoccupied with the germ as a necessary and sufficient cause of disease. The practical triumphs of bacteriology did indeed tend to oversimplify the problem and to cause medical men for nearly half a century to ignore the true many-sidedness of disease. It is well that today we recognize once more —as in the pre-Pasteurian era—the importance of such factors as diathesis and nutrition and climate and season in the prevalence of even germ diseases. No clinical case of any disease is caused solely by the entrance of a germ. Smallpox and measles approach such a situation most nearly; but even here, variations in seasonal prevalence show that other factors are at work.

Pettenkofer was right in maintaining that some factors other than the presence of "comma bacilli" in a town were necessary to produce an epidemic. He forgot, however, that the doctrine of multiple causation implies a corollary. If we are not to attribute disease to one single unique cause, it is illogical to conclude because one cause does not account for all observed facts, that that cause is unimportant. This is essentially what he implied with regard to contagion. Furthermore, he did not limit himself to saying "There are y factors which influence the causation of a cholera epidemic by the germ x." That conclusion would have been justified. What he said was, "There is *one* factor, y, and that factor is the ground-water level." Here, so far as we can see today, he was in error; and his arguments on this point have been very thoroughly confuted.

In the spirit of Pettenkofer's philosophy of multiple causes but in the light of modern knowledge, we may rewrite his famous equation with different symbols as follows:

$$A(a_1 a_2 \ldots a_x) - B(b_1 b_2 \ldots b_x) = C$$

Letting A = the power of the germ to produce disease

$a_1 a_2 \ldots a_x$ = various factors increasing the transmissibility (polluted water or milk, flies, mosquitoes, etc.), or the virulence of the germ.[8]

B = the power of the human host to resist disease

$b_1 b_2 \ldots b_x$ = various factors increasing the resistance of the host (age, specific immunity, nutrition, etc.).

C = a clinical case of a germ disease (or the absence of such a case if the resultant of the factors in the opposite half of the equation falls below zero).

The factors involved may vary enormously in different diseases and at different places and different times. The chain may be broken at any

[8] But soil decomposition does not appear as an a-factor in the light of modern knowledge.

point; and the practical test of any epidemiological theory is the power it gives us of breaking the chain. Chadwick and his associates were dealing with only one "a-factor" in the chain; but their procedures of empirical sanitation were sufficiently effective to eliminate the widespread epidemics of cholera and typhoid which had prevailed for centuries. Pasteur and Koch revealed the nature of the "A-factor" and Pasteur's studies on chicken cholera and anthrax led on to the control of the "b-factor" of specific immunity. It was these revelations which brought about the astounding triumphs of the past half-century; while the ground-water theory, in the hands of Pettenkofer's pupils, led only to a philosophical fanaticism which blinded their eyes to the most obvious facts.

CHAPTER XVI

THE CONCEPT OF THE CARRIER

"Virulent diphtheria bacilli were apparently present in about one per cent of the healthy throats in New York City at the time of these examinations."—
PARK AND BEEBE

As THE long-continued influence of the Pettenkofer school made clear, the demonstration that communicable diseases were caused by living microorganisms was not—by itself—sufficient to establish a consistent and convincing basis for epidemiology. Two major unexplained phenomena continued to vex the critical student, as they had done since the days of ancient Greece. These phenomena were the occurrence of new cases in individuals known to have had no direct contact with previous cases of the disease in question; and the complete absence—in certain diseases—of new cases among groups of people who had experienced such exposure. Additional discoveries with regard to the actual sources and modes of microbic infection were essential before the germ-theory of disease could really come of age.

An eminent New York physician, Dr. Beverley Robinson, in 1893, while recognizing the Klebs-Loeffler bacillus as the normal cause of diphtheria and emphasizing the importance of cultural diagnosis and isolation, went on to say, "On the other hand, we find evidences of diphtheria taking place in a most virulent form, repeated epidemics occurring, indeed, when no such primary case was revealed, at least if this primary cause—or diphtheria bacillus—takes its origin, as is now often assumed, from a previous case from which contagion, either directly or indirectly, is carried. Diphtheria has arisen in small villages, in isolated farmhouses, in palatial country dwellings, where no case of this disease had previously been known to exist. We must admit, therefore, that ill ventilated areas or rooms where dampness and dirt are present, where mold fungi appear upon the walls, that cellars which are wet and contain decaying vegetable or animal matter, are quite sufficient at times to bring this poison into active existence."

This was an argument which was very hard to meet until the discovery was made that human beings, themselves in good health, could serve as the "carriers" of the germs of disease.

As early as 1884 Loeffler described the isolation of diphtheria bacilli from the throat of a well person. In 1890 Escherich noted the persistence of diphtheria bacilli during convalescence, and in 1892 Guttmann, Rommelaere and Simonds noted the persistence of infecting organisms in convalescence after cholera. It was, however, in connection with the study of the cholera epidemic of 1892-1893 by Koch and his associates that the importance of the human carrier as a source of infection was first generally recognized. In 1893, in a paper "On the Present State of the Bacteriological Diagnosis of Cholera" Koch emphasized the significance of the convalescent carrier; "it has been ascertained that the excrements may contain cholera-bacteria a good while after the actual attack of the disease." He also recognized the role of the well carrier, although he considered such individuals as mild cases of the disease and did not emphasize their importance. He says, "These mildest cholera cases, in which cholera-bacteria were found in the solid excreta of apparently healthy persons, occurred only among groups of persons who were equally exposed to infection, and some of whom had the disease in a severe form. . . . One must therefore regard these cases as genuine cases of cholera, and cannot use them as arguments against the specific character of the cholera-bacteria."

In a second contribution of the same year, "Cholera in Germany during the Winter of 1892-93," Koch carries this idea a little further. He says, in this communication, "We know now that some cases of cholera are so mild that they generally escape recognition; we know also that the attack of cholera, strictly so called, is only the most striking part of the illness, and that the infectious matter may be contained in the evacuations of the patient both before and after it, that is, at a time when his intercourse with others is not yet, or no longer, regarded as dangerous." He states that the Hamburg winter epidemic of cholera in 1892-1893 was the first in which systematic examination had been made of the feces of persons with no clinical symptoms but "etiologically suspicious" on account of their contact with cholera cases. It was this procedure which revealed "the extremely important fact that the latter [etiologically suspicious cases] too include a certain number of cases of cholera-infection which can be detected as such only with the aid of bacteriological investigation." He declares, "It is now certain that among a number of persons who have been exposed to cholera-infection, the resultant cases may show the whole scale from the severest and rapidly fatal cases down to the mildest imaginable, demonstrable only by bacteriological investigation. I regard this experience as one of the most important additions to our knowledge of Asiatic cholera, both from the practical and from the theoretical point of view." From the standpoint of practical control he cites two ships in the harbor of Hamburg. On each of these ships two cases of cholera developed; and there were found eight other persons, without recognizable clinical symptoms, but with cholera organisms present in their feces. From the standpoint of epidemiological theory, Koch has this to say: "We now know that a not inconsiderable number, nay, if we take the case of the two ships as typical, the majority of persons infected by cholera, show so insignificant symptoms of disease that under ordinary circumstances, that is, without bacteriological investigation, they would certainly be regarded as in good health. This disposes at once of all the difficulties which have hitherto been found in the fact that human intercourse can propagate cholera, even when only healthy persons are in question. It really not rarely happens that no notoriously sick people, or inanimate articles, such as linen, etc., laden with infectious matter have come, or at least can be proved to have come, to the infected place. Such cases have been interpreted as indicating that, if cholera can be carried without cholera-patients or their feces, a cholera-patient is no more fitted to propagate pestilence than any other type of human intercourse, and such interpreters have then quite consistently gone the length of declaring cholera-patients and their feces comparatively harmless. How overhasty this interpretation of the transmission of cholera by apparently healthy persons is, must now be obvious."

In the next few years a number of German investigators (cited by Simon) presented evidence of the carrier state in cholera; but it was Koch's second 1893 paper which marks the first recognition of the fundamental importance of the phenomenon.

In the same year, 1893, a series of investigations was made by Park and Beebe, establishing the carrier principle in the case of diphtheria in an even more striking fashion. The fact that Koch was a year ahead and, even more, the circumstance that the New York work was published in a Health Department bulletin and not in a regular medical periodical, has caused the importance of this study to be overlooked; but it was one of the most significant contributions in the history of epidemiology— more complete and convincing, indeed, than any of the contemporaneous communications of the Koch school.

We have pointed out above that Loeffler in 1884 reported diphtheria bacilli in the throat of a well person. Roux and Yersin in 1889 noted the persistence of the specific organisms on the mucous membranes of convalescents. These were, however, merely isolated observations which led to no fundamental generalizations. It was in New York City that the new knowledge of bacteriology was first really applied in administrative health practice.

It is interesting to note that progress in America, as in Germany, was the direct outcome of the Hamburg cholera epidemic of 1892. It was the threat of imported cholera from Hamburg which was used by Hermann M. Biggs to force the establishment in the New York City Health Department of a Division of Pathology, Bacteriology and Disinfection, described many years after by C. V. Chapin as "perhaps the most important step in modernizing public health practice in the United States." In 1893, Biggs persuaded a young physician, William H. Park, to organize a bacteriological laboratory for this new division.

Park was born in New York City in 1863. He graduated at the College of Physicians and Surgeons of Columbia University in 1886 and studied at Vienna in 1889-1890. Returning to New York (and looking forward to a career as a practitioner) he became associated with T. Mitchell Prudden, and worked with Prudden on the new European methods for the bacteriological diagnosis of diphtheria. Biggs perceived the possibilities of the young man and invited him to apply these methods to the administrative control of the disease. Park, many years later, said, "Although I had not the slightest idea of doing public health work, his personality and enthusiasm so impressed me that I promised to undertake the technical control of the laboratory if he succeeded in persuading the Board of Health to establish it. His views prevailed with the Board, as they had with me, and the first municipal bacteriological laboratory in the world was established to investigate and utilize whatever measures seemed valuable in the diagnosis, control and prevention of communicable diseases."

Park was to continue as director of this pioneer laboratory until he was made director emeritus in 1936, three years before his death. For forty-three years he made this institution not only the outstanding example of practical applications of bacteriology to administrative public health but a center of notable scientific research. In the bacteriology and serology of diphtheria, in the study of scarlet fever, tuberculosis, meningitis and poliomyelitis, in milk bacteriology and the control of infant diarrhea, Park and his associates made contributions of the first order.

None of these contributions was more notable than the very first of the series. Park began service with the Health Department on May 4, 1893; and a report on the first eight months' studies by Park and his associate, A. L. Beebe, dated January 1, 1894,[1] is included in the *Annual Report* of the Department for 1893 (unfortunately not published till 1897). A review of this work by Biggs, Park and Beebe was, however, issued as a special scientific bulletin of the department in 1895.

The first major point emphasized by Park and Beebe was the basic fact that the disease, diphtheria, was caused by the diphtheria bacillus. It is true that the studies of Roux and Yersin in 1888 had demonstrated this conclusion by animal experimentation to the satisfaction of open-minded investigators. In the United States, Prudden and Welch in 1891 had concluded that "we are now justified in saying that the name diphtheria, or at least primary diphtheria, should be applied, and exclusively applied, to that acute infectious disease usually associated with a pseudo-membranous affection of the mucous membrane which is primarily caused by the bacillus called the bacillus diphtheriae of Loeffler." The fact was, however, by no means generally accepted by the medical profession; and, even from this standpoint, the New York studies were of importance. Park and Beebe reported the application of the bacteriological test to 2,623 cases, clinically reported as diphtheria, and found the bacillus in only 68 per cent of them. In 23 per cent, careful swabbing under the most favorable conditions failed to reveal the organism, while in 8 per cent the negative results obtained might have been due to unsatisfactory sampling. Thus, it appeared that between one-quarter and one-third of the cases of "clinical diphtheria" were not the true disease. On the other hand, 80 per cent of a series of cases of "membranous croup" proved on culture to be true laryngeal diphtheria. The value of the bacteriological criterion was further demonstrated by epidemiological studies, which showed the fatality of culturally-proved diphtheria to be 27 per cent, of "false diphtheria" to be less than 3 per cent.

So far as persistence of the organism in the throats of convalescents was concerned, Park and Beebe cite the work of Loeffler, Roux and Yersin, Koplik, Tobiesen and Escherich (between 1890 and 1893). These investigators had all demonstrated the Klebs-Loeffler bacillus after subsidence of acute symptoms (in one of Roux and Yersin's cases up to two months); but only in isolated instances, except in the case of Tobiesen who reported 24 such isolations. The New York observers report on

---

[1] The report, as finally printed, was obviously written after this date since it contains references to 1894 papers. The actual work, however, was done in 1893.

careful studies of 605 cases. Of these, 176 were positive for 7 days after the disappearance of exudate from the throat; 64, for 12 days; 36, for 15 days; 12, for 21 days; 4, for 28 days; 4, for 35 days; and 2, for 63 days. Again, this bacteriological evidence is supported by epidemiological studies of new infections actually caused by convalescent carriers. The authors conclude that "Individuals who have suffered from diphtheria should be kept isolated until cultures prove the bacilli to have disappeared from the throat for, not only are the bacilli which persist in the throat virulent, but they are not infrequently the cause of diphtheria in others."

Even more significant were the New York studies on well carriers. Park and Beebe cite here the isolated observations of Loeffler, Escherich and Fraenkel between 1890 and 1893, half a dozen cases in all. They themselves examined 48 well contacts in families where there were diphtheria cases and demonstrated the diphtheria bacillus in 24 cases (most of whom later developed the disease). Furthermore, they tested 330 well children who had had no known contact with diphtheria and found 8 carriers of virulent bacilli, of whom 2 later developed the disease. They conclude that "Virulent diphtheria bacilli were apparently present in about 1 per cent of the healthy throats in New York City at the time of these examinations. Diphtheria was, however, rather prevalent in the city at this time. Most of the persons in whose throats they exist have been in direct contact with cases of diphtheria. Very many of those whose throats contain the virulent bacilli never develop diphtheria. We must, therefore, conclude that the members of a household in which a case of diphtheria exists should be regarded as sources of danger unless cultures from their throats show the absence of diphtheria bacilli."

The results reported in this remarkable communication of 1894 have been amply confirmed by all subsequent investigations. It has been shown by Doull and Lara and others, however, that the actual danger from random carriers in the general population is not nearly so great as that from carriers who have been immediately exposed to clinical diphtheria. Among the former, while virulent strains of bacilli may be present, they rarely cause new cases; but the latter distribute enough active organisms to do major damage. Zinsser and Bayne-Jones conclude that "indirect and direct contact with carriers is probably the most common method by which the disease is kept going in modern communities."

The third disease in which the importance of the carrier was demonstrated was typhoid fever.

The studies made in the last decade of the nineteenth century had already suggested the importance of the carrier state in this disease. Reed, Vaughan and Shakespeare in 1900 in their study of camp typhoid during the Spanish War pointed out that "more than 90 per cent of the volunteer regiments developed typhoid fever within eight weeks after going into camp." They found that "the stool of a man in the incubation period of typhoid fever may be laden with the bacilli of this disease"; that "persons who have recovered from this disease may for a long time continue to carry and excrete the specific poison"; and that "the specific germ of this disease may be transported from one place to another in the intestines of an immune man, and when cast out in the stools may become a source of danger to others. It is probably in some such way as this that epidemics of typhoid fever may sometimes appear to originate *de novo*."

Here, then, in essence, was the whole theory of the typhoid carrier. The general acceptance of this theory was, however, due—as in the case of cholera—to Robert Koch. Two years after the American report he published a paper on "The Control of Typhoid Fever" which, on account of his commanding scientific position, had widespread influence. In this paper, Koch first reviews the success attained in the control of cholera by substituting for the "negative" defense procedures of general sanitation the "positive" attack upon all discoverable human sources of infection. He then cites experience with malaria, where control can be accomplished by finding infected persons through the taking of blood smears and the sterilization of carriers by the use of quinine. He calls for a similar procedure with regard to typhoid, and refers to the bacteriological media recently developed by Drigalski and Conradi as providing the necessary techniques for this purpose. By the use of such bacteriological tests, he reports, "it has repeatedly been possible to discover very light cases containing typhoid bacilli in their discharges but displaying scarcely recognizable clinical symptoms. In some cases, typhoid bacilli were found in individuals with no clinical symptoms whatever." To test the practical possibilities of bacteriological control, Koch undertook a special investigation in the neighborhood of Trier. Here he found a group of villages from which, in a period of several months, eight typhoid cases had been reported. By systematic routine examination of family members, contacts, members of the insurance funds, school children and the like, Koch and his associates found 72 persons infected with typhoid bacilli—instead of the 8 reported cases. Fifty-two of the cases found were children, of which only 3 had been reported by physicians. The isolation of a large proportion of the newly-discovered cases in an emergency hospital where their excreta could be disinfected proved effective in stamping out the epidemic. Wider application of the same procedure to other diseases, particularly dysentery, diphtheria and tuberculosis is advocated in conclusion: "What we have already found to hold true for cholera, what is proved for malaria, and what has now found application for typhoid, may be applied to all other diseases which we can diagnose with promptness and certainty and in which it is possible to render the carriers of infection harmless."

What Koch was interested in—here, as in the case of cholera—was not so much the carrier as a philosophical concept as the practical utilization of laboratory methods for the detection of sources of infection. Most of his infected persons at Trier were merely mild cases of disease which had not come to medical attention. What he did, however, was to focus attention on the individual infected human being, sick or well. In the next few years, the various types of "carriers" of typhoid bacilli were promptly discovered and described, and both feces and urine were shown to be involved. Aside from individuals acutely or mildly sick at the moment, Reed, Vaughan and Shakespeare in 1900 had, as we have seen, fully recognized the importance of the carrier state. Dönitz in 1903 gave convincing data on the convalescent carrier. Drigalski and Conradi in 1902 and Klinger in 1906 proved the existence—among contacts—of carriers who apparently had been and were to remain quite well. In 1907 Soper described the exploits of Typhoid Mary, the classic case of a chronic carrier, spreading devastation over a period of years, although with no known record of illness on her own part. In 1909, Rosenau, Lumsden and Kastle reported the examination of about 1,000 well persons tested at random in the city of Washington with the detection of one urinary and two fecal carriers.

The next disease in which the importance of the carrier was demonstrated was epidemic cerebrospinal meningitis. In 1905 and 1906, von Lingelsheim, Weichselbaum and Ghon and Ostermann in Germany described the isolation of meningococci from convalescent and well carriers. In 1907-1908 Bruns and Hohn presented an illuminating study of the proportion of carriers in the normal population during the course of an epidemic. The peak of carrier incidence was reached in March and declined thereafter; while the peak of clinical cases was reached only in May. Finally, during the First World War, British bacteriologists suggested that the proportion of well carriers in a military command could be used for prediction of an epidemic, clinical cases beginning to appear when the carrier rate reached about 16 per cent. Pringle in England has recently pointed out that it was once "accepted *that the cases were the epidemic.* Modern epidemiology recognizes that there are innumerable immunes in densely populated areas who have never had the disease and that the real fact is that the cases are the *evidence* of the *epidemic state.*"

In the middle of the first decade of the present century the carrier state in poliomyelitis was described by Wickman and in the second decade American and Swedish observers demonstrated its importance. Here, as in epidemic cerebrospinal meningitis, the carrier is undoubtedly the chief factor in the transmission of the disease.

The same sort of evidence is, of course, now available for many other communicable conditions. The evidence, as a whole, was reasonably complete by 1910. In that year, Chapin in *The Sources and Modes of Infection* introduced his chapter on "Carriers and Missed Cases" as follows:

"That there are occasionally seen mild cases of the infectious diseases difficult or impossible to recognize, has long been known. That such cases are rare has always been generally believed. That the germs of disease can maintain themselves and increase in number in a person without causing any symptoms at all, was until recently scarcely thought possible, and the idea that such latent infections are extremely common would have been scouted as preposterous. Even today the facts are denied by many sanitary officials, and there are comparatively few who recognize the frequency with which mild atypical forms of disease and healthy 'carriers' of germs are found, or realize the tremendous importance which such cases have in the spread of the contagious diseases. Undoubtedly the most fruitful medical discovery of the last century, and perhaps of all time, was the discovery of the parasitic nature of the infectious diseases. Probably the most important discovery bearing on preventive medicine since the demonstration of the bacterial origin of disease, is that disease germs frequently invade the body without causing disease."

After discussing all then available evidence, Chapin draws the following highly significant conclusions—which will stand excellently as a summary of the present status of the situation:

"We are justified from the evidence presented in coming to the following conclusions:

"1. Mild atypical and unrecognized cases of the infectious diseases are often extremely common. In many diseases they may be more numerous than the recognized cases.

"2. Disease-producing microorganisms, whether bacteria or protozoa, frequently persist in the body without causing symptoms.

"3. Sometimes the germs remain only a few weeks or months after convalescence, and sometimes they may persist for years, perhaps for life. Sometimes these carriers give no history of ever having been sick.

"4. While the bacteria found in carriers are sometimes lacking in virulence, many times they show the highest degree of virulence.

"5. There is ample epidemiological evidence that healthy carriers as well as mild unrecognized cases are the source of well-marked outbreaks.

"6. The number of carriers varies greatly in different diseases. From 20 to 50 per cent of the population are carriers of pneumococci.[2] It seems probable that the influenza bacillus is as widely distributed. During outbreaks of cerebrospinal meningitis the number of carriers may be from 10 to 30 times as numerous as the number of cases. Even when diphtheria is not prevalent 1 per cent of the population may be carrying the bacilli, and during outbreaks the number may be several times greater. Probably 25 per cent of all typhoid fever cases excrete bacilli for some weeks after convalescence, and it is estimated that from 1 in 500 to 1 in 250 of the population are chronic carriers. What little evidence there is indicates that carriers are as numerous in dysentery and cholera as they are in typhoid fever. In yellow fever, sleeping sickness, and particularly in malaria, carriers are very numerous. There is no evidence that there are any carriers of measles or smallpox.

"7. Any scheme of prevention which fails to take into account carriers and missed cases is doomed to partial and perhaps complete failure."

[2] All Chapin's quantitative figures should be materially scaled down for present-day conditions, since the proportion of carriers drops along with the reduction in cases. On the whole, however, the picture given was remarkably accurate for 1910.

CHAPTER XVII

THE INSECT HOST

"Our actual knowledge of the insect carriers of disease has all been acquired during the last fifteen or twenty years, and marks as brilliant and successful an epoch in the history of medicine as did the phenomenal development of bacteriology in the years immediately preceding."—C. V. CHAPIN (1910)

As WE have seen, the spread of disease germs by contact and by articles of food and drink had been clearly elucidated during the latter half of the nineteenth century. In the closing decade of that century and the first decade of the twentieth, a series of brilliant investigations cleared up the mystery which had shrouded such diseases as malaria and yellow fever and closed one more important gap in our basic theories of epidemiology.

As early as 1879 Manson had demonstrated the presence of the parasite of filariasis in mosquitoes; but in this case the germ in question was a parasitic worm and the phenomenon was regarded as an isolated one, without appreciable influence on general epidemiological thinking. The wider problem of the secondary host was opened up only in 1889 by the studies of Smith and Kilborne on Texas cattle fever.

The problem with which Theobald Smith was presented in the study of this disease was an extremely puzzling one. The first basic fact which had been observed was that the development of Texas fever among cattle in the northern states was clearly associated with the transportation to those states of apparently well cattle from a certain rather sharply defined southern area. An epidemic in Pennsylvania had been attributed, as early as 1796, to the arrival of a herd from South Carolina. New cases among the northern cattle did not, however, arise at once from direct contact with the southern herd but after an interval—commonly about one month—and from grazing on an area which had been occupied by the southern herd. This phenomenon occurred only in summer; and only within a moderate interval after the arrival of the southern cattle, which appeared gradually to lose their infective power.

This strange chain of events was explained in every detail by a series of the beautifully planned and controlled experiments carried out, checked and repeated by Smith and Kilborne during the years 1889-1892 and finally summarized in full in 1893.

With regard to the causative agent of the disease, earlier claims by Billings and others of the discovery of responsible bacterial parasites were negatived by competent studies. Since the major characteristic of the malady was a far-reaching destruction of blood corpuscles, Smith and Kilborne looked to these cells for the source of infection and found it in a protozoan parasite which they clearly described and figured and named *Pyrosoma bigeminum* (1889).

As to the mechanism of transmission, Smith and Kilborne almost at once followed up a lead given by the suspicion of cattlemen that ticks played a part in the process (a hypothesis which had been generally ignored or ridiculed by medical authorities). After a long series of experiments they demonstrated the following major results:

a.   Northern cattle placed in the same field with recently-imported southern cattle developed the disease some weeks after their introduction to the area.

b.   If this procedure were modified by removing all ticks from the southern cattle before they were brought in, the associated northern cattle remained unaffected.

c.   If northern cattle were grazed on a field sown with young ticks brought up from a southern grazing area, they promptly became infected.

These three types of experiment really proved the case. They were reenforced through the production of Texas fever by the bites of young ticks reared in the laboratory from eggs laid by parent-ticks which had lived on southern infected cattle; and by successful infection in the north during the winter season in a heated stable (in which the ticks remained viable). The presence of the causative organism was easily demonstrated in the blood of southern cattle, apparently well but functioning as chronic carriers of the *Pyrosoma*.

Thus, the following conclusions were amply demonstrated.

"Texas cattle fever is a disease of the blood, characterized by a destruction of red corpuscles."

"The destruction of the red corpuscles is due to a micro-organism or micro-parasite which lives within them."

"Cattle from the permanently infected territory, though otherwise healthy, carry the micro-parasite of Texas fever in their blood."

"Texas fever in nature is transmitted from cattle which come from the permanently infected territory to cattle outside of this territory by the cattle tick."

"The infection is carried by the progeny of the ticks which matured on infected cattle and is inoculated by them directly into the blood of susceptible cattle."

The soil of a northern area can thus become infectious only when mature female ticks from infected cattle drop off and lay their eggs on the soil. The young which hatch from these eggs carry the germ of the disease and, when they attach themselves to susceptible cattle and bite them, convey the infection. The period needed for the completion of the life history of the tick explains the time phases of the disease. The high temperature required by the tick prevents spread in the northern winter season; and the loss of infective power by southern cattle in northern territories where ticks are rare is due to the fact that all the females they brought with them have matured and dropped off.

Here was the first clear demonstration of a protozoan disease of the higher mammals whose causative agent was transmitted in roundabout fashion by an intermediate host belonging to the group of the Arthropoda (to which the true insects, as well as the ticks, belong). The way was clear for the elucidation of similar relationships in other diseases.

The next application of the theory of the insect carrier was made in the case of tsetse-fly disease by Bruce in 1894; but it was the revelation of the secret of malaria which brought this type of transmission into a field of world-wide interest.

It is fascinating to look at a standard nineteenth century medical text, such as Quain's *Dictionary of Medicine* (1894 ed.) and see how many facts had been observed in regard to the bad-air disease (mal-aria) and yet how puzzling and mysterious was the general picture presented. "An earth-born poison"; evolved from marshes "when the water level is lowered and the saturated soil is exposed to the drying influence of a high temperature"; frequently resulting from "the disturbance of soil that has long been fallow"; as in the construction of the fortifications of Paris under Louis Philippe; "freely generated at the bases of mountain ranges in tropical climates"; "it drifts along plains to a considerable distance from its source, when aided by winds sufficiently strong to propel, but not to dispel it"; and "under the influence of currents of heated air it can ascend in dangerous concentration, far above its source." Here was a typical example of a miasmatic disease, definitely associated not with human contact or water or milk but with particular local geographical conditions. The elucidation of its mystery did more than anything which had gone before to complete the transition from miasms to germs.

The leading figure in this scene of the drama of epidemiology was as different as possible from that of the discoverer of the cause of Texas fever. The latter, Theobald Smith (1859-1934) was called from the Bureau of Animal Industry to the chair of comparative pathology at Harvard and, finally, to the directorship of the Department of Animal Pathology of the Rockefeller Institute for Medical Research. He was the typical scientist, slender and bearded in person, cold and precise in manner, completely absorbed in his researches,[1] accurate and meticulous in his work to the last degree. He was a pioneer in the study of immunology and anaphylaxis, in the study of tuberculosis, in sanitary water analysis, and in a dozen other fields of bacteriology. When the writer was beginning his career, it was a somewhat rueful jest in the laboratory that if you had a new idea you always found that Theobald Smith had had it first. When the International Congress for Microbiology met in New York in 1939, it was natural that the commemorative medal should bear the profile of Smith, as America's most distinguished representative of this field of research.

On the other hand, Ronald Ross (1857-1932) the pioneer of malaria, was burly, red-faced, hot-tempered, emotional, aggressive and egoistic. He was a dreamer and a poet, with passionate curiosity but little basic scientific training. As an officer in the Indian Medical Service he had been impressed with the vital problem of malaria. He examined the blood of patients and concluded that Laveran (1845-1922), who had described the malarial parasite in the blood, in 1880, was in error. Malaria was not a germ disease at all. On a furlough in London, he met Manson who showed him how to recognize Laveran's germ and advanced the guess that the disease was spread in some way by mosquitoes. Ross' imagination was fired by the idea and he returned to India to work passionately on its demonstration. After two years, in 1897, he actually did see the human malaria parasite in the stomach of the mosquito, as we can recognize from his description today. That it really was the parasite was, at that time, however, only a surmise as was clearly acknowledged in the brief formal paper published in December 1897, "On Some Peculiar Pigmented Cells Found in Two Mosquitoes Fed on Malarial Blood."

Ross, however, demonstrated the germ of bird malaria in infected birds and in mosquitoes which had bitten such birds. Finally, in the sum-

---

[1] He forgot to appear for an honorary degree to have been awarded by one of America's most distinguished universities.

mer of 1898, he achieved the final demonstration—so far as bird malaria was concerned—by actually producing the disease in sound birds by the bite of mosquitoes which had fed on infected birds. His, then, was the really basic work in this field; but Ross was denied the final triumph of proving the transmission of human malaria—a fact which he bitterly resented and dealt with in highly controversial fashion for the rest of his natural life. It was an Italian zoologist, G. P. Grassi (1855-1925) who was to complete the argument. Recognizing that there were always mosquitoes where there was malaria, but that mosquitoes might also abound where there was no malaria, he sought for a particular species of mosquito which might be incriminated and—with the advantage of the entomological knowledge which Ross had lacked—he quickly picked out a common local mosquito of the genus *Anopheles* as the probable suspect. In urgent haste and on such rather slender grounds, he and Bastianelli and Bignami of the Hospital of the Holy Spirit in Rome in the fall of 1898, actually produced the first experimental cases of malaria in human beings by the bite of *Anopheles* mosquitoes. The demonstration of the intermediate insect carrier was thus completed in a disease so important that Osler described it as "the greatest single destroyer of the human race."[2] The mysterious malady which had hung like a pall over wide regions of the earth's surface—which, according to Ross, was responsible for the downfall of Ancient Greece—was now controllable by the simple expedient of eliminating its mosquito carrier.

No problems are, however, as simple as they seem at first; and, to realize the complexities involved in the insect-borne diseases, it is well to note two later discoveries in the field of malariology.

Since the anopheline mosquitoes breed in stagnant water, drainage of marshy lands seemed the obvious method of control; and in the United States, this procedure was highly successful. In southern Europe, however, the success attained by the construction of drainage canals was only partial. Malaria persisted in Italy and Albania in the neighborhood of natural rivers and of the drainage canals themselves. European malariologists became highly sceptical as to the whole procedure and suggested that we in the United States really did not know what serious malaria was. The answer to this contradiction was found in the fact that the particular species of *Anopheles* involved on the two continents differed in their breeding habits. The American species bred only in warm

---

[2] It must be acknowledged that Osler said almost exactly the same thing about syphilis in another place; but he picked two excellent contenders for the prize.

water; when drainage removed the small pools warmed by the sun, they disappeared. The European species, on the other hand, preferred cool water and when a large drainage canal was built they continued to breed among the aquatic weeds along the shores of the canal itself. Thus, the difference in experience was explained; and, fortunately, the discovery that dusting Paris green on the surface would destroy the larvae of the mosquitoes made control under European conditions possible.

There remained one mysterious anomaly. In certain parts of Europe —as in the neighborhood of Naples—*Anopheles* mosquitoes were common but there was no malaria. "Anophelism without malaria" remained an outstanding challenge to the imagination. L. W. Hackett of the Rockefeller Foundation in 1931 solved this problem by showing that, in such regions, the anophelines were concentrated in stables and not in houses and had the habit of biting cattle and not men. The adults of human and bovine feeders were alike, apparently belonging to the same species of mosquito; but entomological studies showed differences in the marking of the eggs. Today, half a dozen varieties of the same species can be recognized, some biting men only, some cattle only and some either men or cattle. This discovery threw a flood of light on the history of malaria, showing how the presence of stabled cattle in a fixed agricultural population tended to favor the presence of the bovine feeders; while the driving off of cattle and the abandonment of drainage following a war must favor the replacement of the harmless bovine feeders by the more dangerous malaria-bearing types. Successive cycles of this kind —of periods of intensive cultivation and health, alternating with periods of war and devastation/and disease—may be clearly traced in the history of many parts of Italy. It is clear that the theory and practice of epidemiology depends on an intimate knowledge of the life history of species and sub-species of the insect carriers involved.

The next chapter in our story includes the most dramatic episode in the whole history of public health, the conquest of yellow fever. Between the years 1702 and 1800 this terrible disease had appeared in the United States thirty-five times, and between 1800 and 1879 it visited the country at some point in every year but two. We have seen in an earlier chapter how it terrorized Philadelphia in 1793 and how strong an argument its incidence presented for the localistic, as opposed to the contagionistic theory of disease.

In 1898 the United States was brought face to face with yellow fever on its own ground by the problems associated with the military occupation of Cuba. Yellow fever had killed an average of 750 persons a year in Havana for the previous half-century for which records were available. In 1900, therefore, a commission of army surgeons was sent to Cuba to study the disease, under the chairmanship of Walter Reed, with James Carroll, James W. Lazear and Aristides Agramonte as his associates.

As in the case of Texas fever, the first task of these investigators was to eliminate certain alleged specific bacteria supposed to be the causative agents of yellow fever, and this they accomplished with competence and dispatch. Almost immediately they then turned their attention to the mosquito as a possible agent in the transmission of the disease. Dr. Carlos J. Finlay of Havana had suggested the mosquito theory very convincingly in 1881, though without complete experimental proof, and the discoveries of Manson and Ross and Grassi and Bignami had recently demonstrated a similar origin for malaria. Reed and his colleagues were fortunate in thus beginning almost at once with a correct hypothesis. They were materially aided in their approach by the earlier observations of H. R. Carter of the United States Public Health Service, who had noted in Mississippi that when a case of yellow fever occurred in an isolated farmhouse those who visited the house at the time did not acquire the disease but those who arrived two weeks later were liable to infection. This circumstance obviously suggested an incubation period in the body of an insect carrier.

At this time the lower animals were not known to be susceptible to yellow fever, so that experiments upon human subjects were essential. In the words of Dr. Kelly's life of Major Reed, "After careful consideration the Commission reached the conclusion that the results, if positive, would be of sufficient service to humanity to justify the procedure, provided, of course, that each individual subjected to experiment was fully informed of the risks he ran, and gave his free consent. The members of the Commission, however, agreed that it was their duty to run the risk involved themselves, before submitting anyone else to it."

The first successful experiment was made with Dr. Carroll, who allowed himself to be bitten on August 27 by a mosquito which had previously bitten four yellow fever patients. Four days later he was taken sick and for three days his life hung in the balance. Both he and Private W. H. Dean, the second case produced experimentally in the same way, recovered. Dr. Lazear, however, who came down with the disease, not as a result of the experimental inoculations, to which he also had submitted, but from an accidental bite, was less fortunate than his colleagues, for a week later he died after several days of delirium.

On the basis of the Carroll and Dean cases, the Commission was able to announce before the American Public Health Association in October 1900 that "The mosquito acts as the intermediate host for the parasite of yellow fever."

Proof based on only two cases and without adequate control could not, however, suffice. To complete the demonstration, an experiment station, named "Camp Lazear" after the first martyred member of the party, was established in the open country; and to the lasting honor of the United States Army, volunteer subjects for the experiments from among the troops were always in excess of the demand. Private John R. Kissinger and John J. Moran, a civilian employee, were the first to volunteer "solely in the interest of humanity and the cause of science," their only stipulation being that they should receive no pecuniary reward.

The result of the experiments carried out at Camp Lazear proved beyond peradventure that yellow fever was transmitted by the bite of a certain mosquito, *Aëdes aegypti*, and in no other way, for non-immunes who lived for twenty days in a small, ill-ventilated room, in which was piled clothing and bedding, loathsome with the discharges of yellow fever patients, all escaped infection, so long as they were protected from the bites of mosquitoes.

On the memorial tablet to Lazear in the Johns Hopkins Hospital is the inscription: "With more than the courage of the soldier, he risked and lost his life to show how a fearful pestilence is communicated, and how its ravages may be prevented." The same risk was taken by each member of the party, from major to private, as is described with dramatic force and essential accuracy in Sydney Howard's thrilling play, *Yellow Jack*. The result of their devotion is indicated in two of Reed's letters to his wife; "six months ago, when we landed on this island, absolutely nothing was known concerning the propagation and spread of yellow fever—it was all an unfathomable mystery—but today the curtain has been drawn"; and later, on New Year's Eve—"Only ten minutes more of the old century remain. Here have I been sitting, reading that most wonderful book, *La Roche on Yellow Fever*, written in 1853. Forty-seven years later it has been permitted to me and my assistants to lift the impenetrable veil that has surrounded the causation of this most wonderful, dreadful pest of humanity and to put it on a rational and scientific basis. I thank God that this has been accomplished during the latter days of the old century. May its cure be wrought out in the early days of the new."

Reed's prayer seemed to be fully answered by the accomplishments of the next few years. The scourge of centuries was promptly wiped out in Havana by the practical control of the mosquito carrier. The construction of the Panama Canal was made possible by the application of similar methods. The International Health Board of the Rockefeller Foundation—on the suggestion of W. C. Gorgas, who had been in charge of the control program on the Isthmus—undertook a campaign for the extermination of yellow fever throughout the world. At Guayaquil, once the chief endemic center of the disease, it was promptly eradicated. During 1921, Honduras, Nicaragua, Ecuador and Costa Rica were immune from the disease; Guatemala and Salvador had no cases later than February; by July, Peru, and by November, British Honduras were free of infection.

By 1929, the last known centers in the Americas were apparently under control. It was true that a disease had been described in West Africa which resembled yellow fever and a Rockefeller Commission was studying the problem at Lagos. Yet all authorities then believed that the complete conquest of yellow fever in the immediate future was a practical certainty.

At the moment when victory seemed assured, disquieting events began to occur. In 1929, there were epidemics in Colombia and Venezuela at points in the interior quite unrelated to any known centers of the disease; and the earlier assumption that yellow fever existed in only half a dozen endemic foci on the seaboard received a shattering blow. Meanwhile, the Lagos studies[3] had yielded results of major importance. In 1927, Adrian Stokes, J. H. Bauer and N. P. Hudson had at last found in the Indian monkey, *Macacus rhesus*, an experimental animal susceptible to the disease. In all such investigations, the discovery of a suitable experimental animal is of enormous significance.[4] In 1929, Max Theiler of Harvard simplified experimentation still further by discovering that white mice were susceptible to infection when inoculated in the brain.

[3] Carried on at great risk to the intrepid investigators: eight members of the collaborating staff lost their lives in the course of their investigations in West Africa and Brazil.

[4] It is interesting to note that the demonstration of the cause of yellow fever was delayed twenty years because Finlay in 1881, although he tried to produce the disease by the bite of *Aedes* mosquitoes, did not allow for a possible incubation period in the body of the insect; and that a similar delay of twenty-five years was due to the fact that Reed, though he experimented with the *Macacus*, in 1900, used a local Havana specimen which had probably already acquired immunity to the disease.

With the possibilities opened up by these experimental animals, the Rockefeller investigators promptly demonstrated that the West African and American diseases were identical and were caused by a filtrable virus. Furthermore, a test involving the protection of the mouse against the virus made it possible to conduct far-reaching surveys of human blood samples to determine whether the individual tested had previously suffered from the disease.

These surveys revealed a totally unexpected and very serious situation. Instead of yellow fever infection being confined to a few seaports, it was discovered that the disease extended—in latent form—over vast belts in the continents concerned, from Senegal to the Upper Nile in Africa and including the whole Amazon basin and adjacent countries in South America. In these wild regions it was found that monkeys and possibly other wild animals were reservoirs of the disease and that it was transferred from them by the bite of a large number of species of mosquitoes, causing what is now known as "jungle fever." This is true yellow fever, but occurs only in the wilds in the form of occasional cases among the hunters who are exposed in the forest. It does not spread further in villages, where the *Aedes aegypti* mosquito is absent; but when infection is introduced into a city where the *Aedes* mosquitoes are present, an outbreak of the classical type will result.

Faced with such vast reservoirs of infection, the hope of "stamping out" yellow fever becomes untenable. The disease in epidemic form can be controlled by eliminating the *Aedes* mosquito from cities; and the Rockefeller workers have produced a vaccine which is effective in protecting against infection. We can look forward, however, to no complete and decisive victory but only to a constantly maintained defense of the major centers of population.

During this same general period, there was gradually revealed the secret of the gravest of all pestilences—bubonic plague. Here there is no single outstanding discoverer, no Theobald Smith, no Ronald Ross, no Walter Reed. The light broke gradually, as a result of glimpses of the truth caught by many independent investigators.

We have discussed in earlier chapters the epidemiological aspects of the first two great pandemics of plague—the plague of Justinian, beginning in the sixth century and the Black Death, which became general in the fourteenth. About 1871 the disease again broke out in the Chinese province of Yunnan-Fu and in 1894 it reached Hong Kong and assumed serious epidemic proportions. It passed to India where 6,000,000 people perished in a period of ten years; and has spread to seaports in all parts of the five continents.

This time, however, the great plague was to meet the resources of modern public health science. The relation of human plague to rodent plague had—as we have seen in earlier chapters—been recognized in early Biblical times. In 1894, during the Hong Kong epidemic, A. Yersin and S. Kitasato independently described the plague bacillus. In 1897, M. Ogata isolated the organism from rat fleas. In 1898, P. L. Simond claimed the demonstration of flea transmission.

It was ten years later, however, that the whole problem was analyzed in a complete and rigidly scientific fashion by a Plague Commission appointed by the Government of India. The report of this Commission on *The Etiology and Epidemiology of Plague* is an admirably planned and thoroughly sound piece of epidemiological research, which the authors modestly describe as "a cope-stone to careful and tedious investigations already carried out in India—and of course elsewhere—rather than an original building."

The first section of this report summarizes a survey in various areas of cases of human plague in relation to the prevalence of the disease in rodents as determined by the trapping and examination of many thousands of rats in the same localities. This study showed a close—and roughly quantitative—relation between the epizootic among rats and the epidemic among human beings, the course of the former preceding that of the latter by one to two weeks.

Next, the Commission proceeded to careful experimental studies on the methods by which the disease could be spread from the rat. The guinea pig was used as the susceptible victim and it was shown that—in the absence of fleas—neither intimate contact between infected and non-infected animals, nor habitation on soil which had been occupied by infected animals, nor consumption of food contaminated with the feces and urine of infected animals could produce new infections. (Under very extreme artificial conditions either contaminated soil or food could cause the disease; but, when this occurred, the local foci of infection were entirely different from those apparent in naturally acquired rodent plague.) On the other hand—in the presence of fleas—infection occurred very readily, when susceptible animals occupied experimental cabins where infected animals had lived; it spread with ease to animals in cages adjacent to those occupied by infected ones or in cages suspended 2 inches above the floor. If, however, adjacent cages were separated by a flea-proof screen or a strip of tanglefoot, no transmission occurred. Finally, fleas taken from infected chambers, placed in test-tubes and allowed to bite healthy guinea pigs through muslin, readily transmitted the disease.

Later sections of the report give epidemiological evidence to show that direct transmission of plague (except in the pneumonic form)[5] from man to man is not an important factor; that insanitary conditions are significant only in so far as they favor breeding and harborage of rats; and that the spread of plague from one locality to another is generally due to imported rat fleas on the bodies or in the luggage of persons who themselves are often in good health. The last conclusion may or may not be sound for India; even there, it is probable that the infected rat (rather than the infected flea) may play a major role in place-to-place dissemination. In transport of the disease by sea, the rat is undoubtedly the chief agent.

So far as the rat-flea-man links in the chain are concerned, this 1908 report, however, established the main facts in the case. The role of wild rodents, particularly the Siberian marmot in Manchuria, was also made clear early in the course of the present pandemic. The researches of the past three decades have given us a far clearer conception of the major importance of this factor in the problem. We now know that—as in the case of jungle fever—the permanent reservoir of plague is to be found as "sylvatic plague" in the form of infection of wild rodents, the tarbagans of Manchuria, the sousliks of the Volga Region, the jerboas of South Africa, the ground-squirrels of California, and many more. There are now known nearly a score of such endemic animal foci of wild plague, where the infection is kept going and from which occasional cases arise among hunters and trappers exposed to infected animals. Where infection is carried by fleas, which have bitten the wild rodents or infected human beings, to rats, a rat epizootic may develop to be followed by an epidemic among men.

Here in the United States, we have to face a serious situation of this kind. Plague was—so far as we know—first introduced at San Francisco in 1900, and by 1940, 499 cases with 314 deaths had been recorded, chiefly in California but with a sprinkling in Louisiana, Texas, and six other states. Since 1930 only a handful of human cases have been recognized; but infection of wild rodents is serious and widespread. By 1910,

---

[5] When the disease assumes the pneumonic form it is, of course, spread directly from man to man by mouth discharges; but this form of plague is relatively rare in India.

such sylvatic plague had been recognized in many counties of California and in the state of Washington. By 1939 it had been reported in every West Coast state and extending east to Montana, Wyoming, Utah and New Mexico. About 30 species or varieties of squirrels, chipmunks, marmots, prairie dogs, wood-rats, field mice and rabbits have been incriminated. We do not know whether the disease is steadily spreading eastward among these rodents or whether a long-standing situation has been gradually discovered. We do know, however, that the condition exists and that there is no apparent possibility of eliminating these endemic foci of sylvatic plague. As in the case of jungle fever, we must face the necessity for a continuing defense against a permanently entrenched enemy. As with yellow fever, however, we may confidently hope to prevent the development of any considerable human epidemic—in this case by the control of the rat in communities where alone such an epidemic could arise.

Before closing this chapter, we must summarize briefly the intriguing situation which has been revealed by recent researches in one other field of epidemiology—that of typhus fever and its allied diseases. Next to bubonic plague, this malady, under the names of "ship fever," "camp fever," "jail fever," "spotted fever," was perhaps the most dreaded of European pestilences. It was clearly described by Fracastorius in 1546; and, eighteen years before, its ravages in the French army besieging Naples had been probably decisive in the battle between Charles V and Francis I for the hegemony of the continent. Professor Curschmann says of this disease, "between 1846 and 1848 more than a million cases of typhus occurred in England and more than 300,000 in Ireland, the outbreak starting after the great famine of the earlier year. In every century typhus fever has followed in the wake of armies. During the Thirty Years War it claimed more victims than did the weapons of the contestants. It was the terror of the Napoleonic campaigns and decimated the French Army, already demoralized physically and morally by the terrible retreat from Moscow. During the Crimean War it decimated both the French and English armies, especially the former." In the Balkan War, prior to 1914, typhus again assumed epidemic proportions in Serbia; and in the late stages of the last World War, and the succeeding years of demoralization in Russia it caused terrible destruction. From 1917 to 1921 it is estimated that there were 25 million cases of typhus in the territories of the Soviet Union.

Meanwhile, however, the basic secret of the disease had been revealed by Charles Nicolle who showed in 1909 that European typhus could be transmitted by the bite of the body louse. In the next years, this was confirmed for Mexican typhus by H. T. Ricketts and R. M. Wilder. The latter investigators also saw what we now know as the causative organism in blood smears from patients and in infected lice. This organism was fully studied and identified by H. da Rocha-Lima in 1916 and named *Rickettsia prowazeki* in memory of Ricketts and the Austrian, S. von Prowazek—both of whom had died of typhus contracted in the course of their investigations. S. B. Wolbach, J. L. Todd and F. W. Palfrey in 1922 definitely clinched the proof that this *Rickettsia* was the cause of the disease in a study of post-war typhus in Poland.

Meanwhile, Ricketts in 1906 had demonstrated that Rocky Mountain spotted fever—a disease resembling typhus, centering in certain areas of our own northwestern states—was transmitted by the wood tick. This disease, too, was found to be caused by a *Rickettsia*; and it began to be suspected that typhus fever was only one member of a group of allied diseases, carried by various types of intermediate hosts.

Even what had been called "typhus fever" was found to include several different varieties of disease. We have had occasional outbreaks of true European typhus in the United States; but the form commonly prevalent had several distinguishing epidemiological characteristics. It was milder than the classical European typhus; it occurred at a different season of the year; and it was definitely not limited to persons infested with body lice. In 1931, R. E. Dyer, A. Rumreich and L. F. Badger of the United States Public Health Service demonstrated that the etiology of this form of typhus was entirely different from that of the European epidemic form, being spread not from man to louse to man but from rat to flea to man.

A recent review by Y. Biraud and S. Deutschman of the Health Organization of the League of Nations lists twenty-two different varieties of typhus-like diseases occurring in various parts of the world. All are caused by some species of *Rickettsia* (or a closely allied form); all are more or less related in the immunological reactions which they provoke; all have certain similarities in symptoms; nearly all (except European epidemic typhus) have rats or other rodents as their primary animal reservoirs; all, again with the exception of European typhus, are conveyed to man either by fleas or ticks or mites. They differ in minor details of symptomatology—and very greatly in virulence; in their quantitative serological interreactions; and in the particular rodent reservoirs and flea or tick or mite vectors concerned.

The evolutionary history of such a complex congeries of diseases is a fascinating subject for conjecture. Zinsser, the most philosophical and one of the most profound students of this problem advanced a plausible hypothesis in this connection. The *Rickettsia* group of organisms as a whole are known to be common and widespread parasites of many insects. Certain species of the genus, inhabiting the flea, probably become adapted to the rat or some other rodent, establishing a flea-rat cycle of infection. Occasionally, fleas infected from rats would bite human beings, producing sporadic cases of human disease, as occurs in our American murine (rat-borne) typhus. Here the cycle becomes rat-flea-man. Zinsser concludes, "The human louse was possibly the last of the series of hosts to acquire the virus—for it had, long before this time, become inseparably dependent upon man. And this surmise is in keeping with the fact that in the louse the *Rickettsiae* are more predatory than parasitic. The infected louse always dies." The louse, however, survives long enough—under conditions of crowding of uncleanly persons—to transmit the infection to a new victim; and from the simple and direct louse-man cycle arise the great epidemics of classical typhus fever.

In rickettsial diseases spread from rodents, as in jungle fever and sylvatic plague, we are faced with ineradicable wild reservoirs of infection; yet substantial and serious epidemics of either disease can be controlled by measures directed against the *Aedes* mosquitoes, and the rats in our cities and the lice upon our bodies.

CHAPTER XVIII

THE MODES OF INFECTION

"The first man to pass from theory to practise, who had the courage to abandon final disinfection as a preventive measure against infectious diseases, appears to have been Charles Chapin, Head of the Department of Public Health at Providence, U.S.A. . . . This, however, is not Chapin's only contribution to this branch of knowledge. In 1910, he published a book called Sources and Modes of Infection, which still remains the most complete and most impartial documentary statement of our knowledge concerning the life and virulence of pathogenic microbes in the external world."—CARLOS CHAGAS[1]

B Y the close of the nineteenth century, the concept of the human carrier had explained the occurrence of isolated cases of disease arising without exposure to an earlier clinical case. Demonstration of water-borne epidemics had made understandable the development of sudden explosive epidemics of typhoid and cholera throughout a whole community. The recognition of the insect vector gave a rational explanation of the endemic prevalence of malaria and yellow fever in certain localities. The germ theory could thus account for all conditions under which disease was actually shown to arise.

There was, however, another aspect of the case, related to the converse side of the problem—the question why disease often failed to spread under conditions which seemed highly favorable to transmission, under the earlier chemical conception of contagion. This question was, of course, partly answered by the gradual recognition that *contagia animata* were particulate and not gaseous in nature and by the discovery that certain of them (as in the case of malaria) were incapable of any direct transmission and dependent on the presence of a suitable insect host.

Before all the facts could be understood, however, it was necessary to realize that the germs of disease were not only particulate but parasitic in nature. The parasite is an organism which has become adapted to life in the tissues and cells of some higher form of life; and in the process of adaptation (like human beings who have become parasites on society) it has lost the capacity to earn an honest living in the world outside. The parasite in passage from one human host to another is exposed to serious

---

[1] Report to Fifth Session of the Health Committee of the League of Nations, Geneva, November 10, 1925. p. 74.

hazards; and the duration of such exposure is a determining factor in disease transmission.

During the first decade of the twentieth century a mass of bacteriological evidence accumulated in regard to the general low viability of disease germs outside the human or animal body. In soil, and even in feces, while intestinal parasites might survive for some time, their numbers steadily decreased. In water, destruction was even more rapid. Jordan and Russell in 1904 suspended typhoid bacilli in collodion sacs in the waters of the Chicago River and found that they survived only for 3-7 days. Houston in London in 1908 inoculated drinking water with the same organisms and reported 99.7 to 100 per cent dead in one week. It became clear that rather *prompt* transfer from a sick person or a carrier to a new potential victim was essential for successful invasion. This was the final discovery which was essential to a really balanced picture of the factors at work in the transmission of communicable disease.

We have noted in earlier chapters that Panum in 1847 had shown how a respiratory infection like measles spreads by direct contact from person to person; and how Budd in 1856 had demonstrated the importance of person-to-person contact in typhoid fever. The dissemination of cholera by water-supplies was fully elucidated by Snow in 1849 and by Koch in 1893. In the United States, W. T. Sedgwick in the Report of the State Board of Health of Massachusetts for 1892 reported classic examples of the transmission of typhoid fever by contact (at Bondsville) by water (at Lowell and Lawrence) and by milk (at Springfield). The third vehicle of transmission—by intermediate insect hosts—had been demonstrated by the brilliant series of investigations reviewed in Chapter XVII. Shortly after the turn of the century a mass of laboratory and epidemiological evidence was available, requiring only critical and comprehensive synthesis to lay a firm foundation for the modern public health campaign. This definitive synthesis was made by a distinguished American health officer, Charles Value Chapin, in 1910.

Chapin was born in Providence in 1856. He graduated at Brown University in 1876 and took his medical degree at Bellevue in 1879, receiving his first glimpse of the dawning science of bacteriology from E. G. Janeway and serving as co-interne with W. C. Gorgas. Five years later he was appointed Superintendent of Health of his native city, succeeding Edwin M. Snow who had served in that capacity since the establishment of the post in 1856. The department in 1884 was made up of the "superintendent and one ex-policeman." Chapin was also appointed city registrar in

1888 and continued to discharge the duties of both offices till his retirement in 1932. He held appointments as professor of physiology (1886-1896) and as director of physical culture (1891-1893) at Brown University and as lecturer at the Harvard School of Public Health. He served as president of the American Public Health Association in 1927. He was awarded the Hartley and Sedgwick and Rosenberger medals and received honorary degrees of Sc.D. from Brown and the Rhode Island State College, and LL.D. from Yale. He died in 1941 at the age of eighty-five.

Chapin's direct public health contributions in Providence were along three main lines. He continued the work of Dr. Snow in making the Registration Reports of the city models of accuracy and completeness. He developed the Providence City Hospital (an institution which now, appropriately, bears his name) as the first institution on this side of the water to apply the new conception that germ diseases were not air-borne but spread by contact. Finally, he established a technique of health administration which for the first time involved conscientious and scientific planning for the application of the principles of the new public health. His colleague, Dr. C. L. Scamman, has summarized this latter achievement as follows: "Dr. Chapin saw the change of emphasis from law enforcement to community education as the primary concern of public health administration; from isolation and quarantine as the methods of communicable disease control to a fundamental attack on causative agents as sources and modes of transmission and infection became known; and from care of children only when ill and convalescing to a whole scheme of prenatal and child hygiene as the foundation of sound health in adult life."

Dr. Chapin's wider influence upon the field of public health began in 1901 with the publication of a bulky volume on *Municipal Sanitation in the United States*. Like the true scientist he was, he began by a comprehensive review of the existing situation, giving a complete picture of what health departments were then doing. In the very next year, 1902, he began his pioneer task of changing that situation. In an address on "Dirt, Disease and the Health Officer," before the American Public Health Association in that year, he delivered his first smashing attack on the conventional theories of sanitation. He says that Reed and Gorgas at Havana had driven "the last nail in the coffin of the filth theory of disease. But it is to be feared that the devotees of this theory are loath to bury it, thus violating one of their cardinal principles." Emphasis in health administration, even in the present century, was still chiefly upon environmental sanitation in the vague and general sense of "pure air, pure water and a pure soil." Yet, Chapin said, "it will make no demonstrable difference in a city's mortality whether its streets are clean or not, whether the garbage is removed promptly or allowed to accumulate, or whether it has a plumbing law." "We can rest assured that however spick and span may be the streets, and however the policeman's badge may be polished, as long as there is found the boor careless with his expectoration, and the doctor who cannot tell a case of sapolio from one of diphtheria, the latter disease, and tuberculosis as well, will continue to claim their victims." "Instead of an indiscriminate attack on dirt, we must learn the nature and mode of transmission of each infection, and must discover its most vulnerable point of attack." "The great problem of sanitation today is how to deal with mild or unrecognized cases of contagious disease and with those persons who, though well, are yet infected. This problem is not likely to be solved so long as physicians trace infection to the class of *things* mentioned, instead of to *persons*."

This was in some degree an overstatement in so far as the minimizing of sanitation was concerned. We paid for too long a swing of the pendulum in this direction by the epidemic of amebic dysentery at Chicago in 1933. But the fundamental emphasis on specific infection rather than indiscriminate dirt was of tremendous importance. In 1902, it was a clarion call for the new public health.

In 1906, Chapin continued the battle with an address on "The Fetich of Disinfection," delivered before the American Medical Association, in which the principles of the young science of bacteriology were applied to the specific problem of communicable disease control. Chapin was discussing in this address what we now know as "terminal disinfection" of premises after death or recovery of a case. This type of disinfection he describes as a cult of purification deriving psychologically from the demonic theory of disease. The only scientific basis for such practices is the concept of fomites infection and "while it is admitted that such infection occasionally takes place, there is no evidence that this is a factor of any moment in the extension of the contagious diseases." The emphasis on fomites infection was chiefly due to the desire to explain the occurrence of new cases with no known exposure to earlier cases. This phenomenon, however, can far better be explained by the role of the missed case and the well carrier. All evidence tends to show that contagion usually extends by "pretty direct contact between the infected and the non-infected." Therefore, terminal disinfection of things is far less important than isolation of persons. It was the point of view advanced in this address which Chapin applied in the open wards for communicable disease of the Providence Hospital and in the abandonment of routine terminal disinfection in the practice of the Providence Health Department; and it was these principles and those of the essay on "Dirt and Disease" which he expanded in his classic work on *The Sources and Modes of Infection*, first published in 1910.

This book we must review in some detail. Before doing so, however, reference must be made to another line of Chapin's activity which was second only in importance to his development of the basic epidemiological principles of the public health campaign. This was his contribution to the evaluation of the actual machinery of public health practice.

The volume on *Municipal Sanitation in the United States* (1901), which has been noted above, initiated this line of approach. Chapin's own point of view was more clearly outlined in an address delivered before the American Public Health Association in 1909 on "The Need of Quantitative Methods in Epidemiological Work." He points out in this essay that "the progress of a science is largely dependent upon the extent to which quantitative methods are employed in research." He notes the importance of accurate quantitative analysis in statistical, bacteriological and epidemiological investigation; and appeals for the same sort of careful study of the costs and results of health department administrative procedures. "We are crowding our hospitals with scarlet fever cases and crying for more buildings, but who has figured the amount of case prevention and the cost per case, and has compared this cost with that of district-nursing of home-treated cases?"

This line of thought was continued in 1913 in an address to the Massachusetts Association of Boards of Health on "How Shall We Spend the Health Appropriation?" Here Chapin again urged the need for evaluating each specific health department procedure so that the health dollar could be expended to maximum advantage. Two years later, in 1915, he published a "Report on State Public Health Work Based on a Survey of State Boards of Health." This study, made under the direction of the Council on Health and Public Instruction of the American Medical Association, was the first comparative analysis of health department procedures in the world. It was the inspiration of the far-reaching program of the Committee on Administrative Practice of the American Public

Health Association initiated in 1921 and laid the foundation for the whole movement along the line of quantitative evaluation of procedures which has transformed American public health during the past twenty years.

Throughout his long life, Dr. Chapin, and the wife who shared with him a companionship of rare intimacy and satisfaction, were regular attendants at the meetings of the Massachusetts and national health associations. Here his personal influence produced a deep and lasting impression upon many hundreds of associates. His personal gentleness and profound modesty were coupled with a passion for rigorous scientific truth which made him an unparalleled champion, in battles which left no wounds but opened the way for continuing expansion of our concepts of public health.

We must now consider in some detail the basic theses of the *Sources and Modes of Infection*, which was Chapin's major legacy to the science of public health.

Chapter 1 of the book deals with the bacteriological evidence which formed the primary experimental basis of his epidemiological thinking. At the outset of this chapter on "Life of Disease Germs Outside of the Body" the author points out that the miasmatic theory implicitly assumed an "extra-corporal origin of disease"; and that this view was at first strengthened rather than weakened by the discovery of bacteria since these organisms as a group were also "extra-corporal" and most obviously abundant in dead animal and vegetable matter. Only by recognition of the parasitic nature of the germs of specific diseases was it possible to "question the belief that these diseases have their origin in the outer world rather than in the bodies of men or animals."

Chapin begins with the disease most unfavorable to his theory, that of anthrax. Even here he gives convincing evidence that the causative organism, although its spores persist, rarely increases in numbers in the soil; and concludes that "the history of this disease is best explained on the hypothesis that the soil is infected chiefly if not exclusively by the spores, which may retain their virulence for years, but which rarely germinate in the earth." Similarly, evidence is reviewed with regard to the survival of typhoid bacilli in soil, sewage, water, ice, oysters and milk, of cholera spirilla in water and milk and soil, of plague bacilli in soil and excrement and to the epidemiological evidence in these and other diseases as to causation by extra-corporal sources. He concludes, on bacteriological grounds, that "so far as experimental evidence is concerned there is no warrant for assuming a source for the common infectious diseases outside of animal bodies. It is only with extreme difficulty that a few of the blood parasites belonging to the protozoa can be cultivated, and the cultivation of many bacterial forms is strictly limited, so that it is hardly possible to imagine their maintaining a saprophytic existence. It is true that the bacteria of typhoid fever and perhaps cholera, dysentery, and diphtheria may be conceived of as growing outside of the body under natural conditions, but such growth, if it ever occurs, must be rare."

The epidemiological evidence indicates that, "In such important diseases as smallpox, measles and scarlet fever, the germs of which have not been isolated, as well as in typhus fever, diphtheria and whooping cough, epidemiological evidence of an extra-corporal origin is entirely lacking. Epidemiological and laboratory evidence are against the growth of disease germs outside of the body under ordinary circumstances. The notion still common, even among physicians and health officers, that these infectious diseases are filth diseases, as that term is ordinarily understood, is absolutely without foundation."

In the case of malaria, yellow fever, sleeping sickness and Texas fever "it is the insects which have an extraneous existence and not the parasite of the disease." He concludes, "In reviewing this subject we are forced to the conclusion that while it is possible that the anthrax and tetanus bacilli and the pus-forming bacteria may develop in the soil, there is no evidence that they commonly do so. It is also possible that the typhoid bacilli, and to a still less extent the bacteria of cholera, dysentery and plague, maintain a limited saprophytic existence, but this is probably very unusual. There is ample epidemiological evidence that in temperate climates such a source for these diseases must be an almost infinitesimal factor in their development. Probably the diphtheria bacillus never has a saprophytic growth of any significance, unless possibly very rarely in milk. As for tuberculosis, pneumonia, influenza, cerebro-spinal meningitis, scarlet fever, typhus fever, smallpox, whooping cough, gonorrhea and syphilis, malaria, yellow fever, and sleeping sickness, there is not the slightest reason for supposing that they ever develop outside of the bodies of animals."

Chapin's discussion of "Carriers and Missed Cases" has been discussed in a preceding chapter, and his analysis of "Limitations to the Value of Isolation" applies his theses to the promotion of efficiency and simplicity in the practices of isolation and quarantine. Chapters v and vi are, however, pertinent to the present discussion since they prepare the way for analysis of the important modes of infection by eliminating two channels by which communicable disease does *not* generally spread.

In discussing "Infection by Fomites," Chapin points out that contact and fomites infection obviously overlap. A drinking cup or a borrowed pencil is merely one form of contact. Infection by fomites is defined as "a transference of infecting material on objects under such conditions that considerable time elapses, days at least, usually weeks, sometimes months." Fomites infection of this sort was once universally assumed for yellow fever, at a cost of untold millions in delay of commerce; yet we now know that such transmission never occurs. Similarly Chapin quotes many twentieth century accounts of the spread of smallpox, scarlet fever, diphtheria and cholera by bedding, clothing, toys and the like. (The writer can see even now in his mind's eye a much worn copy of *Dombey and Son* from the Public Library which was supposed to have given him measles as a child.) Yet recent epidemiological evidence shows that physicians rarely spread disease, that laundry workers do not show a high incidence of infection, that rooms occupied by the sick, rags, money, etc. can rarely be incriminated. Where infection does occur, it is persons, not things, which are generally responsible.

The only two diseases which offer an exception to the general rule are tetanus and anthrax. In these—the only common diseases caused by germs which form resistant spores—epidemiological evidence for fomites infection is clear and overwhelming. Truly, this is a case where "the exception proves the rule." Chapin cites two instances in which typhoid fever and diphtheria cases were caused by unusually heavy soiling of bedding and clothing. The fact that such occurrences must be rare is, however, demonstrated by a mass of bacteriological evidence on the rapid disappearance of various pathogenic bacteria when dried, and on the generally negative results of bacteriological examination of fomites. He reviews the experience of Providence with diphtheria for four years in which terminal disinfection was practiced and five years after terminal disinfection had been abandoned. In the first period, 17 recurrences occurred per 1,000 primary cases; in the second period 21 recurrences, a difference of no statistical significance. Chapin concludes that:

"There is no good epidemiological evidence that any diseases except those due to spore-forming bacteria are to any great extent transmitted by fomites. . . .

"Other modes of transmission so much more satisfactorily account for the spread of disease, that there seems to be really little opportunity for infection by fomites.

"Laboratory investigation shows that fomites infection with spore-forming bacteria is common; that such infection in typhoid fever, tuberculosis, diphtheria and with other resistant organisms doubtless sometimes takes place; that it is possible in cholera and plague, while such infection in gonorrhea, influenza, cerebro-spinal meningitis and pneumonia must be practically impossible."

In Chapter vi on "Infection by Air" Chapin deals with a second bogy of pre-bacteriological epidemiology. Air infection, like infection by fomites, had been invoked to explain the development of otherwise mysterious cases and this theory was naturally reinforced by the fact that "the virus of the infectious diseases was believed to be gaseous, or at least readily diffusible." In smallpox, particularly, much evidence had been offered in England and in this country to show that the disease spreads through the atmosphere from smallpox hospitals and from vessels on which smallpox cases are present. (When the New Haven Hospital isolation ward was built about twenty-five years ago, an agreement was signed with the owners of neighboring property that no smallpox cases would be admitted; and this agreement was only abrogated by mutual consent in the 'thirties.) Chapin shows, however, that the actual distribution of cases in the neighborhood of isolation hospitals does not follow any reasonable laws of atmospheric diffusion, and that contact infection, under primitive conditions of administrative control, offers a far better explanation of the facts. Similar alleged evidence in regard to aerial spread of scarlet fever and diphtheria is reviewed and convincing proof is offered that, under such conditions as those of the Pasteur Hospital in Paris and the Providence Hospital, atmospheric dissemination does not occur in open wards. How could it then operate over much greater distances in the open air? The assumption that intestinal diseases may be spread by sewer air and by air-borne dust is similarly analyzed. Such short-range aerial transmission as that implied by the common practice of hanging a wet sheet over the door of the sick room is not supported by any valid evidence; and even in the case of septic wound diseases contact, rather than atmospheric infection, is the major problem. As in the case of fomites, anthrax is the only disease in which air-borne dust is really a demonstrable mode of infection. Bacteriological evidence is then reviewed, particularly in regard to the Cornet theory of dust-transmission and the Flügge theory of droplet-infection. The rapid mortality of pathogenic bacteria when dried and the limited area over which droplets are discharged seem to Chapin to limit the importance of both processes. (Recent studies of coccidiosis indicate one special exception to the general rule that dust infection is not important.)

In summing up, Chapin draws the following conclusions:

"Bacteriology teaches that former ideas in regard to the manner in which diseases may be air-borne are entirely erroneous; that most diseases are not likely to be dust-borne, and they are spray-borne only for two or three feet, a phenomenon which after all resembles contact infection more than it does aerial infection as ordinarily understood. Tuberculosis is more likely to be air-borne than is any other common disease. . . .

"There is no good clinical evidence that the common diseases are airborne.

"There is considerable clinical evidence that scarlet fever, diphtheria, smallpox, measles, whooping cough, typhoid fever and plague are not easily transmissible through the air.

"Scarlet fever and diphtheria can be cared for in the same ward with other diseases without extension, if cleanliness be maintained and infection by contact avoided."

Finally, he says, "If it should prove, as I firmly believe, that contact infection is the chief way in which the contagious diseases spread, an exaggerated idea of the importance of air-borne infection is most mischievous. It is impossible, as I know from experience, to teach people to avoid contact infection while they are firmly convinced that the air is the chief vehicle of infection.

"While it is not possible at present to state with exactness the part played by aerial infection in the transmission of the different infectious diseases, we are by the evidence forced to the conclusion that the current ideas in regard to the importance of infection by air are unwarranted. Without denying the possibility of such infection, it may be fairly affirmed that there is no evidence that it is an appreciable factor in the maintenance of most of our common contagious diseases. We are warranted, then, in discarding it as a working hypothesis and devoting our chief attention to the prevention of contact infection. It will be a great relief to most persons to be freed from the specter of infected air, a specter which has pursued the race from the time of Hippocrates, and we may rest assured that if people can as a consequence be better taught to practice strict personal cleanliness, they will be led to do that which will more than anything else prevent aerial infection also, if that should in the end be proved to be of more importance than now appears."

In chapters IV, VII and VIII Chapin deals with the other side of the case —with the modes of infection which, in the light of newer knowledge, really seem of major importance.

The first of these, of course, is "Infection by Contact." Here Chapin begins with the simplest problem—that of gonorrhea and syphilis. He reviews the admirable studies by Holt of gonococcus vaginitis in the Babies' Hospital in New York and concludes, "Everyone admits that gonorrhea is frequently transferred by indirect contact infection, as it may be called (syringes, fingers of the nurse, etc.), but it is never suggested that this disease is spread by fomites." He then proceeds to the group of the intestinal diseases, citing the Bondsville epidemic of Sedgwick and the Spanish War experience as indicating the importance of contact in the spread of typhoid fever, in the person-to-person fashion described as "prosodemic" infection. Similar data are presented with regard to cholera, dysentery and diarrhea; and hookworm disease is discussed as a perfect type of contact infection. The following illuminating picture is given of what contact infection, in the case of the intestinal diseases, really means. "An inspection of the privies or water-closets in railway stations, factories, shops and tenement houses shows that they usually present evidence of contamination with feces and urine, and in many instances are constantly in a horribly filthy condition. It is only in the better class of hotels and residences that these apartments are kept in even an apparently cleanly condition, and this is only by dint of constant vigilance and frequent cleansing. There can be no doubt that even very careful people frequently infect the seat, their fingers, the pull, the door, etc., and that in a large proportion of privies and water-closets the users almost certainly infect their fingers with at least traces of their own or others' excremental matter. Yet how many persons are there who invariably wash the hands after the use of a closet? How many make it a rule never to put the fingers in the mouth? Yesterday I saw a workman carrying a can of beer to his friends. His thumb was immersed a couple of inches in the beverage. Had he washed his hands after leaving the barroom water-closet? At a recent sanitary convention I noticed the colored waiter stick his finger into a glass which he, however, did not remove, and which the speaker soon drank from. What was the recent history of that finger? Does the fruit peddler wash his hands after using the tenement privy before he ventures to sort his fruit? Do the waitress, the milk peddler, the candy seller, the Pullman porter, the soda-water clerk, the baker's boy, the delicatessen man *always* wash the hands before taking up their work? Are the toilets in their places of business so cleanly that such a precaution is not necessary? However shocking it may seem, it is certain that it requires only a little observation to demonstrate that the path from intestines to mouth is not always a circuitous one."

Next, Chapin turns to the diseases spread by discharges from the nose and throat, in connection with which he gives us another classic description. "Probably the chief vehicle for the conveyance of nasal and oral secretion from one to another is the fingers. If one takes the trouble to watch for a short time his neighbors, or even himself, unless he has been particularly trained in such matters, he will be surprised to note the number of times that the fingers go to the mouth and the nose. Not only is the saliva made use of for a great variety of purposes, and numberless articles are for one reason or another placed in the mouth, but for no reason whatever, and all unconsciously, the fingers are with great frequency raised to the lips or the nose. Who can doubt that if the salivary glands secreted indigo the fingers would continually be stained a deep blue, and who can doubt that if the nasal and oral secretions contain the germs of disease these germs will be almost as constantly found upon the fingers? All successful commerce is reciprocal, and in this universal trade in human saliva the fingers not only bring foreign secretions to the mouth of their owner, but there exchanging them for his own, distribute the latter to everything that the hand touches. This happens not once but scores and hundreds of times during the day's round of the individual. The cook spreads his saliva on the muffins and rolls, the waitress infects the glasses and spoons, the moistened fingers of the peddler arrange his fruit, the thumb of the milkman is in his measure, the reader moistens the pages of his book, the conductor his transfer tickets, the 'lady' the fingers of her glove. Every one is busily engaged in this distribution of saliva, so that the end of each day finds this secretion freely distributed on the doors, window sills, furniture and playthings in the home, the straps of trolley cars, the rails and counters and desks of shops and public buildings, and indeed upon everything that the hands of man touch. What avails it if the pathogens do die quickly? A fresh supply is furnished each day."

The fact that, without opportunities for contact, disease does not spread, is brought out by Providence experience indicating how rarely diphtheria and scarlet fever actually pass from one family to another in multiple dwellings; and the conclusion is reenforced by the success of the Pasteur Hospital and certain English hospitals in controlling cross-infection by appropriate aseptic nursing. Chapin says, in concluding this discussion, "I have sometimes been told that I lay too much emphasis on contact infection, but if it is the principal way in which disease spreads, too much emphasis cannot be placed upon it, and it seems to me that the evidence is that it is the chief mode of infection."

The chapter on "Infection by Food and Drink" clearly recognizes the importance of this second major mode of transmission, although it tends to minimize its relative importance. Chapin begins with the classic example of the Broad Street Well and then reviews the overwhelming evidence of the relation of polluted water to typhoid incidence in European and American cities and the successful reduction of that incidence by water purification. He cites Whipple's estimate that 40 per cent of the typhoid in American cities was due to water, though Chapin himself believes that for the country as a whole the percentage of water-borne typhoid probably does not exceed 15 per cent. It seems quite possible that this estimate was not far from the truth; and it was certain that in 1910 there was a tendency to regard typhoid fever as too strictly a water-borne disease. On the other hand, the interrelationship between water and contact infection was more fundamental than Chapin realized. In cities like New Haven, a single water-borne epidemic so seeded the community with typhoid carriers that the normal rate of prosodemic contact typhoid remained excessive for twenty years thereafter. It seems certain, therefore, that the purification of public water supplies has been a major factor in the control of this disease during the past thirty years.

Chapin was undoubtedly correct in dismissing ice as a relatively unimportant medium of infection; and he showed discernment in refusing to accept the recent claim of Sedgwick and MacNutt that water played a role in the causation of tuberculosis and pneumonia.[2] He reviews the clear evidence of epidemics of typhoid fever due to milk but believes that its relative importance has been exaggerated and that, actually, milk was

[2] This study is of great interest to the student of epidemiology. Careful analysis of statistics for the cities of Lowell and Lawrence, Mass., showed a sharp reduction in tuberculosis and pneumonia rates following purification of the municipal water supplies; while Manchester, N.H., used as a control, exhibited no similar improvement. The results seemed highly convincing but later studies elsewhere failed to confirm them. It appears probable that the reductions of death-rate (aside from typhoid fever) in Lowell and Lawrence were merely part of a general trend; and he failure of Manchester to follow that trend was an unexplained accident.

probably responsible for less than 10 per cent of the total cases of typhoid fever. He was probably correct—as shown by later studies of Kelley and others in Massachusetts—and was also right in his claim that the proportion of tuberculosis caused by the bovine bacillus from milk was not great. He discusses shellfish infection briefly, and with regard to meat concludes that "The diseases which it is alleged may be transmitted by flesh foods are those caused by animal parasites, of which trichinosis is the most important, diseased conditions produced by the colon group of bacilli, and tuberculosis. The latter is a negligible quantity, the second group probably causes very few deaths in this country, while trichinosis is doubtless the most important disease transmitted in this manner."

On the whole there is in this chapter a certain tendency to "play down" the relative importance of infection by articles of food and drink. This was probably a logical emphasis in 1910, when the problems of milk-borne septic sore throat and undulant fever were unknown. With the elimination of large-scale water-borne epidemics and the near-disappearance of typhoid fever, and diphtheria we would today place much more emphasis on food-poisoning (including that due to staphylococci) as a cause of sickness if not of death. Furthermore, the reduction of human tuberculosis makes tuberculosis infection due to the bovine bacillus of relatively greater importance. This, and our knowledge of septic sore throat and undulant fever, justifies a much stronger emphasis than Chapin placed on the importance of pasteurization.

Finally, Chapin reviews in his discussion on "Infection by Insects" such of the discoveries discussed in our Chapter XVII as were known in 1910. He stresses the great significance of the then new knowledge of malaria and yellow fever and bubonic plague, as outstanding examples of the diseases spread solely by true insect vectors. He closes with a discussion of the adventitious spread of typhoid and other intestinal diseases by mechanical fly transmission; and concludes "It is probable that under certain conditions, as in military and civil camps, and in filthy communities without sewerage, insects, especially flies, may be an important factor in the spread of the fecal-borne diseases, but there is no evidence that in the average city the house fly is a factor of great moment in the dissemination of disease."

Here, then, were all the essential bases of modern epidemiology—boldly stated, and with overwhelmingly convincing evidence. It was clear that:

1. Disease germs are parasites, adapted to life in the human body

(and that of other mammals) and generally dying out rather rapidly in the external environment.

2. The primary source of these disease germs is always the human body (or that of one of the higher animals); but this source may be either a well carrier or a sick individual.

3. In view of their poor survival powers in a non-living environment disease germs (except spore-formers such as anthrax) must be transferred rather promptly from one human being to another, if new infection is to occur.

4. The disease germs are particulate objects and on account of this fact, and of their tendency to die outside the body, aerial dissemination and transmission by fomites are relatively unimportant.

5. The major modes of transmission are
    a. Direct or indirect contact
    b. Articles of food and drink
    c. Insect vectors.

In the years which have passed since 1910, the volume of our knowledge of parasitology and epidemiology has increased by leaps and bounds. We have a hundred times as many proven relationships at our disposal as we had thirty years ago. Yet the modifications which must be made in Chapin's analysis are surprisingly slight.

The most striking development of the last three decades has been the flowering of our knowledge with regard to the virus diseases. The causation of tobacco mosaic by a filtrable element had been demonstrated by Iwanowsky in 1892. Similar proof was presented for foot-and-mouth disease by Loeffler and Frosch in 1898. In 1902, the U.S. Army Commission in Cuba caused yellow fever by injection of a sterile filtrate. Remlinger demonstrated the same thing for rabies in 1906. Paschen in the case of variola brought forward convincing evidence that inclusion bodies were manifestations of the development of a very minute infecting agent. Since 1920, the study of these filtrable bodies has revealed viruses as the causative agents of scores of human diseases, including such important epidemic disorders as measles, mumps, poliomyelitis, dengue fever, psittacosis, equine encephalomyelitis and certain forms of the common cold and influenza.

The discovery by Stanley in 1935 that the virus of tobacco mosaic could be isolated in crystalline form shattered, once and for all, the older theoretical boundaries between chemical and biological "germs" of disease, and made us realize that the distinction between the "living" and the "non-living" world is only a matter of definition—and a definition very difficult to draw. Fracastorius would have accepted this demonstration without surprise; and Liebig would have hailed it with delight.

Yet, on the whole, our knowledge of the viruses has not substantially changed most of the broad conclusions advanced by Chapin in 1910 with regard to the epidemiology of the communicable diseases. The origin of infection in the human or animal body (well or ill); the precarious existence of the parasite in the physical environment; the importance of contact, articles of food and drink and insect vectors in transmission; all these principles are as valid for the virus as for the bacterium. Similarly, tremendous advances in the accuracy of epidemiological technique made possible by the splitting-up of bacterial species into autonomous "types," in the case of the pneumococcus, the streptococcus and the typhoid bacillus, have only added new and more convincing evidence of the validity of our general hypotheses.

In certain directions, new discoveries have indicated modification of Chapin's general emphasis. He recognized the role of the ground-squirrel in plague; but recent work on this disease, on yellow fever and on the rickettsial diseases, has given us a much clearer conception of the far-reaching importance of wild animals as basic sources of infection. Studies on "sylvatic plague" and "jungle fever"—and more recently on psittacosis—have revealed the disturbing fact that such reservoirs of potential human epidemic disease exist in nature to an extent hitherto undreamed of. The fundamental Chapin theses are not contradicted; but they are expanded to include what must be recognized as a major problem of future epidemiology.

In one respect only have the studies of the last twenty years indicated a real modification of Chapin's viewpoint. This is in regard to the importance of aerial dissemination of infection.

The observations of Harries at Manchester and others indicated some years ago that there was a fundamental difference in this regard between the bacterial and the viral diseases. Careful isolation procedures in an open ward were successful in preventing cross-infections in diphtheria and scarlet fever; but where cases of measles and chickenpox (diseases caused by viruses) were admitted to such wards in an actively communicable stage a few cross-infections did occur. It appeared highly probable from such observations that the smaller and lighter viruses could be carried by air currents to a greater distance than the larger and heavier bacteria.

More recently, Wells of the University of Pennsylvania—and, independently, Hart of Duke University—have reopened the whole question of aerial transmission in the case of even the bacterial diseases. Wells showed between 1933 and 1936 that the older conception of infective droplets discharged in coughing, sneezing or loud speaking as particles so large as to fall to the ground within a few feet holds only for droplets of a certain size (over .1 mm. in diameter). Two things happen to a droplet suspended in the air. It tends to fall (with a velocity in proportion to its mass); and it tends to become smaller as it evaporates and decreases in mass. A droplet initially below the critical size of .1 mm. evaporates faster than it falls and before it reaches the floor is so small that it will remain suspended for considerable periods. The latter type, called by Wells droplet nuclei, may, as he has demonstrated, float about in the air currents for hours and even days. Actually, Wells has shown that the alpha-hemolytic streptococci, which may be employed as indices of mouth-spray infection, as the colon bacillus is used to measure intestinal infection, can be demonstrated in considerable numbers in the air of hospitals, clinics and schools. Colleagues of Wells have actually demonstrated infection from droplet nuclei by animal experimentation.

To control such aerial transmission of disease, Wells has urged the disinfection of air by ultra-violet irradiation and this practice has been introduced in the operating rooms of hospitals with apparent success.[3] From such experience it appears that while the disinfection of surfaces, instruments and the like controls the severe types of septic infection, the disinfection of the air is of real value in eliminating air-borne organisms which cause mild infections delaying wound healing. Recently, Wells has made studies in school classrooms and has reported that "For three successive years classes in irradiated rooms of the primary department of the Germantown Friends School have been spared the epidemic spread of mumps or chickenpox suffered by comparable classes in unirradiated rooms."

It will be noted that it is again two virus diseases which offer the clearest evidence of aerial transmission. Allison in England has, however, brought forward suggestive evidence of the aerial transmission of scarlet fever in hospital wards. It seems certain that in the case of the virus

---

[3] The same result can be attained by spraying into the air very finely divided chemical disinfectants (aerosols).

diseases the radius of atmospheric dissemination is wider than Chapin thought; and this is probably also true in the case of certain respiratory infections due to bacteria.

On the whole, however, the broad principles of the epidemiology of 1910 remain unchallenged; and the application of those principles has been attended with phenomenal success. We may cite from a study by Horwood the figures below, to demonstrate what has been accomplished by comparing actual deaths from certain causes in 1935 with the number of deaths which would have occurred if the rates of 1900 had continued to be operative in 1935.

Causes of Death	Actual Deaths 1935	Number of Deaths Which Would Have Occurred in 1935 on Basis of Rates of 1900	Number of Lives Saved	Per cent reduction
Tuberculosis, all forms	51,269	224,384	173,115	77
Influenza and pneumonia	110,191	232,187	121,996	53
Diarrhea and enteritis	17,018	125,448	108,430	86
Communicable diseases of childhood*	13,182	72,127	58,945	82
Typhoid and paratyphoid	2,386	35,652	33,266	93
All other causes	1,013,313	1,285,963	272,650	21

* Measles, scarlet fever, whooping cough, diphtheria.

Thus, it appears that over three-quarters of a million lives a year are being saved in the United States by the application of the principles of modern public health; and that the major part of this saving is in the field of five groups of communicable diseases where those principles have been most specifically put in practice.

This astounding reduction in the major epidemic diseases is likely to be accelerated in the immediate future by the remarkable success of the sulfonamide drugs in the treatment of infections due to the pneumococci, streptococci and gonococci. With progress along such lines, the importance of the germ factor in disease is certain to grow relatively less. There is today a wholesome reaction against exclusive emphasis on the germ and a recognition of the importance—even in many germ diseases—of factors of constitutional resistance (diathesis) and of the influences of climate and season and nutrition upon vital resistance. The outstanding problem of epidemiology today is why colds and other respiratory diseases occur in winter and not in summer. This is almost certainly a physiological rather than a bacteriological problem.

So far as the germ factor is concerned, however, the *Sources and Modes of Infection* marked the close of one of the most brilliant chapters in the history of human thought. We shall never return to the demonic and miasmatic theories of the past; and the practical application of the principles developed by a series of clear thinkers and brilliant investigators—from Fracastorius to Chapin—has forever banished from the earth the major plagues and pestilences of the past. To trace the evolution of the theoretical concepts which have made this triumph possible has been the purpose of the present volume.

REFERENCES AND INDEX

ACKNOWLEDGMENTS

THE author is particularly indebted to the following publishers for their courtesy in permitting him to quote from the works indicated:

George Allen and Unwin Ltd.: L. Lévy-Bruhl, *Primitives and the Supernatural*.

Columbia University Press: A. M. Campbell, *The Black Death and Men of Learning*.

The Commonwealth Fund: *Papers of Charles V. Chapin, M.D.*

Dr. Haven Emerson: G. Fracastoro, *De Contagione et Contagiosis*, etc. (translated by W. C. Wright).

Harcourt, Brace and Company, Inc.: R. S. and H. M. Lynd, *Middletown*; C. Dobell, *Antony Van Leeuwenhoek*.

Harvard University Press: *Procopius*, with an English translation by H. B. Dewing; *Hippocrates*, with an English translation by W. H. S. Jones. (Loeb Classical Library.)

William Heinemann: Fracastoro, G. *Syphilis; or the French disease*. Translated by H. Wynne-Finch.

Little, Brown and Company and the Atlantic Monthly Press: Hans Zinsser, *Rats, Lice and History*.

The Macmillan Company: L. Thorndike, *A History of Magic and Experimental Science*; Cato and Varro, *Roman Farm Management*, etc. (translated by F. Harrison); M. Greenwood, *Epidemics and Crowd Diseases*.

Macmillan and Co. Ltd.: D. McKenzie, *The Infancy of Medicine*.

G. P. Putnam's Sons: M. Jastrow, *Aspects of Religious Belief and Practice in Babylonia and Assyria*.

W. B. Saunders Company: F. H. Garrison, *An Introduction to the History of Medicine*.

Charles Scribner's Sons: T. Gomperz, *Greek Thinkers*.

The Soncino Press Ltd.: A. S. Rappoport, *The Folklore of the Jews*.

Charles C. Thomas: W. T. Corlett, *The Medicine-Man of the American Indian*, etc.

John Wiley and Sons, Inc.: C. V. Chapin, *Sources and Modes of Infection* (now permanently out of print).

Yale University Press: W. Osler, *The Evolution of Modern Medicine*.

REFERENCES

CHAPTER I

Corlett, W. T. *The medicine-man of the American Indian and his cultural background*. Springfield, Ill. Charles C. Thomas. 1935. 369 p.

Garrison, F. H. *An introduction to the history of medicine*. 4th ed. Philadelphia and London. W. B. Saunders Co. 1929. 996 p.

Hippocrates. *The genuine works of Hippocrates*. Translated by Francis Adams. 2 v. London. Printed for the Sydenham Society. 1849.

v. Hovorka, O. and Kronfeld, U. *Vergleichende Volksmedizin*. 2 v. Stuttgart. Strecker and Schröder. 1908-1909.

Jastrow, J. *Wish and wisdom*. New York. D. Appleton-Century Co. 1935. 394 p.

Lévy-Bruhl, L. *Primitives and the supernatural*. Translated by L. A. Clare. London. G. Allen and Unwin, Ltd. 1936. 405 p.

Lynd, R. S. and H. M. *Middletown: a study in contemporary American culture*. New York. Harcourt Brace and Co. 1929. 550 p.

McKenzie, D. *The infancy of medicine*. London. Macmillan and Co. Ltd. 1927. 421 p.

Osler, W. *The evolution of modern medicine*. New Haven. Yale University Press. 1921. 243 p.

Rappoport, A. S. *The folklore of the Jews*. London. The Soncino Press, Ltd. 1937. 276 p.

Reed, L. S. *The healing cults*. Publications of the Committee on the Costs of Medical Care, No. 16. Chicago, Ill. University of Chicago Press. 1932. 134 p.

Sticker, G. Vorgeschichtliche Versuche der Seuchenabwehr und Seuchenausrottung. *Essays on the history of medicine presented to Karl Sudhoff on the occasion of his seventieth birthday, 26th November 1923*. Edited by Charles Singer and Henry E. Sigerist. London, Oxford University Press; Zürich, Verlag Seldwyla. 1924. pp. 3-62.

Thiselton-Dyer, T. F. *The ghost world*. London. Ward and Downey. 1893. 447 p.

Thorndike, L. *A history of magic and experimental science during the first thirteen centuries of our era*. 2 v. New York. Macmillan Co. 1923.

Tylor, E. B. *Primitive culture; researches into the development of mythology, philosophy, religion, language, art and custom*. 7th ed. 2 v. in one. New York. Brentano's. 1924.

Whitebread, C. *The magic, psychic, ancient Egyptian, Greek, and Roman medical collections of the Division of Medicine in the United States National Museum*. No. 2528, Proceedings U.S. National Museum, 65, art. 15. Washington. 1925. 44 p.

Wong, K. C. and Wu, Lien-Teh. *History of Chinese medicine. Being a chronicle of medical happenings in China from ancient times to the present period.* Tientsin, China. Tientsin Press, Ltd. 1932. 706 p.

CHAPTER II

Corlett, W. T. *The medicine-man of the American Indian and his cultural background.* Springfield, Ill. Charles C. Thomas. 1935. 369 p.

Lévy-Bruhl, L. *Primitives and the supernatural.* Translated by L. A. Clare. London. G. Allen and Unwin, Ltd. 1936. 405 p.

McKenzie, D. *The infancy of medicine.* London. Macmillan and Co. Ltd. 1927. 421 p.

Rappoport, A. S. *The folklore of the Jews.* London. The Soncino Press, Ltd. 1937. 276 p.

Singer, J. *Taboo in the Hebrew Scriptures.* Chicago and London. Open Court Publishing Co. 1928. 107 p.

Sticker, G. Vorgeschichtliche Versuche der Seuchenabwehr und Seuchenausrottung. *Essays on the history of medicine presented to Karl Sudhoff on the occasion of his seventieth birthday, 26th November 1923.* Edited by Charles Singer and Henry E. Sigerist. London, Oxford University Press; Zürich, Verlag Seldwyla. 1924. pp. 3-62.

CHAPTER III

Corlett, W. T. *The medicine-man of the American Indian and his cultural background.* Springfield, Ill. Charles C. Thomas. 1935. 369 p.

Garrison, F. H. *An introduction to the history of medicine.* 4th ed. Philadelphia and London. W. B. Saunders Co. 1929. 996 p.

v. Hovorka, O. and Kronfeld, U. *Vergleichende Volksmedizin.* 2 v. Stuttgart. Strecker and Schröder. 1908-1909.

Jastrow, J. *Wish and wisdom.* New York. D. Appleton-Century Co. 1935. 394 p.

Jastrow, M. *Aspects of religious belief and practice in Babylonia and Assyria.* New York. G. P. Putnam's Sons. 1911. 471 p.

Lévy-Bruhl, L. *Primitives and the supernatural.* Translated by L. A. Clare. London. G. Allen and Unwin, Ltd. 1936. 405 p.

McKenzie, D. *The infancy of medicine.* London. Macmillan and Co. Ltd. 1927. 421 p.

Osler, W. *The evolution of modern medicine.* New Haven. Yale University Press. 1921. 243 p.

Pareto, V. *Traité de sociologie générale.* 2 v. Lausanne and Paris. Payot et Cie. 1917.

Preuss, J. *Biblisch-talmudische Medizin.* Berlin. S. Karger. 1923. 735 p.

Rappoport, A. S. *The folklore of the Jews.* London. The Soncino Press, Ltd. 1937. 276 p.

Thorndike, L. *A history of magic and experimental science during the first thirteen centuries of our era.* 2 v. New York. Macmillan Co. 1923.

Whitebread, C. *The magic, psychic, ancient Egyptian, Greek and Roman medical collections of the Division of Medicine in the United States National Museum.* No. 2528, Proceedings U.S. National Museum, 65, art. 15. Washington. 1925. 44 p.

CHAPTER IV

Baissette, G. *Hippocrate.* Paris. Éditions Bernard Grasset. 1931. 273 p.

Brock, A. J. *Greek medicine.* London and Toronto, J. M. Dent and Sons, Ltd.; New York, E. P. Dutton and Co. Inc. 1929. 256 p.

Galenus. *Oeuvres anatomiques, physiologiques et médicales.* Translated by C. V. Daremberg. 2 v. Paris. J.-B. Baillière. 1854-1856.

Galenus. *Opera omnia.* Edited by C. G. Kühn. 20 v. Lipsiae. C. Cnobloch. 1821-1833.

Garrison, F. H. *An introduction to the history of medicine.* 4th ed. Philadelphia and London. W. B. Saunders Co. 1929. 996 p.

Gomperz, T. *Greek thinkers.* 4 v. Translated (Vol. 1) by L. Magnus, New York. Charles Scribner's Sons. 1901; (Vols. 2-4) by G. G. Berry. London. J. Murray. 1905-1912.

Greenwood, M. *The medical dictator and other biographical studies.* London. Williams and Norgate, Ltd. 1936. 213 p.

Hippocrates. *The genuine works of Hippocrates.* Translated by Francis Adams. 2 v. London. Printed for the Sydenham Society. 1849.

Hippocrates. *Hippocrates,* with an English translation by W. H. S. Jones. 4 v. London, W. Heinemann, Ltd.; New York, G. P. Putnam's Sons. 1923-1931.

Osler, W. *The evolution of modern medicine.* New Haven. Yale University Press. 1921. 243 p.

Sticker, G. Vorgeschichtliche Versuche der Seuchenabwehr und Seuchenausrottung. *Essays on the history of medicine presented to Karl Sudhoff on the occasion of his seventieth birthday, 26th November 1923.* Edited by Charles Singer and Henry E. Sigerist. London, Oxford University Press; Zürich, Verlag Seldwyla. 1924. pp. 3-62.

Thorndike, L. *A history of magic and experimental science during the first thirteen centuries of our era.* 2 v. New York. Macmillan Co. 1923.

Wong, K. C. and Wu, Lien-Teh. *History of Chinese medicine. Being a chron-*

icle of medical happenings in China from ancient times to the present period. Tientsin, China. Tientsin Press, Ltd. 1932. 706 p.

CHAPTER V

Cato and Varro. *Roman farm management; the treatises of Cato and Varro done into English, with notes of modern instances, by a Virginia farmer.* (Fairfax Harrison). New York. Macmillan Co. 1913. 365 p.

Cohen, H. The hygiene and medicine of the Talmud. *University of Texas Record, 3,* No. 4, 1901 (?) 16 p.

Galenus. *Opera omnia.* Edited by C. G. Kühn. 20 v. Lipsiae. C. Cnobloch. 1821-1833.

Garrison, F. H. *An introduction to the history of medicine.* 4th ed. Philadelphia and London. W. B. Saunders Co. 1929. 996 p.

Lévy-Bruhl, L. *Primitives and the supernatural.* Translated by L. A. Clare. London. G. Allen and Unwin, Ltd. 1936. 405 p.

Ovid. *The metamorphoses of Ovid.* Literally translated into English prose by Henry T. Riley. London. G. Bell and Sons. 1889.

Preuss, J. *Biblisch-talmudische Medizin.* Berlin. S. Karger. 1923. 735 p.

Procopius of Caesarea. *Procopius,* with an English translation by H. B. Dewing. 7 v. London, W. Heinemann; New York, Macmillan Co. 1914-1940.

Singer, C. *From magic to science; essays on the scientific twilight.* New York. Boni and Liveright. 1928. 253 p.

Sticker, G. Vorgeschichtliche Versuche der Seuchenabwehr und Seuchenausrottung. *Essays on the history of medicine presented to Karl Sudhoff on the occasion of his seventieth birthday, 26th November 1923.* Edited by Charles Singer and Henry E. Sigerist. London, Oxford University Press; Zürich, Verlag Seldwyla. 1924. pp. 3-62.

Thucydides. *Thucydides,* translated into English by B. Jowett. 2 v. Oxford. Clarendon Press. 1881.

CHAPTER VI

Avicenna. *I·bri in re medica omnes.* Liber quartus. Venetiis. V. Valgrisius. 1564.

Avicenna. *A treatise on the Canon of medicine of Avicenna incorporating a translation of the first book.* By O. C. Gruner. London. Luzac and Co. 1930. 612 p.

Campbell, A. M. *The black death and men of learning.* New York. Columbia University Press. 1931. 210 p.

Diepgen, P. Die Bedeutung des Mittelalters für den Fortschritt in der Medizin. *Essays on the history of medicine presented to Karl Sudhoff on the occasion of his seventieth birthday, 26th November 1923.* Edited by Charles

Singer and Henry E. Sigerist. London, Oxford University Press; Zürich, Verlag Seldwyla. 1924. pp. 99-120.

Dinānah, T. *Die Schrift von Abī Ga'far Ahmed ibn Alī ibn Mohammed ibn 'Alī ibn Hātimah aus Almeriah über die Pest. Arch. Gesch. Med., 19,* 27-81. 1927.

Eager, J. M. *The early history of quarantine: origin of sanitary measures directed against yellow fever.* Yellow Fever Institute, Bull. No. 12. Treasury Department Public Health and Marine-Hospital Service. Washington. Government Printing Office. 1903. 27 p.

Ficino, M. *Consiglio di Marsilio Ficino Fiorentino contra la pestilenza.* 1481.

Gasquet, F. A. *The Black Death of 1347 and 1349.* 2d ed. London. G. Bell and Sons. 1908. 272 p.

Hecker, J. F. K. *The epidemics of the Middle Ages.* Translated by B. G. Babington. London. G. Woodfall and Son. (The Sydenham Society). 1844. 418 p.

Jacobi, J. *A litil boke the whiche traytied and reherced many gode thinges necessaries for the . . . pestilence.* London. 1485? Reproduced in facsimile from the copy in the John Rylands Library. With an introduction by Guthrie Vine. Manchester, University Press; London, B. Quaritch. 1910. xxxvi p. 9 l.

Klebs, A. C. *A catalan plague-tract of April 24, 1348 by Jacme D'Agramont.* Communication faite au Sixième Congrès International d'Histoire de la Médecine, Leyde-Amsterdam, 18-23 Juillet, 1927. Antwerp. 1929. 6 p.

Klebs, A. C. and Droz, E. *Remedies against the plague.* Paris. Gaston Jeanbin. 1925. 95 p.

Menche de Loisne, A. C. H. *La maladrerie du Val de Montreuil.* Abbeville. Lafosse et Cie. 1903. 132 p.

Michon, L.-A. J. *Documents inédits sur la Grande Peste de 1348.* Paris. J.-B. Baillière. 1860. 99 p.

Mueller, M. J. Ibnulkhatîbs Bericht ueber die Pest. *Sitzber. kgl. bayer. Akad. Wiss. Muenchen, 2,* 1-34. 1863.

Phillippe, A. *Histoire de la peste noire (1346-1350).* Paris. 1853. 295 p.

Pietro da Tussignano. *Consilium pro peste evitanda.* In Ketham, Johannes. *Fasciculus medicinae.* Venice. Johannes and Gregorius de Gregoriis. 15 Oct. 1495.

Rhazes. *A treatise on the small-pox and measles,* by Abú Becr Mohammed ibn Zacaríyá ar-Rází. (commonly called Rhazes). Translated from the original Arabic by W. A. Greenhill. London. Printed for the Sydenham Society. 1848. 212 p.

Seidel, E. Die Lehre von der Kontagion bei den Arabern. *Arch. Gesch. Med.,* 6, 81-93, 1912-1913.

Sudhoff, K. Mittelalterliche Einzeltexte zur Beulenpest vor ihrem pandemischen Auftreten. 1347/48. In *Historische Studien und Skizzen zu Natur-und Heilwissenschaft. Festgabe Georg Sticker zum 70. Geburtstage darge-boten.* Berlin. Springer. 1930. 152 p.

Sudhoff, K. Pestschriften aus den ersten 150 Jahren nach der Epidemie des "schwarzen Todes" 1348. *Arch. Gesch. Med.,* 4, 191-222; 389-424, 1910-11; 5, 36-87; 332-396, 1911-12; 6, 313-379, 1912-13; 7, 57-114, 1913-14; 8, 175-215; 236-289, 1914-15; 9, 53-78; 117-167, 1915-16; *11-12,* 44-92; 121-176, 1918-20.

Sudhoff, K. Der Ulmer Stadtarzt Dr. Heinrich Steinhöwel (1420-1482) als Pestautor. In *Die ersten gedruckten Pestschriften,* by A. C. Klebs and K. Sudhoff. München. Münchner Drucke. 1926. pp. 169-211.

Trouillard, C. La Seigneurie et la Chapelle de Saint-Jacques-des-Lépreux de Mayenne. *Rev. hist. archéol. du Maine, 2,* 315-334. 1877.

CHAPTER VII

Eager, J. M. *The early history of quarantine: origin of sanitary measures di-rected against yellow fever.* Yellow Fever Institute, Bull. No. 12. Treasury Department Public Health and Marine-Hospital Service. Washington. Gov-ernment Printing Office. 1903. 27 p.

Fracastoro, G. *De contagione et contagiosis morbis et eorum curatione, libri III.* Translated by W. C. Wright. New York and London. G. P. Putnam's Sons. 1930. 356 p.

Fracastoro, G. *Opera omnia.* 3d ed. Venice. Giunti. 1584. 214 p.

Fracastoro, G. *Syphilis; or, the French disease.* Translated by H. Wynne-Finch. London. William Heinemann. 1935. 253 p.

Lersch, B. M. *Geschichte der Volksseuchen.* Berlin. S. Karger. 1896. 455 p.

Paget, S. *Ambroise Paré and his times, 1510-1590.* New York and London. G. P. Putnam's Sons. 1899. 309 p.

Paré, A. *Oeuvres complètes.* Edited by J.-F. Malgaigne. 3 v. Paris. J.-B. Bail-lière. 1840-1841.

Winslow, C.-E. A. The drama of syphilis. *J. Social Hyg., 23,* 57-72, 1937.

CHAPTER VIII

Cohen, B. On Leeuwenhoek's method of seeing bacteria. *J. Bact., 34,* 343-346. 1937.

Dobell, C. *Antony van Leeuwenhoek and his "little animals."* New York, Harcourt Brace and Co.; London, J. Bale Sons and Danielsson, Ltd. 1932. 435 p.

Garrison, F. H. *An introduction to the history of medicine.* 4th ed. Philadel-phia and London. W. B. Saunders Co. 1929. 996 p.

Huxley, T. H. Biogenesis and abiogenesis. In *Discourses: biological and geological.* New York and London. D. Appleton and Co. 1915. pp. 232-274.

Kircher, A. *Scrutinium physico-medicum contagiosae luis, quae pestis dicitur.* Rome. Typis Mascardi. 1658. 252 p.

Redi, F. *Esperienze intorno alla generazione degl'insetti.* Firenze. All'Insegna della Stella. 1668. 228 p.

Sigerist, H. E. *The great doctors; a biographical history of medicine.* Translated by Eden and Cedar Paul. New York. W. W. Norton and Co. 1933. 436 p.

Singer, C. *The development of the doctrine of contagium vivum, 1500-1750.* London. Privately printed. 1913. 15 p.

Torrey, H. B. Athanasius Kircher and the progress of medicine. In *Osiris,* (Bruges, Belgium) 5, 246-275. 1938.

CHAPTER IX

Riesman, D. *Thomas Sydenham, clinician.* New York. P. B. Hoeber, Inc. 1926. 52 p.

Sigerist, H. E. *The great doctors; a biographical history of medicine.* Translated by Eden and Cedar Paul. New York. W. W. Norton and Co. 1933. 436 p.

Sydenham, T. *The entire works of Dr. Thomas Sydenham.* By John Swan. 5th ed. London. F. Newberry, 1769. 666 p.

Sydenham, T. *The works of Thomas Sydenham, M.D.* Translated by R. G. Latham. 2 v. London. Printed for the Sydenham Society. 1848.

CHAPTER X

Leman, T. *Some memoirs of the life and writings of the late Richard Mead.* London. M. Cooper. 1755. 49 p.

MacMichael, W. *The gold-headed cane.* London. J. Murray. 1827. 179 p.

Mead, R. *Authentic memoirs of the life of Richard Mead, M.D.* London. Printed for J. Whiston and B. White. 1755. 64 p. Expanded from an Éloge by Matthew Maty in the Journal Britannique for 1754.

Mead, R. *The medical works of Richard Mead, M.D.* Dublin. Thomas Ewing. 1767. 511 p.

Mead, R. *A short discourse concerning pestilential contagion, and the methods to be used to prevent it.* 2d Dublin ed. George Grierson. 1721. 40 p.

Winslow, C. E. A. A physician of two centuries ago: Richard Mead and his contributions to epidemiology. *Bull. Inst. Hist. Med.,* 3, 509-544. 1935.

CHAPTER XI

Carey, M. *A short account of the malignant fever, lately prevalent in Philadelphia.* 3d ed. Philadelphia. Printed by the author. 1793. 112 p.

Ford, E. E. F. *Notes on the life of Noah Webster.* Edited by E. E. F. Skeel. 2 v. New York. Privately printed. 1912.

Goodman, N. G. *Benjamin Rush, physician and citizen, 1746-1813.* Philadelphia. University of Pennsylvania Press. 1934. 421 p.

LaRoche, R. *Yellow fever, considered in its historical, pathological, etiological and therapeutical relations.* 2 v. Philadelphia. Blanchard and Lea. 1855.

Lersch, B. M. *Geschichte der Volksseuchen.* Berlin. S. Karger. 1896. 455 p.

Rush, B. *An account of the bilious remitting yellow fever, as it appeared in the city of Philadelphia, in the year 1793.* Philadelphia. T. Dobson. 1794. 363 p. Also, *Medical inquiries and observations, 3.*

Rush, B. An enquiry into the causes of the increase of bilious and remitting fevers in Pennsylvania, with hints for preventing them. *Am. Museum, 1,* 138-143, 1787.

Rush, B. *An inquiry into the various sources of the usual forms of summer and autumnal disease in the United States, and the means of preventing them. To which are added, facts intended to prove the yellow fever not to be contagious.* Philadelphia. J. Conrad and Co. 1805. 113 p.

Rush, B. *Medical inquiries and observations.* v. 4. 5th ed. Philadelphia. A. Finley. 1819.

Rush, B. *Observations upon the origin of the malignant bilious or yellow fever, in Philadelphia, and upon the means of preventing it; addressed to the citizens of Philadelphia.* Philadelphia. T. Dobson. 1799. 28 p.

Rush, B. *A second address to the citizens of Philadelphia, containing additional proofs of the domestic origin of the malignant bilious or yellow fever, etc.* Philadelphia. T. Dobson. 1799. 40 p.

Warthin, A. S. Noah Webster as epidemiologist. *J. Am. Med. Assoc., 80,* 755-764. 1923.

Webster, N. *A brief history of epidemic and pestilential diseases; with the principal phenomena of the physical world which precede and accompany them.* 2 v. Hartford, Conn. Hudson and Goodwin. 1799.

Webster, N. *A collection of papers on the subject of bilious fevers, prevalent in the United States for a few years past.* New York. Hopkins Webb and Co. 1796. 246 p.

Winslow, C.-E. A. The epidemiology of Noah Webster. *Trans. Conn. Acad. Arts and Sciences, 32,* 21-109. 1934.

CHAPTER XII

Guyton-Morveau, L.-B. *Traité des moyens de désinfecter l'air, de prevenir la contagion et d'en arrêter les progrès.* 2d ed. Paris. Bernard. 1802. 429 p.

Hawley, K. J. *The contributions of Florence Nightingale to hygiene and sanitation.* Unpublished thesis, Yale University. 1938.

Howard, J. *An account of the principal lazarettos in Europe; with various papers relative to the plague.* Warrington. W. Eyres. 1789. 259 p.

Metropolitan Sanitary Commission. *First Report of the Commissioners appointed to inquire whether any and what special means may be requisite for the improvement of the health of the metropolis.* London. William Clowes and Sons. 1848. 430 p. Second Report, 144 p.

Murchison, C. *A treatise on the continued fevers of Great Britain.* London. Parker, Son, and Bourn. 1st ed. 1862. 638 p.; 2d ed. 1873. 729 p.

Richardson, B. W. *The health of nations: a review of the works of Edwin Chadwick.* 2 v. London. Longmans, Green and Co. 1887.

Simon, J. *Public health reports.* Edited by E. Seaton for the Sanitary Institute of Great Britain. 2 v. London. Offices of the Sanitary Institute. J. A. Churchill. 1887.

Winslow, C.-E. A. *The evolution and significance of the modern public health campaign.* New Haven. Yale University Press. 1923. 65 p.

CHAPTER XIII

Budd, W. Intestinal fever essentially contagious. *Lancet, 2,* 4-5; 28-30; 55-56; 80-82. 1859.

Budd, W. On intestinal fever. *Lancet, 2,* 131-133; 207-210; 432-433; 458-459. 1859.

Budd, W. On intestinal fever. *Lancet, 1,* 187-190; 239-240. 1860.

Budd, W. On intestinal fever: its mode of propagation. *Lancet, 2,* 694-695. 1856.

Budd, W. On the fever at the Clergy Orphan Asylum. *Lancet, 2,* 617-619. 1856.

Budd, W. *Typhoid fever; its nature, mode of spreading, and prevention.* London. Longmans, Green and Co. 1873. 193 p.

Gafafer, W. M. Peter Ludwig Panum's "Observations on the contagium of measles." *Isis, 24,* 90-101. 1935.

Panum, P. L. *Observations made during the epidemic of measles on the Faroe Islands in the year 1846.* Translated from the Danish by A. S. Hatcher. New York. Delta Omega Society. Distributed by American Public Health Association. 1940. 111 p.

Prescott, S. C. and Horwood, M. P. *Sedgwick's principles of sanitary science and public health.* Rewritten and enlarged. New York. Macmillan Co. 1935. 654 p.

Snow, J. *On continuous molecular changes, more particularly in their relation to epidemic diseases.* London. J. Churchill. 1853. 38 p.

Snow, J. *On the mode of communication of cholera.* London. J. Churchill. 1st ed. 1849. 31 p.; 2d ed. 1855. 162 p.

Snow, J. On the pathology and mode of communication of cholera. *London Med. Gazette, 44,* 745-752; 923-929. 1849.

Snow, J. *Snow on cholera; being a reprint of two papers by John Snow, M.D.*; together with a biographical memoir by B. W. Richardson, M.D. and an introduction by Wade Hampton Frost, M.D. New York. Commonwealth Fund. 1936. 191 p.

Stallybrass, C. O. *The principles of epidemiology.* New York. Macmillan Co. 1931. 696 p.

CHAPTER XIV

Duclaux, E. *Pasteur; the history of a mind.* Translated by E. F. Smith and F. Hedges. Philadelphia and London. W. B. Saunders Co. 1920. 363 p.

Harden, A. *Alcoholic fermentation.* Monographs on biochemistry. London. Longmans, Green and Co. 1914. 156 p.

Henle, F. G. J. *Pathologische Untersuchungen.* Berlin. A. Hirschwald. 1840. 274 p.

Huxley, T. H. Biogenesis and abiogenesis. In *Discourses: biological and geological.* New York and London. D. Appleton and Co. 1915. pp. 232-274.

Koch, R. *Gesammelte Werke von Robert Koch, unter Mitwirkung von G. Gaffky und E. Pfuhl, herausgegeben von J. Schwalbe.* 2 v. Leipzig. G. Thieme. 1912.

Lister, J. *The collected papers of Joseph, Baron Lister.* 2 v. Oxford. Clarendon Press. 1909.

Pasteur, L. *Oeuvres de Pasteur réunies par Pasteur Vallery-Radot.* 6 v. Paris. Masson et Cie. 1922-1933.

v. Plenciz, M. A. *Opera medico-physica.* Vindobonae. J. T. Trattner. 1762.

Vallery-Radot, R. *The life of Pasteur.* Translated by Mrs. R. L. Devonshire. 2 v. New York. McClure, Phillips and Co. 1902.

Zinsser, H. and Bayne-Jones, S. *A textbook of bacteriology.* 7th ed. New York. D. Appleton-Century Co. 1934. 1226 p.

CHAPTER XV

Bayne-Jones, S. Reciprocal effects of the relationship of bacteriology and medicine. *J. Bact., 21,* 61-73. 1931.

v. Buhl, L. Ein Beitrag zur Aetiologie des Typhus. *Z. Biol., 1,* 1-25. 1865.

Greenwood, M. *Epidemics and crowd-diseases; an introduction to the study of epidemiology.* New York, Macmillan Co.; London, Williams and Norgate, Ltd. 1936. 213 p.

Hume, E. E. *Max von Pettenkofer, his theory of the etiology of cholera, typhoid fever and other intestinal diseases: a review of his arguments and evidence.* New York. P. B. Hoeber, Inc. 1927. 142 p.

v. Pettenkofer, M. Boden und Grundwasser in ihren Beziehungen zu Cholera und Typhus. *Z. Biol.,* 5, 171-310. 1869.

v. Pettenkofer, M. Jubelband dem Herrn. Geh. Rath. Prof. Dr. M. v. Pettenkofer zu seinem 50-jährigen Doctor-Jubilaum gewidmet von seinen Schülern. *Arch. Hyg., 17,* 1893.

v. Pettenkofer, M. *Künftige Prophylaxis gegen Cholera nach den Vorschlägen in dem amtlichen Berichte des königl. bayer. Bezirks- und Stadtgerichtarztes Dr. Frank.* München. Gotta. 1875. 123 p.

v. Pettenkofer, M. Ueber Cholera, mit Berücksichtigung der jüngsten Choleraepidemie in Hamburg. *Münch. med. Wochschr., 39,* 807-817. 1892.

v. Pettenkofer, M. Ueber die Verbreitungsart der Cholera. *Z. Biol., 1,* 322-374. 1865.

v. Pettenkofer, M. *Untersuchungen und Beobactungen über die Verbreitungsart der Cholera, nebst Betrachtungen über Massregeln derselben Einhalt zu thun.* München. J. G. Cotta. 1855. 374 p.

v. Pettenkofer, M. Zum gegenwärtigen Stand der Cholerafrage. *Arch. Hyg.,* 4, 249-354; 397-546; 5, 353-445; 6, 1-84; 129-233; 303-358; 373-441; 7, 1-81. 1886-1887.

Seidel, L. Ueber den numerischen Zusammenhang, welcher zwischen der Häufigkeit der Typhus-Erkrankungen und dem Stande des Grundwassers während der letzten 9 Jahre in München hervorgetreten ist. *Z. Biol., 1,* 221-236. 1865.

Soyka, J. Zur Aetiologie des Abdominaltyphus. *Arch. Hyg., 6,* 257-302. 1887.

v. Voit, C. Max von Pettenkofer zum Gedächtniss. Rede, im *Auftrage der mathematisch-physikalischen Classe der kgl. bayer. Akademie der Wissenschaften in München.* Nov. 16, 1901. 160 p.

CHAPTER XVI

Biggs, H. M., Park, W. H. and Beebe, A. L. *Report on bacteriological investigations and diagnosis of diphtheria, from May 4, 1893 to May 4, 1894.* Scientific Bulletin No. 1, Health Department, City of New York, from the Bacteriological Laboratories. New York. 1895. 57 p.

Chapin, C. V. *The sources and modes of infection.* New York. J. Wiley and Sons. 1910. 399 p.

Koch, R. *Die Bekämpfung des Typhus.* Berlin. A. Hirschwald. 1903. 22 p.

Koch, R. Die Cholera in Deutschland während des Winters 1892 bis 1893. *Z. Hyg. Infektionskrankh., 15,* 89-165. 1893.

Koch, R. Ueber den augenblicklichen Stand der bakteriologischen Choleradiagnose. *Z. Hyg. Infektionskrankh., 14,* 319-338. 1893.

Oliver, W. W. *The man who lived for tomorrow.* A biography of William Hallock Park, M.D. New York. E. P. Dutton and Co., Inc. 1941. 507 p.

Park, W. H. and Beebe, A. L. Report dated Jan. 1, 1894, to Dr. H. M. Biggs. In *Annual Report of the Board of Health of the Health Department of the City of New York for the year ending December 31, 1893.* pp. 73-115.

Reed, W., Vaughan, V. C., and Shakespeare, E. O. *Abstract of report on the origin and spread of typhoid fever in U.S. military camps during the Spanish war of 1898.* Washington. Government Printing Office. 1900. 239 p.

Rosenau, M. J., Lumsden, L. L. and Kastle, J. H. *Report No. 3 on the origin and prevalence of typhoid fever in the District of Columbia (1908).* Hygienic Laboratory, Bulletin No. 52. Public Health and Marine-Hospital Service. Washington. 1909. 160 p.

Simon, C. E. *Human infection carriers.* Philadelphia and New York. Lea and Febiger. 1919. 250 p.

Winslow, C.-E. A. *The Life of Hermann M. Biggs.* Philadelphia. Lea and Febiger. 1929. 432 p.

Zinsser, H. William Hallock Park, 1863-1939. *J. Bact., 38,* 1-3. 1939.

Zinsser, H. and Bayne-Jones, S. *A textbook of bacteriology.* 7th ed. New York. D. Appleton-Century Co. 1934. 1226 p.

CHAPTER XVII

Biraud, Y. and Deutschman, S. Typhus and typhus-like rickettsia infections. Geographical distribution and epidemiology. *Epidemiol. Rept. Health Section, League of Nations, 15,* 1-16; 99-160. 1936.

DeKruif, P. *Microbe hunters.* New York. Harcourt, Brace and Co. 1926. 363 p.

Hackett, L. W. Recent findings bearing on the epidemiology of malaria in Europe. *Med. Parasitol. and Parasitic Diseases, 4,* 39-44, 1935. Also in *Collected papers by members of the staff of the International Health Division of the Rockefeller Foundation, 13,* Part I, 1935.

Hampton, B. C. Plague in the United States. *U.S. Pub. Health Repts., 55,* 1143-1158. 1940.

Howard, S. and DeKruif, P. *Yellow jack: a history.* New York. Harcourt, Brace and Co. 1933. 152 p.

Jorge, R. *Les faunes régionales des rongeurs et des puces dans leurs rapports avec la peste. Résultats de l'enquête du Comité Permanent de l'Office International d'Hygiène Publique. 1924-1927.* Paris. Masson et Cie. 1928. 306 p.

Kelly, H. A. *Walter Reed and yellow fever.* 3d ed. rev. Baltimore. Norman, Remington Co. 1906. 355 p.

Lamb, G. (Compiler). *The etiology and epidemiology of plague. A summary of the work of the Plague Commission.* Calcutta. Superintendent of Government Printing, India. 1908. 93 p.

Ross, R. *Memoirs, with a full account of the great malaria problem and its solution.* London. J. Murray. 1923. 547 p.

Sawyer, W. A. A history of the activities of the Rockefeller Foundation in the investigation and control of yellow fever. *Am. J. Trop. Med.*, *17*, 35-50. 1937.

Sawyer, W. A. The last twelve years of yellow fever research. *Puerto Rico Health Bull.*, *3*, 39-44. 1939. Also in *Collected papers on yellow fever by members of the staff of the International Health Division of the Rockefeller Foundation*, *5*.

Smith, T. and Kilborne, F. L. *Investigations into the nature, causation and prevention of Texas or southern cattle fever.* U.S. Dept. Agriculture, Bureau of Animal Industry, Bull. No. 1. Washington. Government Printing Office. 1893. 301 p.

Soper, F. L. The newer epidemiology of yellow fever. *Am. J. Pub. Health*, *27*, 1-14. 1937.

Winslow, C.-E. A. *The evolution and significance of the modern public health campaign.* New Haven. Yale University Press. 1923. 65 p.

Wolbach, S. B., Todd, J. L. and Palfrey, F. W. *The etiology and pathology of typhus; being the main report of the Typhus Research Commission of the League of Red Cross Societies to Poland.* Cambridge. Harvard University Press. 1922. 222 p.

Zinsser, H. *Rats, lice and history.* Boston. Printed and published for the Atlantic Monthly Press. Little, Brown and Co. 1935. 301 p.

CHAPTER XVIII

Allison, V. D. Streptococcal infection as ascertained by type determination. *Lancet*, *1*, 840-842; Streptococcal infections, *Ibid.*, 1067-1070. 1938.

Allison, V. D. and Brown, W. A. Reinfection as a cause of complications and relapses in scarlet-fever wards. *J. Hyg.*, *37*, 153-171. 1937.

Brown, W. A. and Allison, V. D. Infection of the air of scarlet-fever wards with *Streptococcus pyogenes.* *J. Hyg.*, *37*, 1-13. 1937.

Chapin, C. V. *Papers of Charles V. Chapin, M.D.* New York. Commonwealth Fund. 1934. 244 p.

Chapin, C. V. *The sources and modes of infection.* New York. J. Wiley and Sons. 1910. 399 p.

Harries, E. H. R. Bed-isolation; with special reference to measles and chicken-pox. *Lancet*, *1*, 491-495. 1924.

Horwood, M. P. An evaluation of the factors responsible for public health progress in the United States. *Science*, *89*, 517-526. 1939.

Sedgwick, W. T. Investigations of epidemics of typhoid fever in Bondsville, Provincetown and Millville, apparently due to secondary infection. *24th Annual Report, State Board of Health of Massachusetts.* Boston. 1893. pp. 732-742.

Sedgwick, W. T. On recent epidemics of typhoid fever in the cities of Lowell and Lawrence due to infected water supply; with observations on typhoid fever in other cities and towns of the Merrimack Valley, especially in Newburyport. *24th Annual Report, State Board of Health of Massachusetts.* Boston. 1893. pp. 667-714.

Sedgwick, W. T. and Chapin, W. H. An investigation of an epidemic of typhoid fever in the city of Springfield in July and August, 1892, due to infected milk. *24th Annual Report, State Board of Health of Massachusetts.* Boston. 1893. pp. 715-731.

Viruses and rickettsial diseases with especial consideration of their public health significance. A symposium held at the Harvard School of Public Health, June 12-17, 1939. Cambridge. Harvard University Press. 1940. 907 p.

Wells, W. F. Studies on air-borne infection. *Science, 92,* 457-458. 1940.

Wells, W. F. and Wells, M. W. Air-borne infection. *J. Am. Med. Assoc., 107,* 1698-1703; 1805-1809. 1936.

Winslow, C.-E. A. *The evolution and significance of the modern public health campaign.* New Haven. Yale University Press. 1923. 65 p.

INDEX OF PERSONS

INDEX OF SUBJECTS